The Life Extension Foundation's

Disease
Prevention and Treatment
Protocols

The Life Extension Foundation's

Disease
Prevention and Treatment
Protocols

1997

❖ Offshore Medical Therapies
❖ Natural Alternatives to Toxic Drugs
❖ Therapies for "Untreatable" Diseases
❖ Based on Thousands of Research Studies

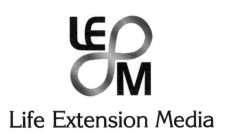

Life Extension Media

Life Extension Foundation books may be purchased for personal, educational, business or sales promotional use. For information, please write: The Life Extension Foundation, P.O. Box 229120, Hollywood, Florida 33022-9120. Website: www.lef.org

FIRST EDITION

Cover design by Roy Rauschenberg
Book design by Jato Design
Set in Korrina

ISBN 0-9658777-0-1

Dedicated to those who needlessly suffered and died.

CONTENTS

Contents

Contents

Contents

Rectifying Missed Opportunities

In 1928, Dr. Alexander Fleming discovered penicillin, and his work was published the very next year in the *British Journal of Experimental Pathology*. Nevertheless, the medical profession did not begin treating humans with this life-saving therapy until 1941, and the general population did not gain access to penicillin until 1946.

Millions of human beings suffered and died from bacterial infectious diseases when a cure had already been discovered, and this cure had already been published in a respected medical journal. It is difficult to describe in words the agony people must have felt as they helplessly watched their loved ones die from a host of bacterial diseases that penicillin could have cured.

The leading cause of death and disability in the United States is ignorance of therapies to prevent and treat the degenerative diseases of aging. This book is dedicated to eradicating the ignorance that is causing humans to suffer and die from diseases that may already have a cure, or at least a palliative therapy. Almost every protocol in this book is extensively substantiated by peer-reviewed, published studies from the most prestigious medical journals in the world. Despite this scientific validation, these therapies are being largely ignored by the medical establishment.

This book will soon be available as a computer program, enabling the user to access more than 2,500 scientific references that substantiate the use of these protocols in preventing and treating disease.

Remember that the information contained in this book is not intended to replace the attention or advice of a physician or other health care professional. Anyone who wishes to embark on any dietary, drug, exercise, or other lifestyle change intended to prevent or treat a specific disease or condition should first consult with and seek clearance from a qualified health care professional.

For additional information on products and treatment protocols, visit our website at www.lef.org.

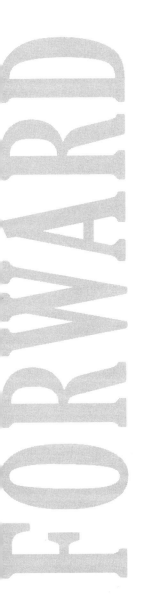

The Life Extension Foundation

Before you consider implementing the aggressive disease prevention and treatment protocols in this book, you should know something about the organization that developed them.

The Life Extension Foundation is the world's largest organization dedicated to investigating every possible method of preventing aging and death. The Foundation funds scientific research aimed at achieving an indefinitely extended lifespan. Foundation members benefit now by obtaining lifesaving therapies that will not be available to the general public for years.

Life Extension Foundation members are people who believe in taking advantage of documented scientific therapies to prevent diseases and slow aging. The medical literature contains thousands of papers on the use of antioxidant supplements, hormone therapies and medications that have been shown to improve the quality and quantity of life. Life Extensionists attempt to use this scientific information to improve their chances of living longer in good health.

The Life Extension Foundation was officially incorporated in 1980, but its founders have been writing about and funding anti-aging research since the 1960s.

Research supported by The Life Extension Foundation has documented the value of antioxidants in preventing diseases and in protecting cells against ischemia (reduced blood flow). Ischemia can be caused by the blockage of a coronary artery which can lead to a heart attack, or a cerebral artery which can lead to a stroke. The Life Extension Foundation is the world's leader in preventing cellular damage and death from ischemia. The Foundation supports a full-time research facility that has broken all world records in protecting against ischemia-induced free radical damage.

The Life Extension Foundation maintains the highest quality-control standards in the world by offering only those products that contain pharmaceutical-grade nutrients. The purity of your supplements is critical if you plan to take them for the rest of your life. Many discount products use low-grade vitamin C imported from China that contains traces of toxic arsenic, lead and iron. Since the Food And Drug Administration does not believe anyone should take more than 100 mg a day of vitamin C, the FDA permits the importation of this contaminated vitamin C. Life Extensionists take 3,000 to 20,000 mg a day of vitamin C, so it is crucial that they use pharmaceutical-grade vitamin C that has gone through 18 purification steps to remove contaminants.

Forward

Since the FDA does not properly regulate dietary supplement manufacturing, the Foundation employs an independent quality-control expert to verify that only pharmaceutical-quality nutrients are used. No other organization in the world does this. The reason you take nutrients is because of published research indicating specific health benefits. In these studies, only pharmaceutical-grade nutrients are used. If you expect to obtain the same health benefits, you need to take the exact same pharmaceutical-grade nutrients used in these scientific studies.

Members of The Life Extension Foundation receive discounts that enable them to purchase premium-grade supplements at prices that are often 50% less than health-food store prices.

The Foundation analyzes thousands of scientific studies every week to make sure its disease-preventing formulas include the most effective life-extending ingredients in the world. The Foundation interacts with the world's foremost anti-aging researchers in order to obtain inside information about anti-aging breakthroughs. The Foundation operates the most advanced anti-ischemia laboratory in the world, where antioxidant nutrients, hormones, and drugs are used to prevent free radical induced cellular damage due to reduced blood flow. Foundation members gain access to the benefits of disease-preventing, anti-aging findings before they are published in science and medical journals.

- ✔ In 1980, the Foundation recommended antioxidants to prevent disease.
- ✔ In 1981, the Foundation introduced DHEA as a disease-preventing therapy.
- ✔ In 1983, the Foundation recommended aspirin to prevent heart attacks
- ✔ In 1983, the Foundation introduced coenzyme Q10 to prevent and treat heart disease.
- ✔ In 1983, the Foundation warned that excessive iron causes cancer and heart disease.
- ✔ In 1985, the Foundation made lycopene available to prevent cancer.
- ✔ In 1986, the Foundation recommended deprenyl as an anti-aging drug.
- ✔ In 1988, the Foundation made phosphatidylserine available to slow brain aging.
- ✔ In 1991, the Foundation sued the FDA for quicker approval of lifesaving drugs.
- ✔ In 1992, the Foundation introduced melatonin for sleep, and the prevention of disease.
- ✔ In 1995, the Foundation introduced the first anti-aging drug formula in the world.
- ✔ In 1996, the Foundation published 110 disease prevention and treatment protocols based upon published medical research.
- ✔ In 1997, the Foundation introduced to Americans a safe and super-effective anti-depressant used in Europe.

The Life Extension Foundation can assist you in finding offshore pharmacies that will sell you advanced European and Asian medications that are usually five or more years ahead of FDA approved drugs. The Foundation is the only organization that actively fights for the right of all Americans to import lifesaving medications for their own personal use.

Call the Life Extension Foundation today for membership information: 1-800-841-5433.

PROTOCOLS

Acetaminophen (Tylenol) Poisoning:
Acute and Chronic

All over-the-counter (OTC) pain remedies cause potentially lethal side effects. People in chronic pain often abuse OTC pain medications. The drug acetaminophen is sold under many brand names, the most popular being Tylenol. One result of acetaminophen injury is the generation of toxic free radicals in the liver.

If a person attempts to commit suicide by taking an entire bottle of acetaminophen, the emergency room doctor will administer an antioxidant drug called Mucosil (Mucomyst). If administered in time, Mucosil can save the patient's life by inhibiting the free radicals.

The active ingredient in Mucosil is the nutrient n-acetyl-cysteine, also known as NAC. N-acetyl-cysteine suppresses the toxic free radicals generated by the ingestion of acetaminophen. If you have to take acetaminophen, we suggest you take the amino acid n-acetyl-cysteine or cysteine along with at least one gram of vitamin C with each dose of acetaminophen.

Additional antioxidants such as glutathione will further protect the liver against acetaminophen-induced free radical injury. A simple approach to protect against acetaminophen-induced free radical liver damage is to take one capsule of a multi-nutrient formula that contains glutathione, vitamin C and cysteine with each dose of acetaminophen. This antioxidant formula will provide significant protection to the liver.

Acetaminophen also can cause permanent kidney damage when taken over extended periods of time. This damage can be lethal to those with underlying kidney disease. There are no nutrient supplements known to protect against acetaminophen-induced kidney damage, although the amino acid taurine (1,000 mg two to three times a day) and some forms of dietary fiber might be helpful.

The FDA does not require the manufacturers of Tylenol and other brands of acetaminophen to warn people with kidney disease to avoid this class of pain medication. However, for those in chronic pain who cannot find relief from natural pain relief therapies (see protocols for Pain and Arthritis), it is suggested that Tylenol and other brands of acetaminophen be used sparingly.

Some people alternate other types of OTC pain-relieving drugs such as Advil, high-dose aspirin and Naprosyn to avoid using acetaminophen on a daily basis. Although these drugs also have dangerous side effects, alternating their use may help to reduce their toxicity. However, one study showed that people who use acetaminophen with other pain relievers on a regular basis have a three- to eight-fold increase in their risk of kidney cancer, which is very difficult to treat. The liver/kidney/heart muscle toxicities and the cancer risks of analgesic drugs have not been revealed by the media, which reap tremendous profits from the advertising of pain relief products.

Product availability: glutathione, vitamin C and cysteine capsules, NAC (n-acetyl-cysteine) Caps, taurine and vitamin C caps are available from The Life Extension Foundation, singly or in a Protocol Pak. To order, phone 1-800-544-4440.

Adrenal Disease

Aging and the diseases of aging can cause a decline in critical hormones produced by the adrenal glands. The most important hormone produced primarily in the adrenal glands is pregnenolone. Pregnenolone cascades down into crucial anti-aging hormones such as DHEA (dehydroepiandrosterone), estrogen, progesterone and testosterone.

Pregnenolone supplementation may help restore hormone balance caused by aging-induced adrenal insufficiency, which can cause life-threatening conditions. One of these imbalances involves over-production of the hormone cortisol, which has been called the "death hormone" because it is a cause of immune suppression, atherosclerosis, brain cell injury and accelerated aging. Pregnenolone or DHEA supplementation may protect against the over-production of cortisol from the adrenal glands. Vitamin C and aspirin may block excessive cortisol production.

A protocol to treat adrenal disease includes one 50-mg pregnenolone capsule once a day for one week. Increase to two capsules a day the second week and then three capsules a day the third week. During week four, have DHEA sulfate and cortisol blood tests to help determine your state of adrenal function. If your cortisol levels are elevated, one-quarter tablet a day of aspirin taken with a heavy meal and 3,000 mg of vitamin C a day could suppress your cortisol levels. The European drug KH3 can block some of the cell-damaging effects of cortisol. To help protect against cortisol toxicity, take one to two KH3 capsules in the morning on an empty stomach and one to two KH3 capsules in mid-afternoon on an empty stomach.

CAUTION: Some adrenal diseases such as Addison's disease involve under-production of cortisol. This is a potentially acute life-threatening condition that requires expert physician intervention. Glucocorticoid and mineralocorticoid drugs will be prescribed for Addison's disease. Once cortisol levels are stabilized, serum levels of DHEA should be evaluated to determine if DHEA replacement therapy is warranted. Addison's disease is caused by autoimmune attack on the adrenal glands in 80% of cases. Before taking DHEA or pregnenolone, refer to the Foundation's DHEA Precautions. Also refer to the Autoimmune Disease protocol for additional suggestions.

Product availability: Pregnenolone capsules, DHEA, vitamin C powders and capsules, and ¼ aspirin tablets (Healthprin) can be ordered singly or in a Protocol Pak by phoning 1-800-544-4440. KH3 is not available from The Life Extension Foundation. Call 1-800-544-4440 for a list of companies that sell KH3 to Americans for personal use.

Age-Associated Mental Impairment (Brain Aging)

Aging causes a progressive decline in overall cognitive function. Aging causes us to lose our ability to store and retrieve short-term memories and to learn new information. Our neurological functions are regulated by the complex interaction of hormones, such as pregnenolone and estrogen, and neurotransmitters such as acetylcholine on brain cell function. Hormone imbalances play a direct role in the decline of cognitive function that occurs with aging.

There are several classes of agents that enhance cognitive function and protect against neurological aging. The most commonly used memory-enhancing nutrients are choline, lecithin and DMAE. These nutrients boost acetylcholine levels in the brain. Acetylcholine is a neurotransmitter that helps brain cells to communicate with each other. Acetylcholine deficiency can predispose a person to a wide range of neurological diseases including Alzheimer's disease and stroke. Suggested dosage ranges are:

- ❖ 2,500 to 10,000 mg a day of choline
- ❖ 10,000 to 15,000 mg a day of lecithin
- ❖ 200 to 1,000 mg a day of DMAE

Take these acetylcholine precursors early in the day for maximum improvements in brain productivity throughout the day.

Another mechanism of memory enhancement involves boosting the energy output of brain cells. Aging causes a decline in the ability of neurons to take up glucose and to produce mitochondrial energy. This decline in energy production causes memory and cognitive deficits and results in the accumulation of cellular debris that eventually kills brain cells. When enough brain cells have died from accumulated cellular debris, senility is usually diagnosed. Therapies that fit into the category of brain cell energy enhancers include:

- ❖ 2,400 to 4,800 mg a day of piracetam
- ❖ 1,000 to 2,000 mg a day of acetyl-L-carnitine
- ❖ 120 mg a day of ginkgo biloba extract
- ❖ 5 to 10 mg a day of NADH (nicotinamide adenine dinucleotide)
- ❖ 100 to 200 mg a day of coenzyme Q10
- ❖ 250 to 1,000 mg a day of centrophenoxine
- ❖ 100 to 300 mg a day of phosphatidylserine
- ❖ 100 to 300 mg a day of Picamilon

Phosphatidylserine also plays an important role in maintaining the integrity of brain cell membranes. The breakdown of brain cell membranes prevents glucose and other nutrients from entering the cell.

Free radicals have been implicated as an initiator of DNA damage that results in the breakdown of brain cell metabolism. Scientists suggest that the consumption of antioxidants, especially vitamin E, can reduce the risk of senility. The daily dose of the 52-ingredient Life Extension Mix provides broad-spectrum antioxidant protection for brain cells. The standard dose of Life Extension Mix tablets is three tablets, three times a day.

In order to take advantage of increases in brain cell energy, elevated levels of acetylcholine, and enhanced brain cell membrane function, hormone imbalances have to be corrected to restore the synchronization of youth within the aging brain. Two hormones that help to re-synchronize brain cell activity are DHEA and pregnenolone.

New studies show that pregnenolone is a potent memory-enhancing hormone. Pregnenolone is converted into DHEA within the body. DHEA helps to preserve youthful neurological function. Together, pregnenolone and DHEA help to maintain the "program" brain cells need to store and retrieve short-term memories. Pregnenolone initiates the memory storage process by stimulating adenylate cyclase activity, which is needed to activate and regulate other critical enzymes required for cellular energy production.

Pregnenolone then regulates the sequential flow of calcium ions through the cell membrane. The pattern of calcium ion exchange has great informational content and may determine how memories are encoded by neurons. Pregnenolone also modulates chemical reactions, calcium-protein bindings, gene activation, protein turnover, and enzymatic reactions involved in the storage and retrieval of memory. Aging results in a severe deficiency in pregnenolone and DHEA. Without adequate pregnenolone and DHEA, we gradually lose the neuronal synchronization required for optimal cognitive function.

The dosage range for pregnenolone is 50 to 150 mg in three divided doses. The recommended dosage for DHEA is 25 mg three times a day for men, and 15 mg three times a day for women. Anyone planning to take pregnenolone or DHEA should have a DHEA-S blood test six weeks after initially taking the hormone to help evaluate the correctness of the dosage.

A convenient way of taking pregnenolone, along with phosphatidylserine and choline is to take five capsules a day of the nutrient formula Cognitex. Five capsules of Cognitex contain the suggested daily doses of pregnenolone, choline, vitamin B5 and phosphatidylserine.

Another hormone that may help prevent age-associated mental impairment is melatonin, which is secreted by the pineal gland. Melatonin is a powerful antioxidant that also plays a role in brain cell synchronization. The suggested dose of melatonin for neurological function for people over age 35 is 500 mcg to 3 mg a night. For people already afflicted with an aging-related degenerative brain disease, 3 to 10 mg a night of melatonin is suggested.

Refer to DHEA Precautions before using DHEA or Pregnenolone.

Product availability: Cognitex, pregnenolone, DHEA, acetyl-L-carnitine, ginkgo biloba, DMAE, lecithin, NADH, coenzyme Q10, Life Extension Mix, and melatonin are available singly or in a Protocol Pak from Life Extension Buyers Club by calling 1-800-544-4440. Piracetam and centrophenoxine are available from overseas companies for personal use only. A list of these companies can be obtained by phoning 1-800-544-4440 .

Alcohol-Induced Hangover: Prevention

The consumption of alcohol results in the formation of two very toxic compounds: acetaldehyde and malondialdehyde. These compounds generate massive free radical damage to cells throughout the body. The free radical damage generated by these alcohol metabolites creates an effect in the body similar to radiation poisoning. That is why people feel so sick the day after consuming too much alcohol. If the proper combination of antioxidants are taken at the time the alcohol is consumed or before the inebriated individual goes to bed, the hangover and much of the cellular damage caused by alcohol may be prevented.

Aging makes us increasingly vulnerable to alcohol-induced hangover, liver injury, and damage to the central nervous system. In the elderly, alcohol and drug-induced injury are more common, more serious, and recovery is more difficult.

Nutrients that neutralize alcohol byproducts and protect cells against the damaging effects of alcohol include vitamin C, vitamin B1, the amino acids cysteine and glutathione, along with vitamin E, and selenium. There are several commercial formulas that can be taken at the time the alcohol is consumed and/or before bedtime to help prevent a hangover. One of these formulas is called Anti-Alcohol Antioxidants. Six capsules of this formula contains the proper amounts of antioxidant nutrients for a hangover.

Another product drinkers use is Kyolic Garlic Formula number 105. Garlic contains s-allyl-cysteine and this particular formula also contains vitamin C and vitamin E, beta-carotene and selenium. Since the heavy consumption of alcohol produces many deleterious effects on the body, including an increased risk of cancer, liver disease, and neurological disease, it is suggested that hangover prevention formulas such as Kyolic Garlic Formula number 105 and Anti-Alcohol Antioxidants be taken any time alcohol is consumed.

Product availability: The Anti-Alcohol Antioxidant formula and Kyolic Garlic Formula number 105 can be obtained singly or in a Protocol Pak from Life Extension Buyers Club by calling 1-800-544-4440.

Allergies

Allergies are abnormal hypersensitive reactions to toxic substances (toxins). Allergic reactions occur when our immune system turns against our own cells (autoimmunity), which often involves the creation of damaging free radicals. Toxins are normally handled within the body by detoxification systems. When the toxic load overwhelms these systems, the "gates" to our bodies that interface with the environment (the skin, lungs and GI tract) close down. This stimulates the release of histamine and other inflammatory agents that generate the rashes, hives and other symptoms that plague allergy sufferers.

Allergic reactions can be suppressed by reprogramming immune cells not to react against us. Allergic reactions can be mitigated and sometimes eliminated by maintaining high levels of antioxidants in the body to suppress the effects of an autoimmune attack. For allergy sufferers who are not taking high doses of vitamins, we suggest that three tablets, three times a day, of Life Extension Mix be taken for five weeks. If Life Extension Mix does not suppress the allergic reactions adequately, then the following additional steps should be considered:

1) Five capsules a day of borage oil, which provides 1,500 mg of the essential fatty acid gammalinolenic acid (GLA), which has been shown to suppress some autoimmune reactions. In addition to borage oil, for long-term essential fatty acid balance and additional protection against allergic attacks, three to six capsules of concentrated fish oil (Mega-EPA) should be taken every day.

2) DHEA can modulate immune system cytokines that causes autoimmune, allergic reactions. The dose of DHEA required to suppress autoimmune cytokines varies, but 25 mg three times a day for men and 15 mg three times a day for women are suggested.

Refer to DHEA precautions before using DHEA.

3) Vitamin C can act as a natural antihistamine in doses of 2,500 to 12,000 mg a day. Bioflavonoids such as the proanthocyanidins found in grape seed extract can work with vitamin C to further suppress allergic reactions. The recommended dose of proanthocyanidins (grape seed extract) to combat allergies is 100 to 300 mg a day.

Product availability: Life Extension Mix, Mega-GLA (concentrated borage oil), Mega-EPA (concentrated fish oil), DHEA, vitamin C and grape seed extract can be obtained singly or in a Protocol Pak by calling 1-800-544-4440.

Alzheimer's Disease

Aging causes deficits in short-term memory and other cognitive functions, deterioration of brain cell structure, the degradation and death of brain neurons, and sporadic pathological lesions such as senile plaques and neurofibrillary tangles. Alzheimer's disease is an accelerated form of aging characterized by the widespread distribution of senile plaques and neurofibrillary tangles, the progressive loss of short-term memory and other cognitive functions, major brain cell structural deterioration, major behavioral disorders, and the eventual loss of one's identity—all of which leads eventually to death.

Alzheimer's disease involves damage to cholinergic neurons in the basal forebrain, resulting in a decline in the secretion of the neurotransmitter acetylcholine, which plays a critical role in learning, memory and other cognitive functions.

Among the proposed causes of the destruction of cholinergic neurons in Alzheimer's disease are the intracellular accumulation of beta-amyloid protein, aluminum, lipofuscin (cellular debris), and the generation of excessive free radical activity. One of the biochemical effects of beta-amyloid protein deposition is the inhibition of mitochondrial succinate dehydrogenase enzyme activity, which leads to a marked decrease in ATP formation, and a resulting decline in energy production.

Although several therapies can produce minor improvements in Alzheimer's patients, none of them can produce major therapeutic benefits when used alone. As a result, the Life Extension Foundation suggests a multi-modal approach to the treatment of Alzheimer's disease. This approach is based upon numerous published studies on the synergistic ability of nutrients, hormones and drugs to help protect brain cells from the deficits of normal aging, including the deposition of cellular debris in neurons, as well as the improvement of cognitive function in subjects of various ages.

Our approach also is based upon clinical results with multi-modal therapies in Alzheimer's patients in medical centers in the U.S. and Europe, including a highly successful program at the Alzheimer's Prevention Foundation in Tucson, Ariz.

The Foundation recommends that several or all of the protocols below be used together in Alzheimer's disease patients for the best possible results. It is imperative that regular biochemical and functional tests be administered to the patient under the supervision of a knowledgeable physician to assess the effects of the treatment program selected, and to determine changes that may be required in the program for optimal results.

❖ **Protocol Number One:** To boost acetylcholine levels in the brain, enhance brain cell uptake of glucose, preserve the integrity of brain cell membranes, and synchronize neuronal activity.

   1) The nutrient-hormone formula Cognitex. The suggested dose is five capsules of Cognitex in the morning and five Cognitex capsules in the afternoon. Cognitex provides potent doses of two forms of the acetylcholine pre-

cursor choline and vitamin B5 to convert choline into acetylcholine, phosphatidylserine to maintain the integrity of brain cell membranes and boost brain cell energy metabolism, and pregnenolone, a hormone that dramatically improves memory by synchronizing neuronal activity in the brain.

2) One capsule of DMAE/Ginkgo caps in the morning and one in the afternoon.

❖ **Protocol Number Two:** To combat excessive free radical activity with potent combinations of antioxidants and antitoxins, take Life Extension Mix, three tablets, three times a day, with meals: Life Extension Mix — Three tablets, 3 times a day, with meals

❖ **Protocol Number Three:** To boost brain cell energy levels necessary for healthy metabolic activity take:

1) Acetyl-L-carnitine — 1,000 mg in the morning and 1,000 mg in the afternoon.

2) Piracetam — 1,600 mg in the morning and 1,600 mg in the afternoon.

3) Hydergine — 5 mg in the morning and 5 mg in the afternoon.

4) NADH — 5-20 mg daily in the morning on an empty stomach.

5) Coenzyme Q10 — 200 to 400 mg daily with or after meals.

❖ **Protocol Number Four:** To elevate dopamine levels, improve cellular communication, and enhance neurological function:

1) Deprenyl — 5 mg, twice a week.

2) NADH — See Protocol Number Two.

3) Vitamin B12, which is often deficient in elderly people suffering from neurological diseases, e.g. Alzheimer's disease: 2,000 mcg a day in sublingual (under the tongue) form.

❖ **Protocol Number Five:** To remove cellular debris including lipofuscin caused by the breakdown byproducts of cellular metabolism and strengthen neuronal membrane structure:

1) Centrophenoxine — one tablet in the morning and one in the afternoon.

2) DMAE/ginkgo caps — See Protocol Number One.

3) LECI-PS (Phosphatidylserine) — An extra amount of this nutrient (see Protocol Number One) should be taken in a dose of 100-300 mg daily with a meal.

❖ **Protocol Number Six:** To replace critically important hormones that are severely depleted and/or inactive in Alzheimer's disease patients:

1) Human growth hormone — 1-2 units a day injected subcutaneously six days a week, or follow physician's prescribed dose based upon blood levels of somatomedin-C (IGF-1).

2) DHEA — 25 mg three times a day in men or 15 mg three times a day in women, or follow physician's prescribed dose based upon blood levels of DHEA sulfate.

3) Pregnenolone — An extra amount of this hormone (see Protocol Number One—50 mg three times a day), or follow physician's prescribed dose based upon blood levels of DHEA.

4) Melatonin — 3-10 mg nightly.

Important Note: Pregnenolone cascades down into DHEA, estrogen, progesterone, and testosterone. Estrogen has been shown to improve memory and reduce the risk of Alzheimer's disease in women and is being used in some clinics as a treatment for Alzheimer's disease. The above Hormone Replacement Protocol may provide enough estrogen (converted from pregnenolone and DHEA) to have a therapeutic effect. Some female patients may require additional estrogen and some males may require supplemental testosterone.

❖ **Protocol Number Seven:** To inhibit the enzyme acetylcholinesterase, which degrades the neurotransmitter acetylcholine excessively in Alzheimer's patients: THA, also known as Cognex or tacrine — 160 to 200 mg daily. Physician supervision is mandatory to test liver enzymes to make sure THA is not causing liver damage. One tablespoon of lecithin will reduce THA-induced liver toxicity and provide phosphatidylcholine from which the brain can produce the neurotransmitter acetylcholine. A new drug called Aricept may be less toxic than THA.

Product availability: Cognitex, DMAE/ginkgo Caps, Life Extension Mix, Acetyl-L-carnitine, NADH, coenzyme Q10, vitamin B12, phosphatidylserine, DHEA, pregnenolone, lecithin and melatonin can be obtained singly or in Protocol Paks by calling: 1-800-544-4440. THA and Aricept are an FDA-approved prescription drug which must be prescribed by a physician. Piracetam, hydergine, deprenyl and centrophenoxine are available from overseas companies for personal use only. For a list of companies offering these products, call 1-800-544-4440 .

Amnesia

European doctors use the drugs piracetam and vasopressin to help people suffering from amnesia recover their memories. Published studies show that the recovery of memory in the amnesia patients took from several hours to a few days when vasopressin and/or piracetam were used.

The recommended dosage of vasopressin is at least 16 international units (hereafter called IU) a day, usually in the form of a nasal spray, though physicians may prescribe higher amounts to treat acute amnesia. The recommended dose of piracetam is 4,800 mg a day until memory is restored.

Product availability: Vasopressin is a prescription drug produced by the Sandoz pharmaceutical company. You must see a physician and get a prescription for this medication. Piracetam is an unapproved drug that has to be ordered from offshore pharmacies. For a list of such pharmacies, call 1-800-544-4440.

Amyotrophic Lateral Sclerosis (ALS) (Lou Gehrig's Disease)

ALS is a disabling disease involving the breakdown of the neurons leading from the brain and spinal cord to the muscles. The result is the progressive wasting of the muscles that leads to death caused by respiratory complications in 2-5 years.

There is no established therapy to treat ALS, but understanding some of the mechanisms of neuron destruction involved in ALS can enable a person to follow a protocol that, in theory, could slow the progression of the disease.

Acetyl-L-carnitine has produced dramatic results in protecting neurons in a wide range of disease states. We therefore suggest that ALS patients consume 3,000 mg a day of acetyl-L-carnitine.

Neuron damage can be caused by degeneration of the myelin sheath, which is a fatty layer that wraps the signal-moving neuronal fibers. Taking two tablespoons a day of Udo's Choice Essential Fatty Acids will provide omega-3 and omega-6 fatty acids, which may help to repair the myelin sheath required for proper neuron conduction.

Since pregnenolone and DHEA are involved in the regulation of neurologic function, supplementation with 50 mg three times a day of pregnenolone and/or 25 mg three times a day of DHEA should be considered.

Innovative drug therapies for ALS might also include 10 to 20 mg a day of hydergine, 40 mg a day of vinpocetin and human growth hormone replacement therapy.

To protect against respiratory dysfunction, 600 mg of n-acetyl-cysteine (NAC) and 1,000 mg of vitamin C are suggested three times a day.

Free radicals have been implicated in the ALS disease process, so the standard dose of Life Extension Mix, which is three tablets three times a day, might be helpful. While Life Extension Mix contains a considerable amount of magnesium, 500 mg a day of additional magnesium is also suggested.

Alpha lipoic acid is a potent antioxidant, which is especially effective in preventing diabetic neuropathy. We, therefore, suggest a dose of 1,000 mg a day of alpha lipoic acid to protect the neurons affected by ALS.

Product availability: For a listing of physicians in your area who might be knowledgeable in these innovative approaches, call 1-800-544-4440. To order acetyl-L-carnitine, alpha lipoic acid, n-acetyl-cysteine, pregnenolone, DHEA, Life Extension Mix and magnesium singly or in a Protocol Pak, phone 1-800-544-4440. Hydergine is available by prescription in the U.S. or from overseas pharmacies. Vinpocetin is available from overseas pharmacies. For a list of such pharmacies, call 1-800-544-4440.

Anemia-Thrombocytopenia-Leukopenia

Aging, viral infections, blood diseases, cancer chemotherapy and radiation therapy can cause deficits in red blood cell, white blood cell, and blood platelet production. Studies have shown that supplemental melatonin in doses of 10 to 40 mg a night can restore normal blood cell production.

Another therapy to restore healthy blood platelet production is five capsules a day of standardized shark liver oil capsules containing 200 mg of alkylglycerols per capsule. Studies have shown that shark liver oil can boost the production of blood platelets. Shark liver oil capsules should only be taken in high doses for a maximum period of 30 days because too many blood platelets might be produced. Melatonin therapy can be used for an indefinite period of time.

Anemia can be caused by various deficiencies in vitamin B1, vitamin B2, vitamin B6, vitamin B12, folic acid, and iron. Thus, supplementation of these nutrients should be considered when there are deficiencies. Regular blood testing should be done to monitor the effectiveness of these blood cell-boosting therapies.

Product availability: Standardized shark liver oil capsules, vitamin B1, vitamin B2, vitamin B6, vitamin B12, folic acid and pharmaceutical grade melatonin can be obtained by phoning 1-800-544-4440.

Anesthesia and Surgery Precautions

Anesthesia and surgery can cause temporary or permanent brain damage. Surgical complications can be caused by the free radicals that occur during the surgical process or during anesthesia.

Some of the mechanisms of neurologic injury caused by anesthesia and surgical procedures have been identified in the scientific literature, and specific nutrients and drugs can be taken ahead of time to help protect against surgery-induced neurologic injury.

During open heart surgery, free radicals have been identified as a primary culprit in preventing the re-establishment of a regular heart rhythm and in causing the common complication of pancreatitis.

The most convenient way of obtaining high potency antioxidants to protect against free radicals induced by anesthesia and surgery is to take three tablets, three times a day of Life

Extension Mix along with 200 mg a day of Coenzyme Q10 and 2,000 mg a day of acetyl-L-carnitine at least one week prior to surgery.

At least 3 to 10 mg of melatonin should be taken every night for one week before the surgery, and 10 mg of melatonin should be taken just before anesthesia is administered to provide further protection against anesthesia and surgery-induced complications. Recent animal research funded by the Life Extension Foundation has shown that melatonin given prior to anesthesia protects cells throughout an animal's body (but especially in the brain) against ischemic injury caused by lack of blood flow.

In addition to these antioxidants, at least 5 mg a day of the drug hydergine and 2,400 mg a day of piracetam should be taken one week before surgery to protect brain cells against the effects of erratic blood flow that may occur during the surgery.

Some surgeons ask their pre-surgical patients to avoid aspirin and nutrients that may promote excess bleeding during surgery. Ginkgo biloba and some of the nutrients in Life Extension Mix, such as vitamin E, can inhibit abnormal blood clotting and may cause excess bleeding during and after surgery. For some surgical procedures, excess bleeding can be a problem, but experienced surgeons should be able to deal with this.

On the other hand, a significant risk factor during and after surgical procedures and long hospital stays is the development of abnormal blood clots inside blood vessels, which can cause a stroke, heart attack or a lethal pulmonary embolism. The platelet aggregation inhibiting effect of vitamin E and other nutrients in Life Extension Mix could prevent surgically induced blood clots from forming.

Published studies have shown that when open heart surgery patients take antioxidants before surgery, far fewer complications develop. There are contradictions in the scientific literature as to whether or not vitamin E and other antioxidants cause enough excess bleeding to create a problem, but when you consider the neurologic benefits, the protection against free radicals, the protection against abnormal blood clot formation, and the overall health benefits these nutrients provide, you (and your physician) may choose to include Life Extension Mix in doses of three tablets, three times a day, as part of your pre-surgery medication protocol.

Product availability: Life Extension Mix, ginkgo biloba, acetyl-L-carnitine, coenzyme Q10 and melatonin can be ordered singly or in a Protocol Pak by calling 1-800-544-4440. Hydergine can be obtained with a physician's prescription. Piracetam can be ordered from offshore pharmacies. For a list of these pharmacies, call 1-800-544-4440 .

Anxiety and Stress

In today's high-pressure world, it's not surprising that many people suffer from chronic stress and fatigue with associated conditions such as anxiety, phobias, and depression. Vast numbers of Americans use FDA-approved drugs for chronic stress and fatigue. These drugs have adverse side effects and often fail to address the underlying anxiety, irritability, depression, and learning dysfunction associated with stress and fatigue.

Europeans and Japanese are increasingly turning to a natural alternative to drugs to alleviate chronic stress and fatigue. One of these products is now being used by innovative medical doctors in the United States in place of FDA approved drugs such Xanax, Prozac, and Buspar. The name of this therapy is Adapton. It comes from a species of deep sea fish called garum, whose only known habitat is off the coast of England.

Adapton is being used throughout Europe and Japan for the treatment of a wide range of stress-induced disorders. In a recent clinical trial, 20 patients who had been ill with various forms of chronic fatigue were studied. The patient's anxiety, depression, muscle fatigue, mental fatigue, sleep disorders and headache were measured. Placebo capsules were given to these patients during the first two weeks of the study.

After two weeks on the placebo, fatigue symptoms were reduced by an average of 14% and overall symptoms of anxiety, depression, and insomnia were reduced by 4%. Then Adapton was given for the next two weeks of the study. After two weeks of taking Adapton, fatigue symptoms were reduced by 51% and overall symptoms by 65%! These results show broad spectrum benefits in taking Adapton for people suffering from chronic stress and fatigue. Another study involved 40 patients who had been suffering from various forms of chronic fatigue syndrome. Four capsules of Adapton per day was prescribed for two weeks. The results, based upon the Fatigue Study Group criteria, showed benefit in 50% of the subjects for the 10 functions that most accurately measure fatigue and depression. No serious side effects were reported. The researchers concluded that Adapton is extremely well tolerated and is without contraindications.

In a soon to be published study on the treatment of anxiety in college students, Adapton was shown to be safe and effective in reducing anxiety in otherwise healthy subjects. Other studies are showing that, when Adapton reduces anxiety, it results in improved learning, including enhanced EEG brain wave activity. Adapton benefits 90% of patients with chronic stress and fatigue compared to only 30% of patients on placebo.

Adapton is comprised of a standardized dose of polypeptides that exert a regulatory effect on the nervous system, enabling people to better adapt to stressful conditions. These unique peptides act as precursors to endorphins and other neurotransmitters that improve our ability to adapt to mental and physical stress. Adapton also contains an omega-3 essential fatty acid complex that enhances prostaglandins and prostacyclins—the chemical mediators that regulate major biological functions in the body. Omega-3 extract is thought to contribute to the stress reducing effects of this European therapy.

If you suffer from chronic stress-induced anxiety, fatigue, or depression, Adapton could provide you with substantial relief. Hyperactive children with learning disabilities such as attention deficit disorder are being treated successfully with Adapton in Europe in place of drugs like Ritalin.

The recommended dosage is four capsules of Adapton on an empty stomach in the morning for 15 consecutive days. After two weeks, the dose should be reduced to two capsules every morning. If complete relief is obtained, Adapton can be discontinued until symptoms return. Some people take 2-3 Adapton capsules every other day. There is no toxicity risk in taking Adapton every day, although it doesn't have to be taken every day for it to work.

For those who suffer from anxiety attacks, 10 mg of the prescription drug propranolol can provide immediate relief. Propranolol works by blocking beta-adrenergic sites on cell membranes so that cells do not overreact to the increased amount of adrenaline secreted in response to anxiety invoking situations. Propranolol is a cardiovascular drug, and those with very low blood pressure, asthma, or congestive heart failure may not be able to use it. The low dose of propranolol required to prevent or treat anxiety attacks is tolerable by the vast majority of people.

Anxiety and stress can result in the excess production of adrenal hormone cortisol. Cortisol damages the immune system, the arterial system, and brain cells, and causes premature aging. While some people never gain complete control over stress and anxiety, the effects of excessive cortisol production can be mitigated by taking one to two tablets of the European medication KH3 in the morning on an empty stomach, and one to two tablets of KH3 in the mid-afternoon on an empty stomach. People allergic to procaine (the active ingredient in KH3) or on sulfa drugs should not take KH3.

The regulatory hormones melatonin and DHEA may also protect against the effects of stress-induced excessive cortisol production. Suggested dosage for melatonin is from 500 mcg to 10 mg a day. Men should take 25 mg three times a day of DHEA, while women should take 15 mg three times a day of DHEA.

Product availability: Adapton, melatonin and DHEA are available by calling 1-800-544-4440. Ask for a listing of offshore companies that sell KH3 to Americans by mail for personal use. Propranolol can be prescribed by a doctor.

Arrhythmia (Cardiac)

Heart arrhythmia is caused by a variety of medical conditions that have to be identified by a cardiologist before appropriate therapies can be devised. Once the underlying cause of the cardiac arrhythmia has been established, there are a number of natural therapies that may be of help in reestablishing normal heart rhythms. These therapies should be used with a great deal of caution.

Anti-arrhythmia nutrients include the minerals magnesium at 500 to 2,000 mg a day, potassium at 200 to 500 mg a day, and selenium at 300 to 600 mcg a day. Coenzyme Q10 is used in Japan as a treatment for cardiac arrhythmia at 100 to 300 mg a day. Acetyl-L-carnitine is used in Europe to treat cardiac arrhythmia at 1,000 to 2,000 mg a day. Taurine at 1,000-to 2,000 mg a day is used with carnitine and coenzyme Q10 in Japan as a treatment for congestive heart failure.

Forskolin is an Indian herbal extract that improves contractile strength in the heart muscle when taken at 10 to 60 mg a day. Forskolin may alleviate cardiac arrhythmia or, over an extended period of time, exacerbate it. Forskolin is most appropriately used when arrhythmia is accompanied by severe congestive heart failure.

CAUTION: Do not use forskolin if you have prostate cancer.

Vitamin D3 enhances calcium metabolism in the sino atrial node of the heart at 1,000 IU a day. Vitamin E at 400 to 800 IU a day is used to treat coronary artery disease, but also helps to establish normal heart rhythms. Five to eight capsules of fish oil concentrates a day have been shown to regulate cardiac arrhythmias in several published studies.

A novel anti-arrhythmia agent may be vitamin A. In a study in the *Journal of Cardiovascular Pharmacology*, December 1995, retinoic acid, a vitamin A derivative, produced marked anti-arrhythmic effects in rats. Those who want to avoid vitamin A drugs that can produce adverse side effects should use 100,000 IU a day of water soluble vitamin A liquid drops as a potential therapy to restore normal heart rhythms. A complete blood chemistry test battery should reveal if this dose of vitamin A is generating toxic effects.

Important: Refer to the Symptoms of Vitamin A Toxicity, in Appendix A.

The use of any of these natural therapies should be done with the full cooperation of a trained cardiologist, as any errors could result in sudden death from a heart attack. Those with cardiac arrhythmias should avoid caffeine, heavy alcohol intake, and dietary saturated fats.

Product availability: Magnesium, potassium, acetyl-L-carnitine, coenzyme Q10, taurine, Mega-EPA, selenium, vitamin D3, forskolin, and water soluble vitamin A drops can be obtained singly or in a Protocol Pak by calling 1-800-544-4440.

Arthritis

Arthritis is epidemic throughout the world. There are two basic forms of arthritis, osteoarthritis and rheumatoid arthritis.

Osteoarthritis is characterized by the inability of the cartilage in joints to maintain and repair itself. The results of osteoarthritis are cartilage degradation, erosion of joint lining, and eventual loss of mechanical function in the joint, all of which involve chronic pain. The initial symptoms of osteoarthritis are joint pain, stiffness and decreased joint movement. In severe cases, the cartilage in the joint disintegrates entirely, causing the joint bones to rub against each other, which causes severe pain and rapid loss of joint function.

Rheumatoid arthritis is characterized by an autoimmune attack on the linings of the joints, resulting in severe inflammation, joint disfigurement, loss of joint function, and chronic pain. The initial symptoms of rheumatoid arthritis are enlargement of the joints, often in the fingers, with increasing pain and loss of function as the disease flares up.

The Life Extension Foundation recommends natural therapies for arthritis and other inflammatory disorders. Newly published scientific research studies confirm the efficacy of natural therapies in suppressing inflammation and pain without adverse side effects.

Mainstream medicine treats arthritis patients with corticosteroids and nonsteroidal anti-inflammatory drugs. While these drugs can work in the short term, they can produce serious adverse side effects such as gastric ulceration and liver and kidney damage when taken chronically. Estimates are that conventional arthritis drugs kill over 7,000 Americans and are responsible for 70,000 hospitalizations every year. Worst of all, long-term use of many of these drugs results in complete joint immobilization because they fail to treat the underlying cause of most forms of arthritis. FDA approved drugs can exacerbate catabolic cartilage breakdown and prevent the expression of natural anabolic repair mechanisms. Scientists have observed that the higher the dose of FDA-approved anti-inflammatory drugs, the faster the loss of joint function!

European doctors have been using non-toxic, natural therapies to treat arthritis with great success for many years. These natural therapies work because they treat the underlying degenerative process affecting the linings of the joints in osteoarthritis and/or improve the autoimmune disorder that destroys the joint linings in rheumatoid arthritis.

The cartilage in our joints is vulnerable to a wide range of insults that can result in cartilage degeneration. When a joint becomes inflamed, the blood supply is reduced, thereby reducing the ability to repair the cartilage. The attack on the cartilage in our joints intensifies as we grow older. First our vascular system becomes blocked, which prevents normal cartilage repair and maintenance. Then our natural antioxidant enzyme systems break down and free radicals attack joint cartilage. Finally, our immune system becomes disoriented and starts attacking the linings of our own joints.

The initial result of joint injury is the formation of free radicals that attack the cartilage and lubricating synovial fluid within the joint. This free radical activity can trigger a cascade of autoimmune events to cause chronic loss of cartilage structure and function. Conventional doctors usually accept these events as the normal, irreversible progression of arthritis.

Research indicates that a deficiency of antioxidants often is a factor in the development of arthritis. While antioxidants can be of help in some early stage arthritis patients, more direct anti-arthritic therapies are required for those whose joint degeneration has progressed significantly.

In order for osteoarthritis to be treated effectively, the cartilage and synovial fluid in the joint must be protected against further destruction. At the same time, it is desirable to stimulate anabolic restoration of joint cartilage and synovial fluid. Chondroprotective agents are compounds the body manufactures naturally to regenerate cartilage and healthy joint function. Aging and trauma disrupt the body's ability to use its own chondroprotective agents. Here are therapies that have been shown to be helpful for osteoarthritis patients:

❖ **Therapy number one** is glucosamine, which has been used extensively in Europe to treat osteoarthritis. Studies document glucosamine's ability to function as a chondroprotective agent. Glucosamine provides the raw material needed for chondrocytes to regenerate cartilage. A glucosamine deficiency caused by aging and/or trauma leads to osteoarthritis.

In nine European studies, the oral administration of glucosamine produced major reductions in joint pain, joint tenderness and joint swelling. Improvements in joint function and overall physical performance were noted in these studies compared to placebo and/or the drug Ibuprofen. While Ibuprofen worked faster than glucosamine in relieving pain, glucosamine improved overall condition better, without any of the toxic side effects associated with Ibuprofen.

The research and clinical results with glucosamine have been so impressive that it has become a first line therapy against osteoarthritis in Europe. It is only when glucosamine doesn't work that European doctors resort to toxic nonsteroidal anti-inflammatory drugs. Glucosamine salts exhibit no toxicity at doses far higher than patients need to treat their arthritis successfully. Glucosamine salts are easily absorbed and distributed in the joint cartilage matrix.

Studies show that glucosamine takes four to 10 weeks to produce noticeable results. A new arthritis formula, that contains glucosamine, has been producing noticeable reductions in inflammation and pain in most arthritis patients in less than four weeks! This new patent-pending formula, which will be described later in this protocol, contains two forms of glucosamine, chondroitin sulfates and the EPA, DHA, and GLA essential fatty acids.

❖ **Therapy number two** includes the chondroitin sulfates, which provide the structural components of the cartilage found in the joint. Chondroitin sulfate is a constituent of shark cartilage, which helps to explain the beneficial effects that shark cartilage produces in some arthritis patients. The chondroitin sulfates have been tested extensively in humans with outstanding success. The FDA has ruled, however, that, because each chondroitin sulfate molecule is different from all other chondroitin sulfate molecules, it cannot be approved because it is impossible to produce a precisely standardized product. Nevertheless, research studies have provided much useful data on the safety and effectiveness of chondroitin sulfates in arthritis patients. Chondroitin sulfates inhibit enzymes that degrade joint cartilage and collagen.

❖ **Therapy number three** involves the use of essential fatty acids such as GLA (gamma linolenic acid) found in evening primrose oil, borage oil, and black currant seed oil and fish oils rich in EPA and DHA. These essential fatty acids are precursors of prostaglandins, such as PGE1, PGE2, and PGI2, which have known anti-inflammatory and, perhaps, anti-autoimmune effects. Here are findings from some of the new studies documenting the benefits of essential fatty acids in treating arthritis:

In the *Annals of Internal Medicine* (1993, 119/9), the findings of a 24-week, double-blind, placebo-controlled trial with GLA derived from borage oil was reported. The patients receiving the borage oil experienced a 36% reduction in the number of tender joints, a 45% reduction in the tender joint score, a 41% reduction in the swollen joint score, and a 28% reduction in the swollen joint count. The placebo group showed no benefits.

A paper in the *British Journal of Rheumatology* (1994, 33/9) reports the findings of a 24-week, double-blind, placebo-controlled trial in rheumatoid arthritis patients using black currant seed oil, rich in gamma linolenic acid (GLA) and alpha linolenic acid. Patients receiving black currant seed oil showed reductions in the signs and symptoms of the disease. The placebo group showed no change in disease status. The researchers concluded that their study showed black currant seed oil is a potentially effective treatment for active rheumatoid arthritis. No adverse reactions were observed, although some people dropped out of the trial because of the size and number of capsules they were required to take.

In *Seminars in Arthritis and Rheumatism* (1995, 25/2), there was a review of all the published literature on the use of gamma linolenic acid (GLA) for the treatment of rheumatoid arthritis. GLA reduced the effects of autoimmune disease on joint linings, though more research was said to be needed to determine the ideal dose of GLA for arthritis.

A study in the *Journal of Clinical Epidemiology* (1995, 48/11), reviewed all the published studies on the use of fish oil to treat rheumatoid arthritis. They revealed that, in general, after three months of use, there was a significant reduction in tender joint count and morning stiffness in patients receiving fish oils. The placebo groups experienced no relief from pain.

In a study in *Arthritis and Rheumatism* (1995, 38/8), rheumatoid arthritis patients stopped taking non-steroidal anti-inflammatory drugs and switched to fish oil. This placebo-controlled, double-blind study showed that the group receiving the fish oil experienced significant decreases in the number of tender joints, duration of morning stiffness, improvements in the physicians' and patients' evaluation of global arthritis activity, and the physicians' evaluation of pain. Patients receiving fish oil exhibited improvement in clinical functions compared to patients receiving placebo. Some patients were able to stop taking conventional arthritis drugs altogether.

A unique formula called Natural Pain Relief For Arthritis has been developed for the treatment of chronic inflammatory diseases such as osteo- and rheumatoid arthritis and bursitis. This formula combines the most effective anti-inflammatory agents European doctors are prescribing as first-line therapies against arthritis and other chronic inflammatory diseases. Natural Pain Relief For Arthritis may also be effective for many conditions such as tendinitis, sprained ankles and knees, lupus, rheumatism, cancer, and ulcers.

The ingredients in Natural Pain Relief For Arthritis have been shown to:

✔ Relieve the inflammation, stiffness, and pain associated with osteo- and rheumatoid arthritis.

✔ Contribute to the regeneration of joint cartilage and joint lubricating synovial fluid.

✔ Contribute to the suppression of autoimmune components that attack joint linings.

✔ Be almost totally free of adverse side effects, especially those associated with nonsteroidal anti-inflammatory drugs.

In addition to relieving chronic joint inflammation and pain, the natural ingredients in Natural Pain Relief For Arthritis have been shown to:

❖ Reduce the risk of abnormal blood clot formation that can lead to a sudden heart attack or stroke.

❖ Contribute to the alleviation of autoimmune disorders not associated with chronic inflammatory diseases.

❖ Help maintain the health of the endothelial linings of the arterial system.

❖ Contribute to the suppression of common inflammatory skin disorders such as eczema.

❖ Reduce serum triglyceride levels.

❖ Reduce blood pressure in some hypertensive patients.

The recommended dose of this new natural formula is based upon weight. For those weighing less than 150 pounds, one capsule three times a day. For those weighing 150 to 200 pounds, two capsules, three times day. For those weighing more than 200 pounds, three capsules, three times a day.

If reductions in inflammation and pain do not begin to occur within a week after starting Natural Pain Relief For Arthritis, increase your dosage by taking one additional capsule with each dose. Instead of taking one capsule three times a day, increase it to two capsules three times a day.

Natural Pain Relief For Arthritis comes in oil-filled, soft gel capsules. Three capsules contain the following:

- ✔ 400 mg EPA (from fish oil)
- ✔ 300 mg DHA (from fish oil)
- ✔ 300 mg GLA (from black currant seed or borage oil)
- ✔ 500 mg N-acetyl-glucosamine
- ✔ 500 mg glucosamine sulfate
- ✔ 200 mg chondroitin sulfate
- ✔ 1 mg magnesium aspartate
- ✔ 5 mg ascorbyl palmitate
- ✔ 10 IU vitamin E

Product availability: You can order glucosamine-chondroitin sulfate formulas or essential fatty acid concentrates as single products. However, we recommend the Natural Pain Relief For Arthritis formula that combines all the natural pain and inflammation-suppressing therapies. To order any of these products, alone or in a Protocol Pak call 1-800-544-4440.

Asthma

Asthma is characterized by recurrent airway obstructions that may resolve by themselves or may require treatment. Asthma may be a response to inhaled allergens, infectious agents, irritants (such as dust, chemicals vapors, cold air) or emotions. Symptoms may range from wheezing, mild coughing and slight breathlessness to severe attacks that can lead to total airway obstruction and death. The lungs become over-inflated because of impaired emptying and respiratory gas exchange deterioration.

The immune system components histamine and leukotrienes generate free radicals that are involved in the inflammatory process that results in lung irritation and airway obstruction. The same mechanisms that cause allergies can also cause asthma. When Life Extension Mix was introduced in 1983, many asthmatics called the Foundation to report that their asthma unexpectedly went away.

Studies document that asthmatics who take high potency vitamin supplements have a significant reduction in the incidence and severity of asthmatic attacks. They also show that high dietary magnesium intake is associated with improvement in lung function and less wheezing and fewer asthma attacks. Life Extension Mix contains high levels of magnesium, which may partially explain why so many asthmatics no longer have asthma attacks after starting Life Extension Mix.

Asthmatics also should consider taking an additional 500 mg of elemental magnesium a day. Histamine is a major factor in asthmatic attacks and vitamin C is involved in the natural destruction of excess histamine. Asthmatics should take at least two 600 mg capsules of N-acetyl-cysteine (NAC) a day, along with two grams or more of vitamin C to break up mucus that could worsen an asthmatic attack.

Asthmatics should consider taking either the drug hydergine or the herbal extract forskolin to safely boost intracellular levels of the messenger effector molecule, cyclic AMP. Higher levels of cyclic AMP often reduce bronchial constriction.

CAUTION: Those with prostate cancer should not take forskolin. The FDA-approved drug, theophylline, is used to treat asthma by boosting cyclic AMP levels. Cyclic AMP levels can be raised in a safer way by using hydergine or forskolin.

Product availability: Life Extension Mix, forskolin, N-acetyl-cysteine (NAC), magnesium and vitamin C are available by calling 1-800-544-4440. You can also ask for a listing of off-shore pharmacies that sell hydergine to Americans for personal use.

Atherosclerosis

Atherosclerosis is the leading cause of death and disability in the Western world. Atherosclerosis can be defined as the progressive narrowing of the arteries. A heart attack or stroke can occur as a result of a blood clot that forms in an atherosclerotic artery, and/or when the artery narrows to the point of severely restricting blood flow. Restricted blood flow results in cell injury and cell death in the heart, brain, kidneys, and other organs.

Specific diseases caused by atherosclerosis include coronary artery disease, angina pectoris, cerebral vascular disease, thrombotic stroke, transient ischemic attack, and diabetic vascular complications.

Three mechanisms have been identified as possible causative agents in the development of atherosclerosis and ischemia (reduced blood flow):

- ❖ Causative agent number one is the oxidation of LDL cholesterol and other serum lipids. Oxidation of blood fats causes them to attach to the linings of the arteries. Oxidation of LDL, also referred to as "bad cholesterol," renders it "sticky" and causes it to deposit on the internal lining of blood vessel walls. One of the immediate results may be elevated blood pressure.

- ❖ Causative agent number two is homocysteine formation in response to dietary protein. Homocysteine alone will promote atherosclerosis, even if cholesterol and triglyceride levels are not significantly elevated.

- ❖ Causative agent number three is abnormal platelet aggregation onto the arterial wall, which promotes the development of atherosclerotic plaques. This can lead to a blood clot on important arterial walls in the heart, brain or any other organ, resulting in ischemia (reduced blood flow), infarction (heart muscle destruction), disability, and sudden death.

Protocols to prevent the development of atherosclerosis and arterial blockage include supplements to lower and inhibit the oxidation of LDL cholesterol, elevate beneficial HDL cholesterol, and lower serum triglycerides, fibrinogen, glucose, and iron levels. Homocysteine levels have to be kept under control and the propensity of the blood to clot within blood vessels has to be reduced.

To prevent oxidation of serum cholesterol we suggest:

1) Life Extension Mix — Three tablets three times a day, preferably with meals. Life Extension Mix contains a potent spectrum of antioxidants, such as vitamin E, which have been shown to inhibit the oxidation of cholesterol.

2) Coenzyme Q10 — CoQ10 works synergistically with vitamin E to prevent LDL cholesterol oxidation. CoQ10 also enhances heart cell energy function. CoQ10 should be taken in doses of 100 to 400 mg daily. CoQ10 in a base of rice bran oil should be used, based on studies showing superior assimilation and cardiac benefits when using CoQ10 dissolved in an absorbable oil.

3) Life Extension Herbal Mix — This formula contains plant extracts, which have been documented to maintain the health of the vascular system and reduce the incidence of cardiovascular disease. Life Extension Herbal Mix contains pharmaceutical doses of premium grade herbal extracts such as green tea, ginkgo biloba, ginseng, bilberry, and grape seed extract. The suggested dose is one tablespoon mixed with water or juice, early in the day.

To prevent the formation of atherogenic homocysteine:

1) Folic Acid — Folic acid has been shown to significantly lower serum levels of homocysteine. Folic acid only stays in the body for 4-5 hours after oral ingestion, so it is crucial to take 800 mcg of folic acid with every meal in order to keep artery-clogging homocysteine at safe levels.

2) Vitamin B6 — Vitamin B6 reduces homocysteine via a different mechanism than folic acid. There is enough vitamin B6 in Life Extension Mix to keep homocysteine levels under control in most people. In familial homocysteinemia however, folate will not reduce homocysteine levels adequately, but doses of vitamin B6 in excess of 500 mg daily can. Since high doses of B6 have peripheral nerve toxicity, high doses (500 mg of B6 a day and higher) should only be used when a blood test documents the failure of folic acid to lower homocysteine levels.

3) Trimethylglycine (TMG) is the most effective homocysteine-lowering substance known. The suggested dose is 500 mg to 1,500 mg a day.

To prevent the formation of blood clots inside arteries:

1) Aspirin — Take ¼ aspirin tablet every day with the heaviest meal of the day.

2) Fish Oils — Take 8-12 capsules daily of a concentrated EPA/DHA fish oil

supplement. Flax oil may work as well as fish oils.

3) Herbal Cardiovascular Formula — One capsule in the morning, one in the evening.

4) Garlic — Take 800 to 4,000 mg a day.

To lower cholesterol levels:

1) Herbal Cardiovascular Formula — Take one capsule in the morning and one in the evening. If your cholesterol levels are not significantly lowered in 30 days, double or triple this dose.

2) Soy protein — Take a minimum of 20 mg a day of genistein. This can be obtained by taking one heaping tablespoon of Super Soy Extract powder or ten Super Soy Extract tablets a day.

3) Fiber — Take 10 to 30 grams of soluble fibers, including pectins, guar and psyllium.

It should be noted that there is an overlapping beneficial effect in the above recommendations, i.e., folic acid will help to reduce homocysteine levels and reduce the formation of abnormal blood clots inside arteries.

Linus Pauling recommended 500 mg of lysine taken three times a day as a therapy for reversing atherosclerosis. Those with coronary atherosclerosis may want to supplement with this inexpensive amino acid.

Following these protocols involves a lot of pill-taking, but it must be understood that there are many factors that can cause an abnormal blood clot that leads to a heart attack or stroke. If you fail to utilize all the known therapies for preventing atherosclerosis and abnormal blood clotting, one missing link could cause a life-threatening cardiovascular event. Many Foundation members are already following our Atherosclerosis protocol because the same antioxidant nutrients used to prevent cardiovascular disease may also help to prevent cancer, cataract, Alzheimer's disease, Parkinson's disease, and a host of aging-related illnesses.

Product availability: You can obtain Life Extension Mix, coenzyme Q10, Life Extension Herbal Mix, folic acid, vitamin B6, aspirin, fish oils, Herbal cardiovascular Formula, garlic, Fiberfood, Healthprin, Mega-EPA, TMG and Super Soy Extract powder, singly or in Protocol Paks, by calling 1-800-544-4440.

Attention Deficit Disorder (ADD)

Children with learning difficulties often have Attention Deficit Disorder (ADD). ADD can be a symptom of vitamin deficiency. Studies document improvement in cognitive function when children and young adults take vitamin supplements. The most difficult aspect of treating ADD in children is compliance. Chewable vitamin supplements do not taste good, and it is sometimes hard to get children to swallow pills.

Many parents have their children drink a glass of juice spiked with Life Extension Mix powder every morning before school. Life Extension Mix is the most concentrated vitamin supplement in the world. Children should take a proportionally smaller dose than an adult based upon their weight. If the child will not drink Life Extension Mix with juice, then other forms of high potency vitamin supplementation should be tried to correct learning disorders and behavior problems.

If vitamin supplements do not work, try taking 350 mg of DMAE liquid every morning. DMAE needs to be taken for six weeks in order to obtain optimum results. The desired amount for learning disabilities is from 350 mg to 1,000 mg and can be gradually increased. DMAE is an acetylcholine precursor that boosts the level of this crucial neurotransmitter in the brain. About 10 drops of DMAE liquid provide 350 mg of DMAE. Elevating acetylcholine levels in the brain can improve cognitive function and concentration. Cognitex also helps elevate acetylcholine levels in the brain. Try taking 4-6 capsules per day in divided doses.

Udo's Choice Oil Blend can also be helpful for maintaining proper growth, helping to stimulate the production of fat-digesting enzymes, and helping to make prostaglandins that are essential for brain function. Essential fatty acids are a structural component of all brain cells, the blood-brain barrier and cell walls, comprising more than 50% of the brain itself, and help with nerve transmission.

If desired results do not occur with vitamin supplements and DMAE, then the European drug piracetam should be added. Piracetam dosing for adults is 1,600 to 4,800 mg a day. Children should take less piracetam, though piracetam does not appear to be toxic even when children take adult doses. All of these nutrients and drugs should be taken in the morning.

Product availability: DMAE Liquid, Cognitex, Udo's Choice Oil Blend, and Life Extension Mix can be ordered singly or in a Protocol Pak by calling 1-800-544-4440. You can receive a list of offshore pharmacies that sell piracetam to Americans for personal use by calling 1-800-544-4440.

Autoimmune Diseases

A wide range of degenerative diseases are caused by the immune system attacking a person's own cells. Our immune system becomes increasingly defective as we age, though some people suffer from autoimmune diseases very early in life. Immune dysfunction can cause immune responsive cells to manufacture antibodies to attack the linings of the joints, resulting in arthritis, or defectively functioning immune cells to attack the insulin producing islet cells of the pancreas, resulting in insulin dependent diabetes.

A host of diseases can be linked to a defective immune system. Many people find that taking three tablets, three times a day of Life Extension Mix multi-nutrient formula can help to correct a defective immune system.

People with existing autoimmune diseases need more help than just Life Extension Mix. The hormone DHEA can help suppress certain unwanted immune system reactions in autoimmune patients. A recent clinical study showed that DHEA reduced symptoms in patients with lupus, a common autoimmune disease.

CAUTION: Refer to DHEA Precautions for safety and proper dosing information before beginning DHEA therapy.

Fish oils that provide concentrated amounts of the essential fatty acids EPA and DHA, and borage oil that contains gammalinolenic acid (GLA), can be effective in alleviating the symptoms of autoimmune diseases. Suggested doses are five capsules a day of the fish oil concentrate Mega-EPA and four capsules a day of Mega-GLA, along with the standard daily dose of Life Extension Mix.

Product availability: Mega-EPA, Mega-GLA, DHEA and Life Extension Mix can be obtained singly or in a Protocol Pak by calling 1-800-544-4440.

Bacterial Infections

Acute bacterial infections require immediate conventional medical care. If FDA-approved antibiotics fail to work, European antibiotics, which are several years more advanced than American antibiotics, may be effective.

❖ Herbal extracts from goldenseal and echinacea may be effective natural antibiotics. Raw garlic has potent antibacterial effects. Kyolic, an aged garlic product, does not kill bacteria directly, but does boost immune function, thus enabling the body to fight off some chronic bacterial infections.

❖ Shark liver oil capsules containing a minimum of 200 mg of alkylglycerols per capsule, at the dose of five capsules a day, can have a direct antibiotic effect. Do not take shark liver oil for more than 30 days because it may cause the overproduction of blood platelets.

❖ Bromelain can potentiate the effects of conventional antibiotics, making them more effective in killing bacteria. Suggested dose is 2,000 mg of bromelain per day.

❖ Arginine in doses ranging from 6 to 20 grams a day can stimulate antibacterial components of the immune system.

❖ Recent electron microscope studies show that bee propolis has a potent anti-bacterial effect by preventing cell division and inhibiting protein synthesis.

For more information about treating bacterial infections, refer to the Foundation's Immune Boosting protocols.

PRECAUTION: When using any bee products for children, they should not be administered to children under the age of three.

Product availability: For information on European antibiotics, call 1-800-544-4440. Kyolic garlic, norwegian shark liver oil, bromelain, echinacea, arginine, and bee propolis can be obtained singly or in a Protocol Pak by calling 1-800-544-4440.

Balding

Although hair loss is an integral part of the aging process, its impact is most pronounced in young people who suffer from a condition called androgenetic alopecia (AGA), which causes accelerated hair loss. AGA is commonly called male pattern baldness, but, in fact, occurs in both men and women.

The pattern of hair loss varies by gender. With men it usually begins with a receding hair line with further loss at the vertex of the scalp. In women the pattern is more diffuse, typically sparing the anterior hairline and predominately affecting the crown.

Pathogenesis Of Accelerated Hair Loss

The current model of how accelerated hair loss (AGA) occurs involves a combination of genetic, hormonal and immunologic factors.

Despite what some doctors (and TV infomercials) would have you believe, AGA has nothing to do with clogged hair follicles, which has been the basis for many "hair growth" products. Good scalp hygiene will improve the appearance of and can add volume to existing hair, but will do nothing to prevent AGA or actually increase hair counts.

There are at least 20 different products on the market today, which claim, either directly or indirectly, that they will grow hair or prevent baldness by "unclogging" your hair follicles. The effectiveness of virtually all these products can be summed up in three simple words—they don't work!

The only exception to this are the compounds polysorbate 60 and polysorbate 80—both of which are in Life Extension Shampoo sold by Life Extension Buyers Club. Polysorbate 60 and 80 appear to be useful in slowing down hair loss when applied topically because of their ability to emulsify androgen-rich sebum deposits from the scalp. They are rarely able to generate any degree of hair regrowth, however, but may be useful in conjunction with other agents.

There's little doubt that some people are genetically susceptible to accelerated hair loss caused by AGA. Generations of young men with bald fathers have traditionally dreaded the first signs of hair loss, which to them signified the beginning of a process that would inevitably end in baldness at an earlier than normal age.

The latest scientific model to explain baldness involves the action of dihydrotestosterone (DHT)—the major metabolite of the male hormone testosterone. Scientists have found that excessive secretion of DHT stimulates a localized immune reaction, which, in turn, generates an inflammatory response that damages hair follicles, resulting in their miniaturization and eventual loss.

What appears to happen is that DHT (and, perhaps, other androgenic hormones) causes the immune system to react to the hair follicles in the affected areas as foreign bodies. This is suggested by the presence of hair follicle antibodies as well as by the infiltration of immune system cells around the hair follicles of balding men and women.

Successful prevention and treatment of accelerated hair loss necessitates dealing with some, if not all, of these factors involved in the process, except for the genetic component of baldness, which is still in the research phase.

Since the male hormone dihydrotestosterone is involved in premature hair loss, scientists have experimented with a wide variety of anti-androgens in an attempt to prevent or reverse the process. Among the anti-androgens that have been used to treat hair loss are: progesterone, spironolactone (Aldactone), flutamide (Eulexin), finasteride (Proscar), cimetidine (Tagamet), serenoa repens (Permixon) and cyproterone acetate (Androcur/Diane). Of these anti-androgens the most effective have proved to be oral finasteride (Proscar) and topical spironolactone, both of which have been able to grow hair to some degree, with minimal side effects.

In the hair loss process, it is the immune reaction caused by male hormones such as DHT that plays, perhaps, the most significant role in the balding process. Stimulated by androgens, the immune system targets hair follicles in genetically susceptible areas to cause the premature loss of hair characteristic of male pattern baldness.

Among the most potent hair growth stimulators are topical oxygen radical scavengers such as the superoxide dismutases (SODases), enzymes that play a critically important role in countering excessive free radical activity throughout the body.

SODases not only inhibit oxygen radicals, but also may inhibit the localized immune response responsible for so much hair loss, and may offset some of the damage and inflammation already incurred. Unless the immunologic factors involved in the hair loss process are dealt with effectively in treatment, the potential for significant regrowth may be very limited.

A Multi-Modal Approach To Hair Treatment

There are many agents available (such as Rogaine) that can stimulate some degree of hair growth in some people, but cannot by themselves produce the kind of health and cosmetic benefits that balding people desire. What's needed is a multi-modal approach to hair treatment that combines anti-androgens with autoimmune protective agents, oxygen free radical inhibitors, and other hair growth stimulators to halt hair loss and generate hair regrowth to a degree well beyond the abilities of single compounds.

Dr. Peter Proctor is the only hair treatment practitioner in the world who has developed unique, patented multi-ingredient hair formulas that address all the known factors in the balding process. He is the author of more than 30 scientific articles and book chapters, and holds several broad patents for hair loss treatment.

Dr. Proctor's Hair Treatment Formulas

Dr. Proctor offers both prescription and non-prescription hair treatment formulas, which vary both in potency and cost. However, even the least potent of Dr. Proctor's formulas has proven to be superior to Rogaine—the only FDA-approved hair treatment product on the market.

The least expensive of Dr. Proctor's hair growth formulas is sold under the name Dr. Proctor's Hair Regrowth Shampoo. This formula includes an abundant supply of the most potent natural, hair growth stimulator available—NANO (3-carboxylic acid pyridine-N-oxide), which is known as "natural" minoxidil.

Dr. Proctor's Hair Regrowth Shampoo has been shown to work effectively in many people who did not respond to Rogaine. It may be all you need if you have only experienced small to moderate hair loss, or if your primary need is for a prophylactic program that will prevent hair loss in the future. Dr. Proctor's Hair Regrowth Shampoo should be used whenever you shower, or wash your hair (at least three times a week). It should be used just like any other shampoo.

The second formula developed by Dr. Proctor, which is being sold under the name Dr. Proctor's Advanced Hair Regrowth Formula, includes a potent dose of a "natural" minoxidil (NANO) combined with the following natural hair protection and hair growth agents: EDRF enhancers, SODases, and various free radical scavengers.

This multi-agent, natural formula is the most potent natural hair growth formula you can buy. It includes every type of natural hair treatment agent available to counter the DHT, autoimmune, and inflammatory effects that are the root of hair loss and baldness. Dr. Proctor's Advanced Hair Regrowth Formula is a liquid that is applied to the scalp.

Dr. Proctor's Advanced Hair Regrowth Formula should be used in the following manner: 8-10 drops applied to the thinning areas once or twice a day. Its side effects include contact dermatitis, an itchy, scaly rash at the site of application.

If you have a really serious hair loss problem, you may need to try Dr. Proctor's most potent hair growth formula, which uses an array of natural hair growth protectors combined with several drugs compounded into a cream base. The natural agents in Dr. Proctor's European Prescription Hair Regrowth Formula include topical anti-androgens which increase EDRF levels and oxygen free radical scavengers. These agents are combined with the following drugs: minoxidil, phenytoin (Dilantin), tretinoin (Retin-A) and spironolactone.

The protocol for using Dr. Proctor's European Prescription Hair Regrowth Formula is as follows: Apply 1/10 of a teaspoon (a dab on the end of your finger) once a day for eight to 12 months, then every other day for maintenance. Its side effects include contract dermatitis.

Product availability: You can order Dr. Proctor's Hair Regrowth Shampoo Advanced Hair Regrowth Formula singly or in a Protocol Pak by calling 1-800-544-4440. European Prescription Hair Regrowth Formula is available by prescription from his office. For further information, call 1-800-544-4440.

Bladder Conditions

Bladder conditions, benign and malignant, often are treated successfully by innovative doctors with the FDA-approved biological, non-toxic solvent dimethylsulfoxide (DMSO).

For bladder infections, refer to the Foundation's Urinary Tract Infections protocol.

For bladder cancer, refer to the Foundation's Cancer Treatment protocols.

For use of DMSO in interstitial cystitis, you must have your doctor contact Research Industries Corporation at 1-801-972-5500. They have a DMSO product under the name Rimso-50.

Blood Testing

Please refer to the Medical Testing Protocol.

Breast Cancer

In 1971, when President Richard Nixon declared "war on cancer," the chance of a woman getting breast cancer was one in 20. Today, after billions of dollars of government research money has been spent fighting the disease, the odds are a shocking one out of eight women who will develop breast cancer.

According to the American Cancer Society, more than 180,000 women will be diagnosed with breast cancer in the coming year, and about 46,000 women will die from it. Breast cancer has become the second largest cause of cancer deaths in women next to lung cancer, and the leading cause of death for women between ages 35 and 54. Ever since the "war on cancer" was declared, more women have died of breast cancer than the total number of

Americans who lost their lives in World Wars I and II, the Korean war, and the Vietnam war combined!

Clearly, we are in the midst of a breast cancer epidemic. By the time the tell-tale lump is detected in the breast, there are already an average of 45 billion cancer cells present, and some of these malignant cells have been metastasized to other parts of the body. Conventional medicine recommends radiation and chemotherapy after the cancerous lump has been removed in an attempt to kill escaped, metastasized cancer cells. The net effect of radiation and chemotherapy is the weakening of the immune system and the rendering of the cancer patient more vulnerable to the development of metastatic lesions in critical organs of the body.

There are alternative therapies that are crucial to the successful treatment of breast cancer. Breast cancer cells differ from other cancer cells, thus mandating the incorporation of immune and hormone modulating therapies that interfere with breast cancer cell proliferation.

One of the most important supplements for the breast cancer patient is high doses of the hormone melatonin at bedtime. Melatonin blocks estrogen receptors somewhat similarly to the drug tamoxifen without the long-term side effects of tamoxifen. When melatonin and tamoxifen are combined, synergistic benefits occur. For women who are prescribed tamoxifen, it is suggested that the drug not be taken for more than two years. Melatonin can be safely taken for an indefinite period of time. The suggested dose of melatonin for breast cancer patients is 10 to 50 mg at bedtime. Melatonin not only blocks estrogen receptor sites on breast cancer cells, but directly inhibits breast cancer cell proliferation and boosts the production of immune components that kill metastasized cancer cells.

CAUTION: While melatonin is strongly recommended for breast cancer patients, interleukin-2 (IL-2), which is often combined with melatonin, should be avoided by breast cancer patients. IL-2 may promote breast cancer cell division.

Vitamin A and vitamin D3 inhibit breast cancer cell division and can induce cancer cells to differentiate into mature, non-cancer cells. Vitamin D3 works synergistically with tamoxifen to inhibit breast cancer cell proliferation. Breast cancer patients should take 4,000 to 6,000 IU of vitamin D3 every day on an empty stomach. Water soluble vitamin A can be taken in doses of 100,000 IU to 300,000 IU every day. Monthly blood tests are needed to make sure toxicity does not occur in response to these relatively high daily doses of vitamin A and vitamin D3. After six months, the doses of vitamin D3 and vitamin A can be reduced.

Important: Refer to the Symptoms of Vitamin A Toxicity, in Appendix A.

Soy contains phytochemicals called genistein and isoflavones that interfere with breast cancer cell division via several mechanisms. Genistein interferes with the formation of new blood vessels supplying a tumor, thus starving the tumor cells to death. There are now supplements available that contain standardized soy extracts. The most concentrated soy supplement is Super Soy Extract powder or tablets. The powder has a pleasant-tasting peanut butter flavor.

It is suggested that breast cancer patients take two heaping teaspoons of Super Soy Extract powder or take 20 1,000 mg tablets a day.

There are phytochemicals in cabbage and broccoli that interfere with breast cancer cell growth. The daily juicing of fresh organic cabbage and/or broccoli is suggested for breast cancer patients. For those who find it too inconvenient to juice cabbage and broccoli every day, there is a product called Phyto-Food powder that is comprised of potent concentrations of broccoli, cabbage and other cruciferous vegetables that contain phytochemicals that help fight cancer. Breast cancer patients should take two heaping tablespoons of Phyto-Food powder every day.

Preliminary research from Europe indicates extremely encouraging results when breast cancer patients take 300 to 400 mg a day of coenzyme Q10. Breast cancer patients should thus consider taking 300 to 400 mg a day of coenzyme Q10 in oil-filled capsules for maximum absorption.

The most current research shows that some of the ingredients of green tea may have a beneficial effect in treating cancer. While drinking green tea is a well documented method of preventing cancer, it is difficult for the cancer patient to obtain a sufficient quantity of anti-cancer components from drinking green tea. We suggest that a person with breast cancer take four to 10 decaffeinated green tea extract capsules every day. These capsules contain a standardized extract of epigallocatechin gallate, which is the component of green tea that makes green tea an effective adjunct therapy in the treatment of breast cancer.

Breast cancer patients often have elevated levels of the pituitary hormone prolactin. Abnormally high levels of prolactin can interfere with successful breast cancer therapy. If a blood test reveals elevated prolactin levels, the oncologist should be encouraged to prescribe 1.25 to 2.5 mg of the drug Parlodel, also known as bromocriptine. Parlodel must be taken after meals as severe nausea can occur when it is taken on an empty stomach. A better way to suppress prolactin is Dostinex. Just twice a week dosing of 0.25 mg to 0.50 mg is needed, and side effects are rare.

One of the most exciting new therapies in the prevention and treatment of breast cancer is conjugated linoleic acid (CLA). CLA is the component of beef that has direct breast cancer cell inhibitory effects. Since most parts of beef are not healthy to eat in large amounts, it is much safer to take the CLA isolated in the form of CLA capsules. For breast cancer prevention and treatment, it is suggested that six to 10 750 mg capsules of CLA a day be taken. When taking CLA, the breast cancer patient also must take soy.

Lignans are an important class of phytochemicals found in flax seed. When rats are fed a diet containing ground flax seed, it becomes very difficult to develop a breast tumor, even when breast cancer cells have been injected directly into the animal. Rats not given flax seed readily develop breast cancers in response to injections with live cancer cells.

When rats with large breast tumors were fed flax seed, the breast tumors shrunk. In laboratory monkeys who eat lignans in their lab chow, it is very difficult to induce breast tumors.

Ground flax seed (but not flax oil) provides a healthy dose of lignans. The most efficient way of consuming fresh flax seed with other cancer fighting phytochemicals is to consume two to five tablespoons a day of The Missing Link for Humans, a specially designed flax seed based meal replacement food.

Monthly blood tests should include a complete blood chemistry with tests for liver function and serum calcium levels, prolactin levels, parathyroid hormone levels and the tumor marker CA 27-29, and Cancer Profile tests (CA Profile) that includes the CEA or carcinoembryonic antigen test. These tests monitor the progress or failure of whatever therapies are being used, and also are able to detect toxicity from high doses of vitamin A and vitamin D3. The patient should insist on obtaining a copy of their blood workups every month.

Product availability: Melatonin, Phyto-Food, Super Soy Extract, coenzyme Q10, green tea, Water-soluble vitamin A, vitamin D3 caps, LIPAEN (conjugated linoleic acid) and The Missing Link For Humans, can be ordered singly or in a Protocol Pak by calling 1-800-544-4440. Ask for a listing of innovative physicians in your area who may be able to help you implement an alternative therapy cancer program.

Bursitis

The same therapies used to treat arthritis may also be used for the treatment of bursitis and other inflammatory disorders. Refer to the Foundation's Arthritis protocol.

Cancer Chemotherapy

There are nutrient and hormone therapies that can mitigate the toxicity brought about by cancer chemotherapy. In peer-reviewed scientific papers, nutrients such as coenzyme Q10 and vitamin E have been shown to protect against chemotherapy-induced cardiomyopathies. Melatonin has been shown to protect against chemotherapy-induced immune depression.

Product availability: coenzyme Q10, vitamin E, and melatonin can be obtained by calling 1-800-544-4440.

Cancer Radiation Therapy

Cancer radiation therapy inflicts tremendous damage to healthy cells in the body. There are specific nutrients that have been shown to protect the body against cancer radiation therapy.

The amino acid taurine is severely depleted when humans undergo radiation therapy. Supplementation with 2,000 mg a day of taurine is, therefore, recommended to people undergoing cancer radiation therapy. When ginseng was administered with radiation therapy in animal studies, a far greater percentage of the animals survived in the ginseng-supplemented group compared to the group receiving radiation without ginseng. Cancer patients should consider taking two to four capsules daily of Sports Ginseng by Nature's Herbs, which combines Korean and Siberian ginseng.

Shark liver oil containing standardized alkylglycerols can prevent immune impairment and irradiation injury to healthy tissues. Cancer patients should take six 200 mg standardized shark liver oil capsules a day for 30 days. Shark liver oil can cause an overproduction of blood platelets, so high doses should not be taken for more than 30 days.

Antioxidant supplements can reduce the amount of free radical damage produced by cancer radiation therapy. While soy extracts are strongly recommended as an adjuvant cancer therapy, do not take soy or genistein extracts one week before and during radiation therapy because soy may prevent radiation from killing cancer cells.

Product availability: Shark liver oil capsules, taurine, ginseng and melatonin can be obtained by calling 1-800-544-4440.

Cancer Surgery

Most people don't realize that surgery places tremendous stress on the body that causes significant immune depression. This is of particular danger to the cancer patient who undergoes surgery to remove a primary tumor. Billions of cancer cells often remain in the body after the surgery and a strong immune system is required to eradicate these remaining cancer cells.

A study conducted several years ago in Germany showed that for most forms of cancer, surgical removal of the primary tumor did not result in prolonged survival compared to cancer patients who refused surgery. For many forms of cancer, however, the surgical removal of the primary tumor is crucial if long-term remission is to occur. The nutrients and hormones in the Cancer Treatment protocol can help protect against surgically induced immune depression, thus improving the odds of long-term survival.

Cancer Treatment Protocol

Conventional oncologists often fail to recognize that most cancers already have metastasized to other sites in the body by the time the primary tumor is diagnosed.

The Life Extension Foundation's cancer treatment protocol incorporates a wide range of therapies designed to boost immune function, inhibit cancer cell division, induce cancer cells to differentiate into mature cells, inhibit the ability of cancer cells to metastasize, prevent angiogensis, and modulate the effects of hormones on cancer cell growth.

Conventional oncologists deal with tumor metastasis by applying whole-body cytotoxic chemotherapy, which aims to kill the metastasized tumor cells. However, chemotherapy also destroys immune function, thereby condemning the cancer patient to the likelihood of recurrence of the primary tumor or other cancers, along with infections, often leading to death. If the immune system is unable to recognize and destroy metastasized cancer cells, then the chances of achieving a permanent remission are remote.

In the 30 years that cancer chemotherapy has been used, it has proved effective for relatively few cancers. The cancers that chemotherapy can benefit include testicular cancer, choriocarcinoma, Hodgkin's disease and some forms of leukemia and lymphoma. For the majority of cancers, however, chemotherapy has been a failure. Conventional oncology has failed to recognize that cancer is a systemic, whole-body disease. This misconception causes conventional oncologists to continue to use immune system-destroying chemotherapy inappropriately.

When cancer is first diagnosed, the primary tumor is often too large for immunotherapy to be effective by itself. In these cases, conventional cancer therapy (surgery and/or radiation) is often necessary to eradicate the primary tumor. However, surgery and radiation put tremendous stress on the body that severely weakens immune function and can put the body into a catabolic (wasting) state that leads to noticeable weight loss.

Total Nutritional Support is needed to mitigate the damaging effects of surgery/radiation therapy. Unfortunately, conventional cancer therapy seldom includes any kind of nutritional support. We, therefore, include a Total Nutritional Support program in our Cancer Treatment Protocol.

At this time, the Life Extension Foundation does not have a good alternative for conventional therapies when it comes to large primary tumors. Even the advanced therapies used at offshore cancer clinics are usually not potent enough to shrink large, primary tumors. One alternative therapy that is being used at cancer clinics to attack a primary tumor is high doses of pancreatic enzymes. Cancer patients are given 40 to 70 420 mg of pork pancreas enzyme capsules throughout the day for the first month, and lesser amounts in subsequent months. Pancreatic enzymes have been shown in some studies to "digest" primary tumors. The effectiveness of high-dose pancreatic enzyme therapy varies widely from patient to patient.

It is crucial for cancer patients to monitor the effectiveness of any cancer therapy they are using under the care of a physician, preferably an oncologist. Blood tests should be done monthly that measure tumor markers in the blood and measure the effects of immune-boosting therapies on specific immune components of the blood. Dr. Emil Schandl's CA Profile (Cancer Profile), which has an excellent track record for more than ten years, is strongly recommended.

We cannot overemphasize the importance of monthly blood testing for all cancer patients. Every patient responds differently to both conventional and alternative cancer therapies. The results of blood tests provide critically important data to evaluate the effectiveness of these therapies.

Some of the blood tests commonly used by doctors to evaluate different types of cancers are:

Type of Cancer	Blood Test
Ovarian cancer	CA 125
Prostate cancer	PSA and Prolactin

Disease Prevention and Treatment Protocols

Breast cancer	CA 27.29, CEA, and Prolactin
Colon, rectum, liver, pancreatic, stomach and other organ cancers	CEA, CA 19-9, GGTP
Leukemia, Lymphoma, and Hodgkin's disease	Immune Cell Differentiation and CBC with differential

In order to assess the effectiveness of immune-boosting therapies, a complete Immune Cell Subset test could be performed bi-monthly in order to measure CD4 (T-Helper) total count, CD4/CD8 (T-helper to T-suppressor) ratio, and NK (Natural Killer Cell) Activity.

While you may have to rely on conventional cancer therapy to treat a primary tumor, immune-boosting therapies improve the chances of bringing metastasized cancer cells under control. Immune-boosting therapies include drugs such as isoprinosine, thymic hormones in products such as Thymex or Thymus Standardized Extract, plus the adrenal hormone DHEA and melatonin, all of which boost immune function via several mechanisms.

Some doctors are under the impression that ovarian cancer, leukemia, Hodgkin's disease, and lymphoma patients should avoid melatonin until more is known about its effects on these forms of cancer. If melatonin is tried in these types of cancer, tumor blood markers should be watched closely (e.g., if melatonin causes the CA-125 marker to go up in an ovarian cancer patient, it could be a sign that melatonin is promoting tumor growth). The scientific literature, on the other hand, suggests that melatonin warnings are appropriate for multiple myeloma, rather than ovarian and immune cancers, meaning that melatonin may not be contraindicated in ovarian, leukemia, and lymphoma patients.

Those with prostate cancer should avoid DHEA. Generally, it is a good idea to to use any hormone with caution under the direction of a competent physician.

Melatonin may be the single most effective alternative cancer therapy because it boosts immune function, suppresses free radicals, inhibits cell proliferation, and helps to change cancer cells into normal cells.

Nutrients that have an inhibitory effect on cancer cell proliferation include vitamin A (and synthetic vitamin A analogs), and phytochemicals found in cruciferous vegetables (Phytofood) such as sulforaphane, 3-indole-carbinol and isothiocyanate. Soy contains numerous anti-cancer agents such as genistein and other isoflavones. Vitamin D3 inhibits cancer cell growth and induces cancer cells to differentiate into normal cells.

The best example of the effectiveness of vitamin A and beta-carotene in inhibiting cell proliferation is in patients with cancer of the mouth. Vitamin A or beta-carotene supplementation puts most forms of early stage mouth cancer in remission as long as these nutrients continue to be consumed.

The Foundation's Cancer Treatment Protocol is for most forms of cancer, including metastasized prostate cancer.

This protocol assumes that the patient's primary tumor has been eradicated (at least partially) by surgery or some other treatment. However, it may be followed even if the primary tumor has not yet been eradicated.

Here is the Life Extension Foundation's Cancer Treatment Protocol:

❖ **Step One: Arrange for monthly blood tests, to include:**

1) Tumor Marker Test — Type of cancer dictates type of test used. Some cancers do not have a specific tumor marker test available. However, the CA Profile is not organ specific and has been shown to be effective in monitoring the progression and regression of cancer.

2) Immune Cell Subset Test (This is an expensive test.)

3) Complete blood chemistry — to include all standard liver, thyroid, heart, and kidney function tests. This is a low-cost test.

4) Blood PTH test — to help determine if too much vitamin D3 or vitamin A is being taken. The serum calcium test is usually included in the low-cost standard blood chemistry profile. However, it may not accurately reflect calcium status. PTH will be elevated if the bones are losing calcium and osteoporosis development is taking place.

These blood tests must be taken on a regular basis under the supervision of a physician in order to follow our Cancer Treatment Protocol scientifically. It's the only way you'll know if what you are taking is working and if significant toxicity is developing. This is no time to guess!

Since you will be having these tests performed monthly, you should price-shop for the best deal. The Life Extension Foundation now offers these tests at discount prices.

❖ **Step Two: Total nutritional support**

1) Life Extension Mix — tablets, capsules, or powder. The standard daily dose involves three tablets, three times a day. Also available in powder or capsule form to be taken in three divided doses.

2) Life Extension Herbal Mix — powder only. One tablespoon early in the day.

3) Super Selenium Complex. One tablet, two times a day.

4) Super Soy Extract powder or tablets. Two heaping teaspoons of powder (20 grams) or 20 1,000 mg tablets every day.

5) Green Tea Capsules (decaffeinated) — Four to ten capsules a day in divided doses.

6) Coenzyme Q10 — oil filled capsules. 200-400 mg early in the morning.

7) Kyolic Garlic — Formula #105. Four capsules a day with meals.

8) Essential Fatty Acids — Mega-EPA or Udo's Choice Ultimate Oil. Highest tol-

erable doses. Suggested dose is 12 Mega-EPA Caps or two tablespoons of Udo's Choice Ultimate Oil daily. Do not take these oils if you have prostate cancer.

9) Vitamin C — Capsules or powder. Highest tolerable dose of pharmaceutical grade vitamin C to be taken throughout the day. Significant doses of vitamin C are already included in the multinutrient formulas at the beginning of the list.

10) Phyto-food powder. One to two tablespoons daily. Juicing organic vegetables is an alternative to Phyto-Food powder.

11) L-carnitine capsules (600 mg) — Four capsules early in the day. Use acetyl-L-carnitine if affordable.

12) Curcumin — four 500 mg capsules daily.

❖ **Step Three: Boosting immune function**

1) If the immune system is weakened enough, cancer cells can survive and multiply. The most critical part of the immune system is the thymus gland, a small organ just below the breastbone that governs the entire system. There are two products that promote healthy thymic activity:

   a) Thymic Protein A has been shown in laboratory and animal experiments to cause the T-4 lymphocyte to mature, thereby initiating a specific cell-mediated immune response.

   This specific protein has been shown to be a stimulant in animal models for the production of interleukin-2. Interleukin-2 production by T-4 cells is the benchmark measurement for T-cell maturity and initiation of immune response.

   A trial with 22 cats infected with feline immunodeficiency virus (FIV) concluded that this protein enhances immune response to infectious agents measured serologically, diminishes disease symptoms, lengthens survival and increases lymphocyte values.

   A daily dose of four micrograms of this material may make a major difference in longevity by strengthening the immune system through its T-cell "programming" role. The more T-cells that are properly functioning, the more immune response may be mounted against metastasized cancer cells.

   Initial reports from those undergoing chemotherapy indicate that Thymic Protein A has maintained their total white blood count at acceptable levels during the therapy. It is well-known among oncologists that chemotherapy and radiation will often induce a serious drop in white blood count to dangerous levels, which may dictate cessation of therapy. Healthy people can take one packet every day or every other day. Those with disease whose treatment is dependent on a strong immune system may need three packets a day for several months.

b) Thymex provides extracts of fresh, healthy tissue from the thymus and other glands that produce the disease-fighting cells of our immune system.

The primary ingredient in Thymex is immunologic tissue from the thymus gland. Also included in Thymex is tissue from the lymph nodes and spleen which produce the white blood cells that engage in life-or-death combat with invading organisms in our bloodstream under the "instruction" of the thymus gland.

Thymex is a synergistic formula that contains herbal activators and a full complement of natural homeopathic nutrients, in addition to fresh, healthy thymus, lymph and spleen tissues. Thymex is a professional formula normally dispensed through doctor's offices. Thymex has been extensively used to amplify the immune potentiating effect of DHEA replacement therapy. According to a physician most familiar with DHEA, thymus extract is required to obtain the immune system boosting benefit of DHEA.

2) Cancer patients usually have elevated cortisol levels that can suppress immune function. Take 1-2 tablets of KH3 daily on an empty stomach first thing in the morning, and one or two KH3 tablets in the mid-afternoon on an empty stomach to suppress the damaging effects of cortisol.

3) DHEA can also suppress dangerously high cortisol levels. DHEA can boost immune function via other mechanisms. Doctors usually prescribe at least 25 mg per day of DHEA for their male cancer patients and a minimum of 15 mg a day of DHEA for females. Your monthly or bi-monthly DHEA-S and Immune Cell Subset tests and tumor marker tests will determine if DHEA is producing a beneficial effect. Do not use DHEA if you have prostate cancer or estrogen-sensitive breast cancer.

4) Melatonin boosts immune function via several mechanisms of action. It also exerts an inhibitory effect on cancer cell proliferation and induces the differ-

entiation of cancer cells into normal cells. Melatonin should be taken every night in doses ranging from 3 to 50 mg.

5) Show your oncologist information in this book regarding the use of the FDA-approved drugs interleukin-2 or interferon and melatonin. Studies document that low doses of interleukin-2 or interferon combined with high doses of melatonin (10-50 mg nightly) are effective against advanced, normally untreatable cancers. Ask your doctor to prescribe these agents:

    a) Interleukin-2 at a dose of 3 million units injected subcutaneously six out of every seven days for six weeks. And then one month later:

    b) Interferon (alpha and gamma interferon) at a dose of 100,000-300,000 units injected subcutaneously six out of seven days for six weeks.

Subcutaneous injections can be self-administered at home.

CAUTION: Breast cancer patients should not use interleukin-2 (IL-2). While low-dose IL-2 and high-dose melatonin has been shown to be effective against many forms of cancer, interleukin-2 could promote breast cancer cell division. Breast cancer patients are encouraged to take 10 to 40 mg of melatonin nightly (See Breast Cancer protocol).

This protocol should be adjusted if the Immune Cell Subset test or the CA Profile fails to show marked improvement in the patient's immune function. For example, if there are too many T-suppressor cells, 800 mg a day of the drug Tagamet (now available over-the-counter) can lower the T-suppressor cell activity. T-suppressor cells are often elevated in cancer patients, which prevents them from mounting a strong immune response to the cancer.

❖ **Step Four: Inhibiting Cancer Cell Proliferation**

1) Water soluble vitamin A liquid in doses of 100,000 to 300,000 IU a day should be used for several months. Monthly blood tests can help ascertain if toxicity is occurring in response to these high doses of vitamin A.

Important: Refer to the Symptoms of Vitamin A Toxicity, in Appendix A.

2) Melatonin taken to boost immune function also inhibits cancer cell proliferation.

❖ **Step Five: Inducing Cancer Cell Differentiation**

Cancer cells are aberrant, transformed cells that proliferate (divide) more rapidly than normal cells until they kill the patient. Inducing cancer cells to "differentiate" back into normal cells is a primary objective of cancer researchers.

1) The Total Nutritional Support protocol supplies nutrients like beta-carotene and the phytochemicals found in fresh fruits and vegetables that induce cancer cell differentiation into normal cells and inhibit cancer cell proliferation.

2) Melatonin, which boosts immune function and inhibits cancer cell proliferation, also induces cancer cell differentiation.

3) Vitamin D3 and its analogs may be the most effective therapies to induce cancer cell differentiation. Vitamin D3 can cause too much calcium to be absorbed into the bloodstream. As a result, you should take vitamin D3 on an empty stomach with essential fatty acid (fish or flax oil). A daily dosage range of 2,000-3,000 IU of vitamin D3 is suggested. Increase vitamin D3 if blood tests show blood calcium levels are not being affected and parathyroid hormone (PTH) levels are not suppressed. Decrease or eliminate vitamin D3 supplementation if hypercalcemia occurs. Underlying kidney disease precludes high-dose vitamin D3 supplementation.

Note the importance of competent, professional guidance by a physician. Monthly blood testing is mandatory when taking high doses of vitamin A or vitamin D3.

❖ Step Six: Preventing Cancer Cell Metastasis

Modified Citrus Pectin interferes with cancer cell communication, enhances killer cell activity, and inhibits cancer cell metastasis. Suggested dose of this powder is 15 grams a day.

❖ Step Seven: Call The Life Extension Foundation

If following the above protocol does not result in significant immune enhancement, improvements in blood tumor markers, tumor shrinkage, weight stabilization, and an overall improvement in well being within two months, please call the Life Extension Foundation at 1-800-544-4440 for other, more aggressive options.

Product availability: You can order Life Extension Mix, Life Extension Herbal Mix, selenium complex, pork pancreas enzymes, Thymex, DHEA, melatonin, vitamin A emulsified drops, vitamin D3, Super Soy Extract, green tea caps, coenzyme Q10, garlic, vitamin C, Phyto-food, carnitine, acetyl-L-carnitine and modified citrus pectin by calling 1-800-544-4440.

For some forms of cancer, you may be able to get in a free program utilizing experimental cancer therapies that are sponsored by the National Cancer Institute. For information about experimental cancer therapies, call 1-800-4-CANCER. Make sure you do not enroll in a study where you may be part of a placebo group or where the potential toxicity of the drug may kill you before the cancer does.

Candida (Fungal, Yeast) Infections

Chronic fungal infections are often found in the gastrointestinal (GI) tract. Improving the bacterial flora and the overall health of the GI tract can help to prevent recurring candida infections throughout the body.

The intake of bifido bacteria concentrate capsules every day can dramatically increase the quantity of this beneficial bacteria in the gut to help fight candida infections. Acidophilus bacteria can also help to fight candida in the upper intestinal tract. Bifido bacteria feed on a special sugar trade-marked under the name Nutraflora. One teaspoon a day of Nutraflora promotes the proliferation of friendly bifido bacteria in the gut.

Garlic (not Kyolic garlic), biotin and caprylic acid have a direct yeast-killing effect in the intestine. Fiber in the diet can help remove yeast and fungus from the intestines. A product called Yeast Fighters Capsules contains an odorless garlic concentrate, caprylic acid, biotin, acidophilus and a fiber blend to control candida overgrowth in the intestine before it spreads to other parts of the body.

Chronic candida infections can be caused by a deficient immune system. If you suffer from an acute candida infection, or one that has not responded to standard therapy, the most potent FDA-approved drug available is called Diflucan. One month's treatment with Diflucan can temporarily eradicate a systemic candida infection so that anti-candida nutritional supplements like Yeast Fighters, bifido bacteria, and Nutraflora can prevent a new candida infection from occurring.

Shark liver oil has demonstrated an antifungal effect in laboratory studies. Shark liver oil capsules containing 200 mg of alkylglycerol can be taken in doses of five capsules a day for up to 30 days. Dietary modifications should include avoiding sucrose and fructose as these types of sugars can cause yeast overgrowth.

Product availability: Yeast Fighters capsules, bifido bacteria, standardized shark liver oil capsules, and Nutraflora can be ordered singly or in a Protocol Pak by calling 1-800-544-4440. Diflucan is an expensive prescription drug that needs to be prescribed by your physician.

Catabolic Wasting

Cancer, HIV infection, congestive heart failure, aging, surgery, and a host of degenerative diseases can result in the body shifting from a healthy anabolic cell replacement metabolism into a catabolic wasting state, characterized by severe weight loss and muscle breakdown. If untreated, catabolic wasting, also known as cachexia, can result in death.

Catabolic wasting can be counteracted by proper nutrient supplementation. The essential fatty acid conjugated linoleic acid (CLA) has anti-catabolic properties. The suggested dose of CLA for a person in a catabolic state is four 750 mg capsules taken twice a day. Fish oil supplementation is also suggested in a dose of five Mega-EPA fish oil capsules a day.

The standard dose of Life Extension Mix should be given to all people suffering from catabolic breakdown to provide the nutrient building blocks the body needs to start rebuilding the body. The amino acid arginine can induce help to generate anabolic cell replacement throughout the body, and can suppress excess levels of ammonia in the body, a common problem associated with catabolic breakdown. The suggested dose for arginine to counteract catabolism is 5 to 20 grams a day.

Additional amino acid supplementation should include 2,400 mg of L-carnitine, 2,000 mg a day of glutamine, and four capsules a day of the branched chain amino acid complex that includes leucine, isoleucine, and valine.

WARNING: Arginine is not recommended for people who have cancer.

Product availability: Arginine powder, capsules and tablets, Life Extension Mix, CLA, Mega-EPA, L-carnitine, glutamine, and the branched-chain amino acid formula can be ordered by calling 1-800-544-4440.

Cataract

Cataract surgery costs Medicare more money than any other medical procedure. Cataract is epidemic among the aged. It is usually caused by the excessive production of free radicals throughout life.

It is difficult to treat cataract with oral antioxidants because there is only a minimal amount of blood circulation within the eye compared to other parts of the body. Yet, there is evidence that the progression of cataract disease can be slowed by taking nutrients that improve blood circulation to the eye.

Ginkgo biloba extract should be taken at a dose of 120 mg a day by anyone suffering from cataracts. Bilberry extract should be taken at a dose of 150 mg a day by cataract patients. These two flavonoid nutrients may help to restore microcapillary circulation to the eye.

After taking ginkgo and bilberry for a month, add 600 mcg of the mineral selenium, 500 mg of the amino acid glutathione and 1,000 mg of the super-antioxidant alpha lipoic acid every day. Melatonin is a potent antioxidant that may be especially effective in treating cataract. Melatonin production slows down in people over the age of 40, and by age 60 there is virtually no melatonin being produced. It is over the age of 60 when most cataracts develop. The suggested dose for melatonin is 3 mg taken at bedtime.

It is crucial for cataract patients to wear protective eyeglasses to shield against free radical damage induced by ultraviolet (UV) sunlight. If UV blocking sunglasses were to be worn throughout life, the risk of cataract would be reduced greatly. Exposure to sunlight is a major risk factor in the development and progression of cataract disease. Life Extension Buyers Club sells low-cost wrap-around sunglasses called Sun-Shields that fit over regular glasses to provide almost 100% protection against UV penetration to the eye.

Some cataract patients apply vitamin drops to their eyes every day. While there is no published data on whether Viva Drops can slow the cataract disease process, these vitamin drops do provide antioxidant protection directly to the lens of the eye.

Product availability: You can order ginkgo biloba and bilberry, high-potency glutathione capsules,a special selenium complex that contains three different forms of selenium, alpha lipoic acid, melatonin, Sun-Shields, and Viva Drops singly by calling 1-800-544-4440 or in a Protocol Pak.

Cerebral Vascular Disease

For those suffering from hemorrhagic cerebral vascular disease, cerebral hemorrhage or cerebral aneurysm, it is suggested that nutrients that help build collagen and elastin be taken to help rebuild the endothelial lining of the arterial system.

Vitamin C at 5,000 mg a day is suggested along with 300 mg a day of the flavonoid proanthocyanidin (grape seed extract). Magnesium is crucial for arterial structure, and it is suggested that 1,500 mg a day of elemental magnesium be taken along with 1,000 mg a day of calcium, and 500 mg a day of potassium.

Essential fatty acids in the form of fish oil concentrates should also be considered. Mega-EPA enables a person to get pharmacologic doses of fish oils by taking only five capsules a day. Extreme caution should be exercised when taking these supplements because they inhibit blood clotting. There is a chance that a cerebral hemorrhage could occur because of the blood thinning effects these nutrients can produce. Blood tests that measure clotting time can be used to make sure these nutrients are not reducing the clotting factors in your blood too much. Reducing hypertension is crucial when cerebral vascular disease is present.

Refer to Age Associated Mental Impairment and Stroke protocols for additional suggestions.

Product availability: Mega-EPA, Proanthocyanidins (grape seed extract), vitamin C, magnesium, calcium, and potassium are available by calling 1-800-544-4440.

Cholesterol Reduction

Elevated LDL cholesterol is associated with a greater-than-normal risk of atherosclerosis and cardiovascular disease. The objective is to lower total cholesterol to 200 mg/dL or less, and to lower dangerous LDL cholesterol to under 120 mg/dL. The best way of lowering cholesterol is through dietary modification, yet for some people, no matter how little fat and cholesterol they consume, their livers produce too much cholesterol.

FDA-approved cholesterol-lowering drugs can produce serious long-term side effects. There are nutrients that lower cholesterol as well or better than FDA-approved drugs. By having regular blood tests to measure cholesterol levels, you can now choose less costly herbal supplements that produce beneficial side effects.

One newly identified herbal extract that can lower cholesterol levels is curcumin, the yellow pigment of turmeric. Curcumin helps to prevent several diseases. When rats were fed small doses of curcumin, their cholesterol levels fell to one-half those of rats not receiving curcumin (*Journal of Nutrition* 100:1307-16, 1970).

Curcumin's mechanisms of cholesterol reduction include interfering with intestinal cholesterol uptake, increasing the conversion of cholesterol into bile acids, and increasing the excretion of bile acids, according to the *International Journal of Vitamin Nutritional Research* (61:364-9, 1991).

Curcumin inhibits abnormal blood clot formation by blocking the formation of thromboxane, which is a promoter of platelet aggregation. Curcumin increases prostacyclin, the body's natural inhibitor of abnormal platelet aggregation (*Arzneim Forsh* 36:715-7,1986). When 500 mg a day of curcumin was administered to 10 human volunteers, there was a 29% increase in beneficial HDL cholesterol after only seven days. In this study, total cholesterol was reduced by 11.6% and lipid peroxidation was reduced by 33% (*Indian Journal of Physiology* 36(4):273-275, 1992).

If you are taking cholesterol-lowering drugs, you may be able to substitute curcumin and other nutrients that have been combined in a product called Herbal Cardiovascular Formula. In order to document the effectiveness of nutritional cholesterol-reducing formulas, test your cholesterol first, then obtain another cholesterol test 45 days later. If curcumin and other nutrients work for you, you will save money, avoid potential side effects, and obtain additional health benefits.

While FDA-approved cholesterol lowering drugs can cause liver damage and may cause cancer, curcumin has well-documented cancer and viral inhibiting effects. Curcumin also has anti-inflammatory effects. It neutralizes dietary carcinogens and inhibits cancer at the initiation, promotion, and progression stages of development.

Curcumin is a potent antioxidant and an inhibitor of HIV replication. Unlike FDA-approved drugs, curcumin may protect against viral hepatitis-induced liver damage. Do not use curcumin if a biliary tract obstruction exists because curcumin increases the excretion of cholesterol bile acids. High doses of curcumin on an empty stomach can cause stomach ulceration.

Curcumin is in the Herbal Cardiovascular Formula. A small amount of curcumin is also included in Life Extension Booster. Curcumin also is available in 500 mg capsules.

Another cholesterol-lowering herbal extract is gugulipid, an extract from the mukjul tree. In a study in the *Journal of Associated Physicians-India*, 37(5):323-8, 1989, 125 patients receiving gugulipid experienced an average 11% decrease in total cholesterol, and a 16.8% decrease in triglycerides within 3-4 weeks. Patients with elevated cholesterol responded better than normal patients. HDL cholesterol increased in 60% of the patients receiving gugulipid.

In a placebo-controlled study, 205 patients received gugulipid at a dose of 25 mg three times a day. Of the gugulipid-treated patients, 70-80% experienced cholesterol reduction compared to virtually none in the placebo group (*Journal of Associated Physicians-India* 37(5):328-8 1989). In another placebo-controlled trial in 40 patients with high blood fat levels, serum cholesterol declined by 21.75%, and triglycerides by 27.1% after three weeks of gugulipid administration. After sixteen weeks of gugulipid administration, HDL cholesterol increased by 35.8%.

Foundation members who have been following a life extension lifestyle normally have healthy vascular systems. Newly identified herbal extracts may provide further protection against cardiovascular disease risk factors. These herbs have been combined into the Herbal Cardiovascular Formula to provide the ideal potency of each pharmaceutical grade herbal extract at a far lower price than these herbs cost separately.

Each capsule of the Herbal Cardiovascular Formula contains:

Curcumin (97% purity)	250 mg
Bromelain (2000 gdu per gram)	250 mg
Ginger (gingerol standardized)	500 mg
Gugulipid	35 mg

Take one capsule in the morning, one in the evening. Cardiovascular patients should test their cholesterol/fibrinogen levels within 45 days to make sure the formula is providing sufficient cholesterol and fibrinogen lowering effects. Higher doses of Herbal Cardiovascular Formula can be taken to provide additional cholesterol-fibrinogen lowering effects.

Note: for information about fibrinogen, refer to the Fibrinogen and Cardiovascular Disease protocol in this book.

While blood testing is not mandatory for healthy people seeking to reduce their risk of heart attack or stroke, it is recommended that everyone have an annual blood test to fine tune and optimize their life extension program.

You may be able to substitute the Herbal Cardiovascular Formula if you're taking cholesterol-lowering drugs such as:

Mevacor	Lescol
Lopid	Questran
Zocor	Atromid
Pravachol	Lorelco

Another cholesterol-lowering therapy is soy. Phyto extracts from soy can help prevent cancer, and may even be effective in the treatment of certain cancers. The Foundation strongly recommends that members use soy concentrates to reduce cancer risk.

Evidence for the cholesterol-lowering effect of soy protein has been in the medical literature for 80 years. *The New England Journal of Medicine* (Aug 3, 1995) published an analysis of all studies relating to the use of soy to lower blood fat levels. The results of their analysis of 38 controlled studies showed that soy protein produced a reduction of 9.3% in total cholesterol, 10.5% in triglycerides, and 12.9% in dangerous artery-clogging LDL cholesterol. A small increase in beneficial HDL of 2.4% was observed.

The primary mechanism by which soy protein lowers cholesterol appears to be related to the phytoestrogen, genistein, and other isoflavones in soy. It seems that soy boosted thyroxine levels, which caused enhanced metabolism of serum cholesterol. This means that people using FDA-approved cholesterol-lowering drugs might be able to substitute soy extracts to lower their cholesterol-triglyceride levels.

The side benefit of taking soy extracts is cancer prevention, while many FDA-approved cholesterol-lowering drugs produce adverse side effects. In addition to lowering blood fat levels, soy may protect against the development of atherosclerosis and cerebrovascular disease via other mechanisms.

Anyone contemplating using nutrients to replace drugs should have their cholesterol-triglyceride levels checked regularly to make sure the desired blood-fat reducing effect is really occurring. It is advisable to do this under the supervision of a competent physician.

Super Soy Extract and Soy Power are soy concentrates that contain standardized levels of the phytochemical genistein and other isoflavones. These soy extracts contains high standardized potencies of the active phytoestrogens from soy.

The minimum dose for cholesterol reduction is five 1,000 mg tablets a day or one heaping teaspoon (5-6 grams) of powder a day.

For those with elevated cholesterol levels, we suggest one to two heaping teaspoons of powder or 20 to 40 1,000 mg tablets a day. Soy powder is easily dispersed and has a light peanut butter taste. Another cholesterol-lowering nutrient is niacin. The best form of niacin is inositol hexanicotinate, which is sold under brand names such as Flush-Free Niacin. This form of niacin is tolerable for most people in daily doses of 2,400 mg. High intakes of fiber also will facilitate serum cholesterol reduction.

Product availability: Herbal Cardiovascular Formula containing curcumin and gugulipid, Flush-Free Niacin, and Soy Extracts are available by phoning 1-800-544-4440.

Chronic Fatigue Syndrome
(Low Energy)

Chronic fatigue is sometimes an outward manifestation of multiple nutrient deficiencies. For many people, taking high potency vitamin supplements alleviates chronic fatigue and restores youthful energy levels.

However, there are those who suffer from chronic low energy levels who need more than just vitamins. Victims of chronic fatigue syndrome are often helped by taking 100 mg of coenzyme Q10, three times a day. Another energy-boosting therapy involves taking 5 mg of NADH two times a day.

The amino acid L-carnitine has been approved by the FDA as an energy-boosting drug. People with low energy have been helped by taking 1,000 to 2,000 mg a day of acetyl-L-carnitine. A potent antioxidant called alpha lipoic acid has improved energy levels in some people on doses of 500 to 800 mg a day.

Some people's low energy levels are caused by deficiencies of brain hormones and neurotransmitters. The amino acid phenylalanine or tyrosine taken in daily doses of 1,500 mg a day can boost epinephrine and norepinephrine levels. Refer to Phenylalanine Precautions before taking phenylalanine or tyrosine products. Phenylalanine and tyrosine are available in capsule and powder forms.

The European anti-anxiety therapy Adapton has been shown to alleviate chronic fatigue symptoms when two capsules a day are used.

If none of these energy-boosting therapies work, there may be a chronic viral condition causing your chronic fatigue. You should have a medical test for herpes, Epstein-Barr virus and cytomegalovirus antibody activity. If you are infected with a chronic energy-depleting virus, there are conventional and alternative therapies that may be of help. It should be noted that most individuals have been exposed to pathogenic viruses that can be reactivated by adverse environmental conditions and cause chronic fatigue and other diseases.

DHEA has been reported to improve energy levels in chronic fatigue patients. Refer to DHEA Precautions before embarking on this therapy. For those with a viral induced chronic fatigue syndrome, refer the Foundation's protocol on Immune Enhancement.

Product availability: Alpha lipoic acid, acetyl-L-carnitine, NADH, coenzyme Q10, Adapton, DHEA, phenylalanine and tyrosine are available by phoning 1-800-544-4440.

Cirrhosis

Refer to the protocol on Liver for diseases of the liver, and also the Hepatitis B and Hepatitis C protocols.

Cognitive Enhancement

Refer to Age-Associated Mental Impairment and Attention Deficit Disorder protocols.

Common Cold

There are more than 300 viruses that have been identified as causing the common cold. Most cold viruses replicate in the throat.

By dissolving two zinc lozenges in the mouth every few hours, the zinc will help inactivate cold viruses multiplying in the throat. Vitamin C in doses of 5,000 to 20,000 mg has been used by many people as a natural antihistamine and antiviral therapy to treat common colds. Studies document the ability of vitamin C to shorten the duration of cold symptoms.

Echinacea standardized liquid herbal extract is effective at a dose of six full droppers followed by two full droppers every two waking hours until the 2-oz bottle is empty. Astragalus herbal extract at 300 mg a day can boost immune function and produce direct antiviral effects.

The amino acid n-acetyl-cysteine (NAC) helps to break excessive mucous and can have a direct antiviral effect. It is suggested that 600 mg of n-acetyl-cysteine be taken with 2,000 mg of vitamin C three times a day by those who get colds.

Ribavirin is a broad-spectrum antiviral approved in almost every country in the world except the United States. There is evidence that some cold virus strains can be stopped from replicating with ribavirin at a dose of 800 mg a day.

A well-documented, but little used therapy to treat the common cold involves an injection of 500,000 to 3 million IU of interferon (Interferon alpha-2a) combined with 40 mg of melatonin every night. Studies document the ability of interferon to kill many common cold viruses. Interferon is a component of your immune system that kills viruses (and cancer cells). Since it is a prescription drug, you will have to convince your doctor to prescribe and inject the one-time dose of interferon to combat your cold. For additional suggestions, access the Foundation's Immune Enhancement protocol.

Product availability: Zinc lozenges, NAC, echinacea, astragalus, vitamin C, and melatonin are available by calling 1-800-544-4440. Ask for a listing of offshore companies that sell ribavirin to Americans by mail. If you live close to the Mexican border, you can buy ribavirin in a Mexican pharmacy and bring it back into the United States under the FDA's personal use importation policy.

Congestive Heart Failure
and Cardiomyopathy

Energy deficiencies at the cellular level cause a gradual weakening of the heart muscle until a transplant becomes necessary. These energy deficits are often a cause of congestive heart failure and many forms of cardiomyopathy. Some of the energy factors have been identified that may help restore heart muscle function.

We will discuss in detail one of these energy factors and then provide a step-by-step nutritional approach to the treatment of heart muscle energy deficiencies clinically diagnosed as congestive heart failure or cardiomyopathy.

The herbal extract forskolin improves left ventricular function (*Arzheim Forsch* 37:364-7), which confirmed earlier animal studies showing that forskolin increases the contractile force of the heart.

Forskolin given to cardiomyopathy patients reduced systolic and diastolic blood pressure and pulmonary artery pressure with a concomitant increase in cardiac output. Cardiac stroke volume and the stroke volume index were increased by 70% in these cardiomyopathy patients. The authors of the study concluded that forskolin could be used in the treatment of severe heart failure (*Journal of Cardiovascular Pharmacology* [16/1]).

Forskolin's energy-enhancing effects are due to its unique ability to stimulate adenylate cyclase activity and elevate cellular cyclical adenosine monophosphate (cAMP) levels. cAMP regulates and activates critical enzymes required for cellular energy.

If you are going to attempt to use forskolin or any other alternative therapy to replace drugs that strengthen heart muscle contraction, extreme caution is mandatory and physician cooperation essential. Tests should be conducted to make sure forskolin and other nutrients are maintaining sufficient cardiac output.

Forskolin comes in capsules that contain 10 mg of elemental forskolin (extracted from the coleus forskohli herb). One capsule a day is suggested for the first two weeks. Then an additional capsule should be taken for the next two weeks. Up to six capsules a day can be taken.

CAUTION: Do not take forskolin if you have a prostate cancer. Forskolin may lower blood pressure. Use caution if you have low blood pressure.

Those who suffer from cardiac insufficiency diagnosed as cardiomyopathy or congestive heart failure may be substantially helped by taking the following energy-enhancing nutrients:

1) Forskolin — three to six 10 mg capsules daily.

2) Coenzyme Q10 — 100 mg, three times a day.

3) Acetyl-l-carnitine — 2,000 mg daily.

4) Taurine — 2,000 mg a day.

5) Magnesium — 1,500 mg a day.

6) Potassium — 500 mg a day (if needed).

7) NADH — 5 mg, twice a day.

8) Human Growth Hormone — 1-2 IU a day (or as prescribed by your physician). Advise your physician about everything you are doing so he can adjust your treatment program. For additional suggestions, refer to the Foundation's Atherosclerosis protocol.

Product availability: Forskolin, coenzyme Q10, acetyl-L-carnitine, taurine, magnesium, potassium, and NADH are available by calling 1-800-544-4440. Growth hormone has to be prescribed by a knowledgeable physician.

Constipation

Conventional and alternative doctors often recommend fiber supplements to prevent constipation. Yet, published studies show that a significant number of chronically constipated people do not find relief from fiber supplements.

Dietary modifications can help some people, but many people's constipation is caused by insufficient peristalsis, which means that there is not enough colon contractile activity to completely evacuate the bowel. Many chronically constipated people become laxative addicts. However, there are specific nutrients, if taken at the right time, that can induce healthy colon peristaltic action without producing side effects.

Nutrients that induce healthy colon peristalsis work best when taken on an empty stomach. One combination is 4 to 8 grams of vitamin C powder and 1,500 mg of magnesium oxide taken with the juice of a freshly squeezed grapefruit. If that's too tart for you, use vitamin C and magnesium capsules with fresh orange juice. This therapy has to be individually adjusted so it will not cause diarrhea.

Vitamin B5 in a dose of 3,000 mg on an empty stomach will produce a rapid evacuation of bowel contents. Durk Pearson and Sandy Shaw's Powermaker II sugar-free formula contains vitamin B5, vitamin C, arginine and choline—all of which induce significant peristaltic action when one to two tablespoons of the product is taken on an empty stomach. Nutritional laxatives have many health benefits, whereas pharmaceutical laxatives have been linked to the development of cancer.

Product availability: You can order pure ascorbic acid crystals, magnesium oxide powder, vitamin B5 powder, vitamin C caps, magnesium caps, and Powermaker II sugar free by calling 1-800-544-4440.

Deafness

Refer to Hearing Loss protocol.

Depression

Depression is now acknowledged to be an epidemic disease. The most widely sold prescription drug to treat depression in the United States is Prozac.

The safest and most effective antidepressant in the world is the European drug S-adenosylmethionine (SAM), a natural compound found in every cell within the body, which plays an important role in many critical biochemical processes. When compared with other antidepressants, SAM works faster and more effectively, with virtually no adverse side effects. In fact, unlike FDA-approved antidepressants, which have both lethal and non-lethal side effects, SAM produces side benefits such as improved cognitive function, protection of liver function, and potential slowing of the aging process. Some people take SAM for its anti-aging properties alone.

The major drawback of SAM at this time is its high cost. SAM is a difficult-to-produce natural substance, which has high manufacturing and packaging costs. At this time, the retail price of using SAM to treat depression is more than the price of Prozac. The suggested dose of SAM to treat depression ranges from 400 to 1,600 mg a day. In one study, as little as 25 mg a day was used to treat depression, while most have used 1,600 mg a day of SAM.

A more affordable antidepressant being used in Europe, and sold in some American health food stores, is an extract from the herb St. John's Wort called hypericum or hyperforat (St. John's Wort extract). For treating depression we suggest 300 mg, three times a day of hypericum (with a standardized concentration of 0.3% hypericin, the primary active ingredient in hypericum). Small children should be limited to 300 mg a day; larger children may take 600 mg a day; adolescents may take the full adult dose.

Another European antidepressant drug called adrafinil is being successfully used by Europeans and Americans who import it for personal use. The dose of adrafinil is two tablets twice a day. Some people with depression benefit by the inhibition of the enzyme monoamine oxidase (MAO). While MAO-inhibiting drugs have many side effects, the use of the European drug KH3 can safely alleviate depression in some people, without classic MAO-inhibiting drug side effects. KH3 is a mild inhibitor of MAO and is very inexpensive.

The amino acid acetyl-L-carnitine has been reported to safely alleviate depression in some people in doses of 1,000 mg twice a day. Acetyl-L-carnitine has cognitive-enhancing and anti-aging effects. The brain cell energy-enhancing NADH (nicotinamide-adenine-dinucleotide) has alleviated depression in studies where 5 to 10 mg a day was used.

Nutrition plays a critical role in the treatment of depression. The supplementation of specific nutrients can correct an underlying deficiency that may be the cause of some depressive states. The most comprehensive nutrient supplement formula is Life Extension Mix, which contains high doses of of 52 different ingredients. Depressed people who have not taken vitamin supplements before should try three tablets, three times a day of Life Extension Mix, for five weeks, to see if it helps correct their depressive state. If vitamin supplements have already been tried and failed to correct a depressive state, amino acid therapy should begin immediately in conjunction with Life Extension Mix and any needed pharmacologic anti-depressant.

The amino acid dl-phenylalanine, when taken with the nutrients in Life Extension Mix, can boost endorphin levels in the brain to help lift a person out of a depressed state. The suggested dose is to two 500 mg capsules of dl-phenylalanine in the morning on an empty stomach and one 500 mg capsule of dl-phenylalanine in midafternoon on an empty stomach.

Some people use the powder formula Rise & Shine, designed by Durk Pearson and Sandy Shaw, which provides phenylalanine and co-factors. The suggested dose is one tablespoon in the morning and one in mid afternoon. If phenylalanine does not work after several weeks, then the amino acid tyrosine should be tried at the same dose.

There are some people who are genetically sensitive to phenylalanine and cannot take it. Hypertensive people should use phenylalanine with caution because it can elevate blood pressure in people who already have high blood pressure. Cancer patients should avoid taking extra phenylalanine and tyrosine because these amino acids can contribute to cancer cell proliferation.

CAUTION: None of the above natural therapies may be effective in patients suffering from serious clinical depression or manic-depression. Such patients may require FDA-approved antidepressant drugs and/or lithium. Anyone suffering from clinical depression of any type should be under the care of a physician.

Product availability: SAM, dl-phenylalanine, l-tyrosine, Life Extension Mix, St. John's Wort extract, NADH, Rise & Shine, and acetyl-L-carnitine are available by calling 1-800-544-4440. Ask for a listing of offshore companies that sell adrafinil and KH3 to Americans by mail.

DHEA-Pregnenolone Precautions

DHEA replacement is becoming a very popular anti-aging therapy. There are some precautions that should be exercised when taking DHEA. Since the hormone pregnenolone can cascade down into DHEA and estrogen, some of the precautions discussed for DHEA replacement therapy may also apply to pregnenolone replacement therapy.

A DHEA blood test should be taken 3-6 weeks after beginning DHEA (and/or pregnenolone) therapy to help determine optimal dosing. Some people take a DHEA blood test before beginning DHEA replacement therapy, but the Life Extension Foundation has found that every person evaluated over 39 years of age shows marked DHEA deficiency.

For the DHEA test, blood should be drawn between the second and third daily dose of DHEA (or pregnenolone). While this test can be costly, it can save you money in the long-run if it shows that you should take less of the hormone to produce youthful DHEA levels.

Take antioxidant supplements after every DHEA dose. Men with prostate cancer or severe benign prostatic hypertrophy should not take DHEA because it can be converted into the metabolite, testosterone and dihydrotestosterone, which could promote prostate cell proliferation.

Men over 40 who take DHEA should also take 320 mg of saw palmetto extract a day, or another 5-alpha reductase inhibitor to reduce the conversion of testosterone to dihydrotestosterone.

Men over 40 should also consider checking their PSA (prostate specific antigen) level when they have their first DHEA blood test, and every year thereafter. This test can reveal the presence of prostate cancer.

Do not take DHEA if you have prostate cancer.

DHEA can increase serum estrogen levels in women. It could reduce or eliminate the need for estrogen replacement therapy by naturally elevating estrogen levels in the body. To help protect cells (especially breast cells) from excessive proliferation in response to estrogen in the blood, women should consider taking 1-10 mg of melatonin every night, especially if they take DHEA. Soy provides phytoestrogens that also reduce breast cancer risk.

Women with an estrogen-dependent cancer may want to avoid taking DHEA. However, some physicians find physiological DHEA replacement beneficial for patients with such cancers. Women should consider estrogen testing when they take their DHEA blood test in order to evaluate DHEA's effect on their blood levels of estrogen when a follow-up test is performed.

If you have liver disease, it is more important that you take DHEA sublingually (under your tongue) to reduce the amount of DHEA entering your liver. Check your liver enzyme levels to make sure DHEA is not making an existing liver disease worse. Some animal studies suggest the possibility of liver damage from large doses of DHEA. Antioxidants should be taken to protect against DHEA-induced free radical damage to the liver.

Pregnenolone can be taken in doses of 50 to 200 mg a day. If more than 50 mg of pregnenolone is taken, it should be taken in divided doses. Pregnenolone can also be converted into progesterone in the body, which may be beneficial for women.

Product availability: To obtain low cost DHEA and pregnenolone and blood tests to measure these hormones by mail, phone 1-800-544-4440.

Diabetes Type I
(Juvenile Diabetes)

Diabetes type I is caused by the destruction of the insulin producing cells in the pancreas. The resulting insulin deficiency requires the lifelong administration of insulin by injection several times a day in precise doses for improved glucose utilization.

The frequency and dose of insulin used by type I diabetics is determined by the results of blood sugar readings on a glucometer. Type I diabetics should use the glucometer at least three times a day to regulate their insulin dosing. Juvenile diabetes is thought to be caused by an autoimmune or viral attack on the insulin-producing beta cells of the pancreatic islets.

Juvenile diabetes may be prevented or mitigated by following our Autoimmune Disease protocol. Once the insulin-producing cells are destroyed, the best alternative therapy involves protecting against the pathological effects caused by wide variations in blood sugar levels.

Diabetics are at risk of becoming disabled or dying from premature cardiovascular disease. To find out how to prevent diabetic cardiovascular diseases, follow the Atherosclerosis protocol.

To facilitate the cellular metabolism of glucose, diabetics should take 200 mcg of chromium picolinate with every meal. Chromium may reduce the amount of injected insulin required, so using the glucometer can enable the diabetic patient to determine the proper amount of insulin to inject.

Diabetic retinopathy is a leading cause of blindness. Studies show that supplementation with vitamin B6 can help to prevent diabetic retinopathy. The appropriate amount of vitamin B6 is included in the Atherosclerosis protocol. Diabetic neuropathy can cause severe pain throughout the body. The nutrients alpha lipoic acid in doses of 500 to 800 mg a day, and acetyl-L-carnitine at 1,000 to 2,000 mg a day, have been effective for diabetic neuropathies.

The premature aging caused by diabetes is primarily the result of uncontrolled glucose that binds with protein in the blood to form nonfunctioning structures within the body. This devastating process is known as glycosylation. Everyone suffers from glycosylation as a normal consequence of aging. However, diabetics suffer from accelerated glycosylation that causes many of the health problems associated with juvenile diabetes. Vitamin C and chromium may inhibit glycosylation. Juvenile diabetics may want to take five additional grams of vitamin C to further inhibit glycosylation.

The European drug aminoguanidine inhibits an enzyme required for glycosylation. The recommended dose of aminoguanidine is 300 to 600 mg a day. DHEA is an adrenal hormone that may protect against some diabetic complications. Refer to DHEA Precautions.

Product availability: Chromium picolinate, DHEA, alpha lipoic acid, acetyl-L-carnitine, vitamin B6 and vitamin C are available by phoning 1-800-544-4440. Ask for the name of an offshore supplier of the anti-glycosylation drug aminoguanidine.

Diabetes Type II
(Adult Onset Diabetes)

Diabetes Type II is very different from Diabetes Type I. Unlike type I diabetes, which is characterized by a severe insulin deficiency, type II diabetes usually involves normal or overproduction of insulin by the pancreas. Type II diabetes occurs when the cells become resistant to insulin due to receptor malfunction. Insulin is the hormone that normally drives glucose into cells. Insulin resistance causes elevated blood sugar levels because sugar is not able to be absorbed and utilized by the cells. The pancreas may recognize the elevated blood sugar levels and secrete more insulin in a futile attempt to lower the elevated sugar levels.

In order to effectively treat type II diabetes, insulin resistance needs to be alleviated. Chronically elevated levels of serum glucose and insulin predispose a person to premature cardiovascular disease and other diabetic complications.

Aging causes a breakdown in normal glucose metabolism. Dietary fat and obesity can contribute directly to type II diabetes. A possible dietary cure for type II diabetes involves eating a reduced calorie diet comprised of 10% fat that is high in protein and low in carbohydrates. Since most people are unable to restrict their fat intake to only 10%, the Life Extension Foundation has specific nutrient, hormone and drug recommendations to help break down insulin resistance.

Anyone with type II diabetes should follow the Atherosclerosis protocol. To help bring blood sugar levels under control, 200 mcg of chromium picolinate and 7.5 mg of vanadyl sulfate should be taken with each meal. An arginine formula called Powermaker II (Sugar-Free) can be of significant benefit to most adult onset diabetic patients. One of the factors involved in cellular insulin resistance is a deficit of nitric oxide. Arginine induces the production of nitric oxide so sugar molecules can more easily enter cells. Arginine promotes youthful anabolic cell renewal throughout the body that can result in improvements in type II diabetics. The dose of Powermaker II (Sugar-Free) should be one to two tablespoons a day.

CAUTION: For a minority of type II diabetics, arginine can elevate their blood sugar by neutralizing insulin. Therefore, diabetics contemplating using arginine or Powermaker II (Sugar-Free) should check their blood sugar with a glucometer every time they take an arginine supplement during the first three weeks they use arginine.

If following the Atherosclerosis protocol and taking arginine, chromium and vanadyl sulfate does not bring your blood sugar levels under control, then the drug Glucophage, also known as metformin, should be prescribed by your doctor. Glucophage was used in Europe 40 years before it was approved by the FDA for use in the United States. Glucophage can break down insulin resistance so that cells are better able to absorb and utilize glucose. Lower glucose levels in the blood will result in reduced insulin output by the pancreas. The dose of Glucophage most commonly prescribed is 500 mg, twice a day.

In addition to Glucophage, thyroid hormone replacement therapy can further help to drive glucose into your cells. Your doctor should prescribe the proper dose of thyroid hormone if this is required. Blood tests may not always reveal a thyroid hormone deficiency, even though most people over age 40 have altered thyroid hormone metabolism. These people can benefit from some degree of thyroid hormone replacement.

DHEA hormone replacement therapy can also be beneficial in restoring youthful carbohydrate metabolism. See the DHEA Precaution protocol for proper DHEA dosing and safety precautions. The combination of chromium, Glucophage, DHEA and thyroid hormone therapy can slowly produce weight loss, further reducing the risk factors for diabetes type II. Since being overweight is usually a contributing factor in diabetes type II, please check the Weight Management protocols for further suggestions.

A common complication of diabetes is painful peripheral nerve disease. Two nutrients that have been shown to be beneficial in preventing and treating diabetic neuropathy are alpha lipoic acid and acetyl-L-carnitine. Suggested dosing is 500 mg to 1,000 mg a day of alpha lipoic acid and/or 1,000 mg to 2,000 mg a day of acetyl-L-carnitine. In Europe, these nutrients are used as "drugs" to treat neuropathies.

Product availability: Chromium, DHEA, vanadyl sulfate, Powermaker II, alpha lipoic acid, acetyl-L-carnitine, and arginine can be ordered by calling 1-800-544-4440. Your doctor can prescribe Glucophage and thyroid hormone replacement therapy.

Digestive Disorders

Aging causes a decline in our natural production of digestive enzymes, thereby making the efficient processing of our food more difficult. Digestive enzyme deficiencies can cause our liver and pancreas to be overworked and become pathologically enlarged. There are specific enzymes and acids that are needed to break down proteins, carbohydrates, and fats.

Many people over age 40 begin using digestive enzymes when eating a heavy meal. The enzymes quicken the digestive process so that the feeling of being bloated, heavy and tired after eating does not occur. There are many enzyme products available, but most people choose a multi-enzyme formula called Super Enzyme Caps that contains a concentrated standardized pancreatin enzyme, along with enzymes to break down every food group. Super Enzyme Caps also contain hydrochloric acid and ox bile. For people seeking a vegetable derived multi-enzyme supplement without pancreatin, hydrochloric acid and ox bile, a product called N-Zymes is often used. For heartburn problems refer to the Esophageal Reflux protocol.

Product availability: You can order Super Enzyme Caps and N-Zymes by calling 1-800-544-4440.

Down Syndrome

Until recently, the birth defect that causes severe mental retardation, known as Down syndrome, was thought to be untreatable. A search of the scientific literature, however, indicates that high potency vitamin supplements, along with the European drug piracetam, can be effective in treating children with Down syndrome.

Desperate parents have been using high-potency vitamin supplements and piracetam to treat Down syndrome with astonishing results. News reports have documented the before-and-after effects when Down syndrome children followed this protocol.

The Life Extension Foundation suggests that children with Down syndrome be given Life Extension Mix powder in doses slightly below the adult dose. We suggest that a teaspoon of choline bitartrate powder be added to the Life Extension Mix powder to potentiate the neurologic-enhancing effect of this vitamin formula.

Piracetam should be administered in doses beginning at 800 mg a day, and then working up to as high as 4,800 mg a day for short periods of time. Small children should be given lower doses of all the above.

Daily compliance is the most difficult aspect of the protocol. Children do not like the taste of vitamins. Life Extension Mix powder, choline chloride liquid or choline bitartrate powder, and crushed piracetam tablets can all be administered together in juice to help improve the palatability of the mixture.

Product availability: Life Extension Mix powder and choline are available singly or in a Protocol Pak by phoning 1-800-544-4440. When calling the Foundation ask for a listing of offshore suppliers of piracetam.

Emphysema and Chronic Obstructive Pulmonary Disease

Emphysema is a pulmonary deficiency usually caused by years of uncontrolled free radical damage resulting in degenerative changes in the air sacs of the lung. Emphysema patients suffer shortness of breath, congestive heart failure, cough, and increasingly troubled breathing. Chronic obstructive pulmonary disease (COPD) is a disease of the bronchi in the lungs characterized by the production of large amounts of thick mucus, which causes difficulties in breathing. The Life Extension Foundation's protocol for these diseases involves the regular intake of high potency antioxidant supplements to inhibit free radical lung damage.

The suggested daily dose of high-potency vitamins for patients with these lung diseases is three tablets three times a day of Life Extension Mix and one capsule a day of Life Extension Booster. In order to help break up the thick mucus, 600 mg of N-acetyl-cysteine should be taken three times a day along with two grams of vitamin C.

If the combination of these nutrients does not sufficiently break up the mucus, a drug used to treat cystic fibrosis called Pulmozyme can be prescribed by your doctor. Pulmozyme is the most effective mucous-eradicating drug available. However, it is only approved for cystic fibrosis, and, as a result, physicians often fail to prescribe it for acute mucus problems. To restore energy production to damaged cells in the lungs, the following nutrients are suggested:

1) Coenzyme Q10 — 100 mg three times a day
2) Forskolin — 10 to 60 mg a day
3) Acetyl-L-carnitine — 1,000 mg twice a day
4) NADH — 5 mg twice a day
5) Taurine — 1,000 mg twice a day
6) Magnesium — 500 mg of elemental magnesium once a day
7) Potassium — if needed

CAUTION: Do not use forskolin if you have prostate cancer. Forskolin may lower blood pressure.

Product availability: Life Extension Mix, Life Extension Booster, n-acetyl-cysteine, vitamin C, coenzyme Q10, forskolin, acetyl-L-carnitine, NADH, taurine, magnesium, and potassium can be obtained by phoning 1-800-544-4440.

Esophageal Reflux (Heartburn)

About 40% of Americans suffer from heartburn to one degree or another. Heartburn is caused by an incomplete closure of the sphincter muscle at the end of the esophagus, causing stomach acids to wash up against the relatively delicate esophageal lining, resulting in the pain and discomfort of heartburn. This is technically known as esophageal reflux.

Conventional therapy involves sleeping with two pillows to keep stomach acid out of the esophagus at night, taking antacids after each meal, avoiding certain foods, not eating before bedtime, and using acid suppressing drugs such as Zantac, Tagamet and Pepcid.

The constant irritation of stomach acids on the lining of the esophagus can result in an increased risk of esophageal cancer and esophagitis. Antioxidant nutrients can protect against esophageal inflammation and, according to published studies, they may lower the risk of esophageal cancer. If you suffer from heartburn, you should consider taking three tablets of Life Extension Mix with each meal to help reduce your risk of esophageal cancer and esophagitis.

Product availability: Life Extension Mix can be ordered by phoning 1-800-544-4440. Zantac, Tagamet and Pepcid are now sold over-the-counter.

Estrogen Replacement Therapy

Few gynecologists are using estrogen replacement therapy safely to help prevent osteoporosis, heart disease, and premature aging. A recent study in *The New England Journal of Medicine* showed that women taking estrogen and a synthetic progestin had a 32% to 46% increase in their risk of breast cancer. The most popular estrogen drug in the United States is Premarin, which contains estrogens derived from the urine of pregnant mares. Provera is the name of a popular synthetic progestin, that, when taken with Premarin, helps to prevent estrogen-induced uterine cancer, but does not prevent estrogen-induced breast or ovarian cancer.

The mechanisms by which estrogen causes cancer are well documented in the scientific literature. Yet the profits generated by Premarin sales have enabled its manufacturer to create the impression that Premarin is the only therapy for menopausal and post-menopausal women.

Although estrogen increases the risk of some types of cancer, it also has critical anti-aging benefits, including the prevention of osteoporosis and heart disease, and the reversal of some aspects of neurologic decline.

Many doctors don't believe that estrogen causes cancer at all, while others believe that combining estrogen with a synthetic progestin neutralizes the cancer causing potential of estrogen. The scientific facts are obscured by studies that appear to contradict each other about estrogen's carcinogenic potential. Some studies show that estrogen may not cause cancer in the short-term. However, in women taking estrogen and/or a synthetic progestin for more than 10 years, there appears to be a significantly elevated risk of breast, ovarian, and uterine cancer.

The Life Extension Foundation bases its warning about the carcinogenic risk of estrogen-progestin replacement therapy on these longer term studies. *The New England Journal of Medicine's* report that women using estrogen alone, or estrogen and a synthetic progestin, had an increased risk of breast cancer of 32% to 46% was based upon data from the famous Nurses' Health Study conducted at Harvard Medical School. The nurses participating in this study represented 725,550 person-years of follow up. Because of the sheer size of this study, its findings are persuasive. They showed that women who took estrogen plus a synthetic progestin actually had a higher rate of breast cancer than women who took estrogen alone!

The authors of the study concluded as follows:

> "The addition of progestins to estrogen therapy does not reduce the risk of breast cancer among post-menopausal women. The substantial increase in the risk of breast cancer among older women who take hormones suggests that the trade-offs between risks and benefits should be carefully assessed."

The New England Journal of Medicine's report about the elevated risk of breast cancer from hormone therapy obscured another recent report in the *American Journal of*

Epidemiology showing that long-term estrogen replacement therapy increased the risk of fatal ovarian cancer. This seven-year study included 240,073 pre- and post-menopausal women. After adjusting for other risk factors, women who used estrogen for 6-8 years had a 40% higher risk of fatal ovarian cancer, and women who used estrogen for 11 or more years had a shocking 70% higher risk of fatal ovarian cancer! The increased ovarian cancer risk from estrogen is a serious concern. Cancers of the breast, uterus, and ovary account for 41% of cancer incidence in U.S. women. Breast cancer is running at epidemic levels, striking one in eight women, up from one in 30 women in 1960. Conventional hormone replacement therapy and oral contraceptives have been used since 1960. Clearly, an alternative is needed to provide the anti-aging benefits of these youth hormones, while protecting against their potential cancer-causing effects.

In addition to increased cancer risks, some of the risks of estrogen/progestin therapy include:

- ✔ weight gain,
- ✔ abnormal blood clot formation,
- ✔ increased risk of gallstones, fibroid tumors, headaches,
- ✔ premenstrual type symptoms (irritability, fluid retention)

Some of these side effects may be attributable to the synthetic progestins prescribed with estrogen, and not necessarily to estrogen itself.

It is important to note that dangerous forms of estrogen can be produced naturally within the body, so avoiding FDA-approved drugs like Premarin does not always protect against estrogen-induced cancer. Estrogen may increase the risk of cancer, yet it is an important anti-aging hormone that provides us with many health benefits. This creates a dilemma that conventional medicine admits it has yet to resolve.

Estrogens are steroid hormones that promote youthful cell division in target organs of the body. The benefits of maintaining this youthful cellular division with the proper estrogen replacement therapy include:

- ❖ enhanced skin smoothness, firmness, and elasticity
- ❖ enhanced moistness of skin and mucus membranes
- ❖ enhanced muscle tone
- ❖ reduced genital atrophy and enhanced sex drive in women
- ❖ reduced menopausal miseries
- ❖ reduced risk of heart disease and osteoporosis
- ❖ reduced risk of colon cancer
- ❖ improved memory and overall neurologic function
- ❖ protection against Alzheimer's disease
- ❖ enhanced immune function
- ❖ a greater feeling of well-being

Given all this, it is no wonder that Premarin is the number one prescription drug in the United States.

Despite conventional medicine's enthusiastic endorsement, Premarin is not for everyone. According to a 1987 survey, more than 50% of women quit estrogen therapy after a year because they didn't feel right, or were concerned about the long-term cancer risks. On the other hand, many women feel wonderful on estrogen replacement therapy and plan to take it for the rest of their lives.

The primary forms of estrogen are estradiol, estrone and estriol

Estradiol and estrone are potent estrogens and are thought to be the estrogens that increase the risk of cancer. Estriol is a weak estrogen that provides anti-aging benefits with minimal risk of cancer.

Your objective should be to follow a program that produces high levels of estriol and relatively low levels of estradiol and estrone.

Blood tests can measure the relative levels of these forms of estrogen within your body. Every woman is different, which means that for some women, Premarin may produce high levels of safe estriol, while other women may find that Premarin elevates their estradiol and estrone levels. The same may be true for DHEA replacement therapy. In some women, DHEA may cascade down to safe estriol, or it could convert into the more dangerous estradiol and estrone.

DHEA replacement therapy may be a safer and more natural way of replacing estrogen levels diminished by the aging process than taking FDA-approved estrogen drugs. Most women take 15 mg of DHEA three times a day. DHEA is naturally converted to estrogen compounds within the body. Refer to DHEA Precautions for proper DHEA dosing and safety precautions.

Eating soy products, like miso, is another natural way of boosting estrogen levels. There are soy extracts now available in tablet and powder form that contain standardized phytoestrogens. Phytoestrogens are weak estrogens that protect against cancer and provide some anti-aging benefits.

Cruciferous vegetables protect against estrogen-induced cancers. Many women take a tablespoon of Phyto-Food powder every day to obtain the vegetable concentrates of broccoli and cabbage that contain breast-cancer-preventing phytochemicals. Flax seed and fish oils may lower production of toxic estrogens and may block some of their tumor-initiating effects.

Vitamin E supplementation may boost estriol levels in the body. The B-complex vitamins may protect against some of the toxic effects of estrogen. Estrogen may produce some of its toxicity by binding to vitamin B6 in the body, thus causing a vitamin B6 deficiency.

If pregnenolone, DHEA and/or soy extracts fail to provide you with enough estrogen, estriol should be considered as the ideal form of estrogen for supplementation. While it may not be available at your corner drug store, doctors are free to prescribe it, and there are European pharmacies who sell it.

Women using estriol replacement therapy should do so in conjunction with the regular application of topical progesterone cream (not Provera) and the nightly intake of one to 10 mg of melatonin.

Blood tests may not accurately reflect a women's individual need for hormone replacement. Some clinicians believe that hot flashes, dry skin, and vaginal dryness during and after menopause may be better indicators of the need for estrogen replacement therapy than blood tests. However, blood tests can be important indicators for dosage determination.

The symptoms of progesterone deficiency may manifest themselves as depression, irritability, mood swings, and insomnia.

There are several mail order pharmacies that custom-compound the estriol form of estrogen used in Europe to treat estrogen deficiency safely.

Estriol can be obtained in capsule form, or as a topical transdermal cream. The dosage range is 0.05 to 10 mg, twice a day.

One protocol to treat vaginal dryness is to use one gram of low potency estriol cream for seven continuous days, and then drop back to two to three applications a week.

If low potency estriol cream does not work, then order a more potent concentration. The objective is to provide the minimum estrogen replacement therapy your body needs for optimal, overall anti-aging benefits.

For some women, estriol is too weak an estrogen to provide relief from hot flashes and the other symptoms of estrogen deficiency during menopause. A popular cream or capsule used in this case is called TriEst (which stands for triple estrogen). It comes in a wide range of strengths. TriEst contains 10% estrone estrogen, 10% estradiol estrogen, and 80% estriol estrogen

To treat mild to moderate hot flashes and vaginal dryness, capsules or cream containing 1.25 mg of TriEst should be used twice a day. For moderate to severe estrogen deficiency symptoms, 2.5 mg of TriEst capsules or cream should be used twice a day.

Estriol and TriEst can be ordered from offshore pharmacies that ship European medications to Americans for personal use.

A newly available product is Natural Estrogen, which is a combination of highly potent plant estrogens, or phytoestrogens. Among the ingredients of Natural Estrogen are extracts with high phytoestrogenic activity from Himalayan yams, angelica, and glyrrhetic acid (from licorice root).

A recent study with Natural Estrogen in 381 menopausal women by Dr. Barry Gushleff of Lakeside Medical Center in Lake St. Louis, Missouri, showed improvement in symptoms in 87-92% of the women using Natural Estrogen.

Women who want to use Natural Estrogen should first undergo testing to determine their baseline hormone levels, and then should be tested again after therapy has begun (see

Medical Testing Protocol). Although patients can go "cold turkey" from estrogen drugs to Natural Estrogen, Dr. Gushleff suggests that women who have been using estrogen drugs gradually wean themselves off. The following program is suggested:

1st month — Natural Estrogen every other day
2nd month — Natural Estrogen two days in a row
3rd month — Natural Estrogen three days in a row, continuing until
estrogen drugs are completely eliminated.

Calcium and vitamin D augment estrogen's ability to prevent osteoporosis. The suggested doses are 1,500 to 2,000 mg of calcium and 400 IU of vitamin D, along with Natural Estrogen and a progesterone cream.

To reiterate, the objective is to use the minimum amount of estrogen replacement to achieve anti-aging benefits, without increasing the risk of cancer. That is why it is imperative that women using any form of estrogen replacement therapy use a topical progesterone cream and take melatonin to protect against the side effects of estrogen.

Women should try soy-derived phytoestrogens first to see if these safe forms of natural estrogen will provide the desired anti-aging benefits of estrogen.

You might consider a complete blood hormone profile that includes estrogen, progesterone, testosterone, and DHEA.

Members of the Life Extension Foundation can have total estrogen, progesterone, testosterone and DHEA-S tests performed by mail. To inquire about these tests, call the Foundation at 1-800-544-4440.

Product availability: Soy extracts, pregnenolone, DHEA, vitamin E, melatonin, Phytofood and progesterone cream, and Natural Estrogen are available singly or in a Protocol Pak by calling 1-800-544-4440. When calling the Foundation, ask for a listing of offshore companies that sell estriol and TriEst.

Fibrinogen and Cardiovascular Disease

Blood clots that form inside arteries are the leading cause of death in the Western world. Most heart attacks and strokes are caused by a blood clot that obstructs the flow of blood to a portion of the heart or the brain. No blood flow means no life to heart or brain cells deprived of oxygen. Blood clots kill more than 600,000 Americans every year, yet conventional medicine has largely ignored well-documented methods of reducing abnormal blood clot formation.

Low dose aspirin and certain nutrients provide partial protection against abnormal blood clots, but a newly identified clotting factor mandates that additional measures be taken to prevent heart attack and stoke. Fibrinogen is a component of blood involved in the clotting process. High levels of fibrinogen predispose a person to coronary and cerebral artery disease, even when other known risk factors such as cholesterol are low.

Cigarette smoking increases cardiovascular disease risk. Cigarette smoking also raises fibrinogen levels in the blood. Published studies documenting the dangers of cigarette smoking show that cigarette smokers who suffer from cardiovascular disease also have high fibrinogen levels. Fibrinogen elevation in cigarette smokers has been identified as a primary mechanism causing heart disease and stroke. In fact, high fibrinogen levels may be a more powerful predictor of cardiovascular mortality than cigarette smoking itself.

The role of fibrinogen in the development of cardiovascular disease has been fully confirmed by the results of all relevant studies conducted during the past 10 years. High fibrinogen levels have at least as great a predictive value as any other known risk factor, such as elevated LDL cholesterol, elevated triglycerides, obesity, and diabetes.

In persons with a family history of heart disease, fibrinogen levels are high. Fibrinogen levels are primarily genetically inherited, meaning that fibrinogen may be the genetic factor causing familial premature heart disease. Exposure to cold increases fibrinogen levels by 23%, and mortality from heart attack and stroke are higher in winter than in summer.

Fibrinogen hinders blood flow and oxygen delivery by deforming red blood cells, causing red cell aggregation, and thickening the blood, all of which lead to diminished circulation. Fibrinogen binds blood platelets together, thus initiating abnormal arterial blood clots. Fibrinogen is then converted to fibrin, which is the final step in the blood clotting cascade.

Fibrinogen contributes to the development of atherosclerosis by incorporating itself into the arterial plaque. Fibrinogen and LDL cholesterol work together to generate atherosclerotic plaques. Fibrinogen initiates the atherosclerotic plaque. Fibrinogen then converts to fibrin and serves as a scaffold for LDL cholesterol in the atherosclerotic plaque that slowly occludes an artery. Fibrinogen and its derivatives trigger a variety of other mechanisms thought to be involved in the atherosclerotic process. Fibrinogen and LDL cholesterol have a synergistic effect in promoting atherosclerosis, though fibrinogen may play a more important role in the development of atherosclerotic lesions.

Most heart attacks occur because a blood clot forms inside a coronary artery and chokes off the blood supply to the heart. Most strokes occur because a blood clot forms inside a cerebral artery and blocks the blood supply to the brain. Therefore, it is crucial to take steps to reduce the risk of fibrinogen causing an abnormal arterial clot.

Platelet aggregation inhibitors reduce the risk that fibrinogen will cause an abnormal blood clot. Platelet aggregation inhibitors include aspirin, green tea, ginkgo biloba, and vitamin E. For optimal protection against the formation of arterial blood clots, it makes sense to utilize therapies that lower elevated fibrinogen levels.

High vitamin A and beta-carotene serum levels have been associated with reduced fibrinogen levels in humans. Animals fed a vitamin A-deficient diet have an impaired ability to break down fibrinogen. When animals are injected with vitamin A, they produce tissue plasminogen activator (tPA), which breaks down fibrinogen. Both fish and olive oil have been shown to lower fibrinogen in women with elevated fibrinogen levels. The daily amount of fish oil required to produce a fibrinogen-lowering effect was 6 grams, which equals about five capsules of Mega-EPA fish oil concentrate capsules.

Elevated homocysteine levels have been shown to block the natural breakdown of fibrinogen by inhibiting the production of tissue plasminogen activator (tPA). Folic acid and vitamin B6 help to reduce elevated homocysteine levels.

One of the more interesting studies involved the use of vitamin C to break down excess fibrinogen. The FDA has stated that Americans only need 60 to 100 mg of vitamin C a day, while a government report published in the beginning of 1996 says that Americans need only 200 mg of vitamin C a day. This report received widespread media support. The media used this government report to ridicule the use of vitamin C supplements in excess of 200 mg.

However, in an earlier report published in the journal *Atherosclerosis*, heart disease patients were given either 1,000 or 2,000 mg a day of vitamin C to assess its effect on the breakdown of fibrinogen. At 1,000 mg a day, there was no detectable change in fibrinolytic activity or cholesterol. At 2,000 mg a day of vitamin C, however, there was a 27% decrease in the platelet aggregation index, a 12% reduction in total cholesterol, and a 45% increase in fibrinolytic (fibrinogen breakdown) activity. Again, the U.S. government and the medical establishment tried to convince Americans that they do not need vitamin supplements. Those Americans who believe the government are dying of artery disease.

For maximum fibrinogen-lowering effect, the proteolytic enzyme bromelain may be the most effective nutrient supplement. For those seeking to lower elevated fibrinogen levels, 2-6 capsules a day of Herbal Cardiovascular Formula containing a standardized bromelain concentrate should be considered.

Some non-pharmacologic ways of lowering fibrinogen include stopping smoking, avoiding obesity, lowering LDL cholesterol and avoiding exposure to cold

Don't depend on FDA-approved drugs to lower fibrinogen levels. The popular cholesterol lowering drug Lopid (gemfibrozil) increases fibrinogen levels by 9 to 21%. Other FDA-approved heart medications have shown little effect on fibrinogen levels.

A European drug called Bezafibrate has been shown to lower fibrinogen levels by 25% in patients with fibrinogen levels between 300 and 415 mg/dL. In patients whose fibrinogen levels were over 600, Bezafibrate lowered fibrinogen levels by 45%. Bezafibrate has been used extensively in Europe since 1978 to lower LDL cholesterol by 20 to 30%, and increase beneficial HDL cholesterol. It has over nine million patient-years of safety documentation. The fact that Bezafibrate is still not approved by the FDA reflects a serious lack of care by our government about the healthcare of its citizens. For those with vascular disease, please access the Foundation's Atherosclerosis protocol for additional suggestions.

Product availability: Healthprin (aspirin), green tea, ginkgo biloba, vitamin E, Mega-EPA, folic acid, vitamin C, vitamin B6, and Herbal Cardiovascular Formula can be ordered singly or in a Protocol Pak by phoning 1-800-544-4440. Call for a list of offshore pharmacies if you are interested in obtaining the drug Bezafibrate.

Fibromyalgia

Refer to the Depression protocol for suggested therapies. Consideration should be given to the European antidepressant drug S-adenosylmethionine (SAM), as published studies indicate that SAM may be the most effective therapy available to reduce the chronic pain and depression associated with fibromyalgia.

Product availability: S-adenosylmethionine is available through an overseas company. Call 1-800-544-4440 for further information.

Flu-Influenza Virus

Flu viruses temporarily disable most Americans every year, and at least 60,000 elderly Americans can die in a year when there is a flu epidemic. If you have the flu, there are alternative therapies that can shorten the duration of your illness and, if you are elderly, possibly save your life.

Ribavirin is a broad spectrum anti-viral drug that is especially effective against influenza-like viruses. Ribavirin is approved in almost every country in the world. If you have Ribavirin on hand when you first develop the symptoms of the flu, you should take 200 mg of Ribavirin every three to four hours. In many cases, this can prevent the full development of the flu because of Ribavirin's ability to interfere with influenza virus replication.

There are herbal extracts that have anti-viral effects. When flu symptoms occur, it is suggested that you take echinacea liquid herbal extract at a dose of six full droppers in a small amount of water, followed by two full droppers every two waking hours until the two oz. bottle is gone.

Another alternative is 300 mg of astragalus extract and four capsules a day of Sports Ginseng, which is a standardized extract containing both Korean and Siberian ginseng.

A new extract from the elderberry called Sambucol has been shown to keep the influenza virus from entering the cells. Sambucol should be taken in doses of one tablespoon four times a day.

DHEA is an adrenal hormone that has shown anti-viral and immune-boosting benefits. When flu symptoms occur, 100 mg of DHEA should be taken three times a day until flu symptoms subside. Refer to DHEA Precautions before taking DHEA. Melatonin has immune-enhancing benefits, possible anti-viral effects and helps you to get the sleep you need to fight the flu virus. Melatonin should be taken in doses of 10 mg before going to sleep for the duration of the flu attack.

High potency vitamin formulas such as Life Extension Mix and other nutrients in the Immune Enhancement protocol should be considered. Also refer to the Common Cold protocol for additional suggestions.

Product availability: Ribavirin can be obtained in Mexico or you can call 1-800-747-0149 for a list of offshore suppliers who will mail it to you. If you have the flu, it will take too long to obtain Ribavirin by mail to be of any help. Echinacea liquid herbal extract, elderberry (Sambucol) astragalus extract, Sports Ginseng, DHEA, melatonin, and Life Extension Mix can be ordered for overnight delivery, singly or in a Protocol Pak, by phoning 1-800-544-4440.

Gingivitis

Gingivitis is characterized by inflammation, swelling, irritation and redness of the gums. If left untreated, it will result in tooth loss. Gingivitis is the most common cause of tooth loss. Modern dentistry has succeeded in preventing most problems associated with chronic gingivitis by encouraging daily flossing, regular brushing, and professional teeth cleaning every three to six months.

Gingivitis can be an underlying symptom of diabetes, leukemia, or a vitamin deficiency. Vitamin supplements, coenzyme Q10 and green tea can alleviate the symptoms of gingivitis. However, proper dental hygiene is still required for optimal oral health.

The standard dose of Life Extension Mix (3 tablets, three times a day) can improve the health of your gums. Life Extension Mix provides over 2,500 mg of vitamin C. Coenzyme Q10 in oil-filled capsules should be taken in 100 to 200 mg daily doses. Green tea beverages provide direct bacteria-killing, plaque-inhibiting effects for the gums. Two standardized green tea capsules providing 200 mg a day of polyphenols can be used to help deliver gingiva-protecting nutrients.

For people suffering from chronic gingivitis, the regular use of Life Extension Mouthwash provides every nutrient shown to be of benefit topically for the health of your gums. One study showed that zinc and folic acid can inhibit gingivitis. Life Extension Mouthwash contains the identical amount of zinc and folic acid used in this study. Life Extension Mouthwash also contains a chlorophyll extract, sanguinaria extract, vitamin E, aloe vera, and caprylic acid—all of which contribute to the health and healing of the gums via different mechanisms.

Product availability: Life Extension Mouthwash, coenzyme Q10, Life Extension Mix, and green tea capsules can be ordered singly or in a Protocol Pak by calling 1-800-544-4440.

Glaucoma

Glaucoma is a condition in which the pressure within the eye becomes elevated. If not brought under control, glaucoma will cause visual defects leading to blindness. Glaucoma is caused by blockage of the normal flow of fluid between the cornea and lens of the eye. Conventional ophthalmologists will prescribe eye drops that are usually highly effective in controlling intraocular pressure.

If conventional anti-glaucoma eye drops are not successful, or if you wish to attempt to address the underlying cause of glaucoma, it is suggested that you try the herbal extract forskolin at a dose of 10 to 60 mg a day. Forskolin lowers intraocular pressure by enhancing the energy cycles that are necessary to move fluid into and out of the eye. Check your blood pressure to make sure that forskolin is not causing low blood pressure.

CAUTION: If you have prostate cancer, do not use forskolin.

Hydergine also improves energy factors via the same mechanism as forskolin. A dose of 5 to 20 mg a day of hydergine could be effective in lowering intraocular pressure. It is mandatory that you have regular intraocular pressure tests administered by an ophthalmologist if you are trying to use forskolin or hydergine as a treatment for glaucoma.

Product availability: You can order forskolin by calling 1-800-544-4440. Call for a list of offshore suppliers who sell high-potency hydergine tablets by mail order for personal use, or ask your physician to prescribe hydergine for you.

Refer to the protocol for Balding.

Hair Loss

Refer to the protocol on Balding.

Hearing Loss

Aging produces a consistent reduction in the ability to hear sounds. Deafness is a common ailment associated with normal aging. The drug hydergine may help restore hearing in some cases of deafness. While the FDA has only approved doses of three mg a day of hydergine, doses of 12 to 20 mg a day may be required to help restore hearing. The best form of hydergine to take is enterically coated liquid capsules made by Sandoz. These are expensive because they only come in one mg strength. Many people choose to obtain low-cost 5 mg hydergine from overseas pharmacies.

Ginkgo biloba has helped some people with the hearing disorder tinnitus, and it also improves neurological function. Ginkgo provides a wide range of health benefits. People with hearing loss should consider taking 120 mg a day of ginkgo extract.

Product availability: Hydergine is a prescription drug in the United States. For a list of suppliers that sell low cost, high potency hydergine from offshore pharmacies, phone 1-800-544-4440. You can also order pharmaceutical ginkgo biloba extract at that number.

Hemochromatosis

A genetic defect can predispose some people to build up toxic levels of iron in their body. Conventional medicine's solution to this problem is to have these people donate blood regularly to purge their bodies of excess blood.

If affordable, the Life Extension Foundation recommends that hemochromatosis patients have their blood frozen for future use. An interesting anti-aging and immune-boosting therapy involves the administration of one's own youthful blood during a state of disease or severe aging.

Iron is a catalyst for many enzymatic reactions as well as for massive free radical damage to cells. The chronic high iron levels that hemochromatosis patients suffer from predisposes them to a host of free radical generated diseases including cancer and heart disease. It is crucial to inhibit these free radicals by consuming large amounts of antioxidants on a regular basis.

One problem that hemochromatosis patients must face is that the potent antioxidant, vitamin C, when taken in the presence of iron-containing foods, can dramatically increase the absorption of iron from the digestive tract into the bloodstream. Therefore, hemochromatosis patients should take a 500 mg buffered vitamin C capsule three times a day between meals.

Hemochromatosis patients should take, with meals, a total of 800 IU of vitamin E, 400 mcg of selenium, the complete vitamin B-complex, including at least 800 mcg of folic acid, 60 mg of zinc, 100 mg of grape seed extract, 120 mg of ginkgo extract, 2,000 mg of garlic, 1,200 mg of n-acetyl-cysteine, 500 mg of alpha lipoic acid, and 3 mg of melatonin.

Melatonin should be taken at bedtime only. The other nutrients should be taken in two or three divided doses. The most potent iron chelating agent is green tea extract. Green tea is a potent antioxidant and helps to remove excess iron from the liver. Hemochromatosis patients should take four to 10 green tea extract capsules that provide at least 100 mg of active polyphenols per capsule. Hemochromatosis patients may also consider intravenous chelation therapy administered by a knowledgeable physician.

Product availability: Vitamin C, vitamin E, selenium, folic acid, zinc, grape seed extract, n-acetyl-cysteine, garlic, ginkgo biloba, alpha lipoic acid, B-complex, green tea, and melatonin can be ordered by calling 1-800-544-4440. Call for a list of physicians in your area who are knowledgeable in the administration of chelation therapy.

Hepatitis B

Hepatitis B is a viral disease characterized by inflammatory necrosis of the liver. The symptoms of hepatitis include anorexia, malaise, flu-like conditions, nausea, vomiting, fever, hives, joint pain, dark urine and a distaste for tobacco. Jaundice often appears if the disease is well advanced. Liver function blood testing and a specific test for hepatitis B can determine if hepatitis B is active and causing liver damage. The blood tests that monitor viral hepatitis liver damage include AST (SGOT), ALT (SGPT), alkaline phosphatase, and GGTP. The hepatitis B antibody test together with the hepatitis surface antigen (HBsAg) test can provide a definitive diagnosis. The presence of HBsAg refers to the viral surface coat.

Hepatitis B is most often spread by contact with contaminated blood via the sharing of unsterilized needles or sexual contact. Treatment by an infectious disease specialist is essential. One-third of all people infected by this virus can expect total remission after two to four months of treatment with alpha-interferon. Of the remaining two-thirds, 10% to 15% will become lifelong carriers of the disease. It is this group that is at greatest risk of hepatocellular carcinoma. Cirrhosis is also a great risk, and many of these patients will find themselves future candidates for liver transplants.

In Europe, isoprinosine, a powerful immune-stimulating drug, which is unapproved in the U.S., has been found to be effective in treating hepatitis B. Also in Europe, the herb silybum marianum (milk thistle) has been given German Commission E status as a supportive agent in the treatment of inflammatory liver diseases (hepatitis and cirrhosis). In Japan, glycyrrhiza glabra (licorice root) has found widespread use in the treatment of hepatitis B. This herb has the ability to decrease serum liver enzymes, aspartate aminotransferase (AST) and alanine aminotransferase (ALT).

The Life Extension Foundation's protocol for hepatitis B includes:

1) The standard dose of alpha-interferon (3 million IU injected subcutaneously, three times a week) for four months, prescribed by your infectious disease physician. (Interferon is FDA-approved therapy to treat hepatitis B. It works only in one-third of patients.)

2) Isoprinosine at a dose of 2,000 to 3,000 mg per day for two months on and two months off (continue for two rounds).

3) Milk thistle extract, 150 mg, three times per day. Licorice root extract 500 mg three times a day. Green tea extract, 10 capsules in three divided doses, to reduce serum iron levels that may facilitate liver injury.

4) The standard doses of Life Extension Mix and Life Extension Herbal Mix to further reduce free radical damage, along with 2,000 mg per day of garlic and 5,000 to 20,000 mg of vitamin C. Please note that some hepatitis patients cannot tolerate beta-carotene. If liver enzyme levels increase in response to Life Extension Mix, discontinue it and take most of the nutrients

separately, avoiding vitamin A, beta-carotene and niacin. Beta-carotene has potent immune-boosting properties that can be beneficial for hepatitis B patients, but it may not be tolerated by some people.

5) Reduce serum and liver iron levels to a minimum. Green tea, garlic and chelation therapy may facilitate this. Iron promotes hepatitis virus-induced liver injury and precludes successful treatment with interferon. Verify that liver iron levels have been reduced before commencing interferon therapy.

Please refer to the Hepatitis C protocol for additional suggestions.

Product availability: Milk thistle extract, green tea extract, Life Extension Mix, Life Extension Herbal Mix, Kyolic garlic, vitamin C, licorice can be ordered singly or in a Protocol Pak by phoning 1-800-544-4440. Call for a list of offshore companies that sell isoprinosine to Americans by mail for personal use. Interferon is a drug that should be prescribed by a knowledgeable physician.

Hepatitis C

Infection with the hepatitis C virus occurs from blood transfusions, needle sharing, working in a medical environment, and sexual contact. Often, the infected individual does not know how he/she acquired this potentially lethal virus that has a high affinity for liver cells.

Hepatitis C used to be called non-A/non-B hepatitis and was not considered a significant health risk. There is now more research being conducted on hepatitis C than any other cause of liver disease. New data indicates that those infected with the hepatitis C virus are likely to develop hepatocellular carcinoma, a primary cancer of the liver with a very low cure rate. If the hepatitis C victim does not develop liver cancer, there is still a great risk that he/she will develop cirrhosis of the liver, which may require a transplant. There also are other, non-liver diseases associated with hepatitis C viral infection.

The hepatitis C virus does most of its damage by latching on to molecules of iron and then delivering massive free radical damage to liver cells. These free radicals can mutate DNA to cause hepatocellular carcinoma, and can kill large numbers of liver cells, causing havoc throughout the body. Successful eradication of the hepatitis C virus from the body requires that iron levels in the liver and blood be at very low levels. High stores of iron in the liver precludes successful therapy against the hepatitis C virus.

The blood test that can identify the hepatitis C virus and measure overall viral load is the polymerase chain reaction test (PCR). Standard tests to measure hepatitis C activity include the liver function tests SGOT, SGPT, GGTP, and alkaline phosphatase. Hepatitis C antibody tests can accurately diagnose hepatitis C infection, but are not always precise in evaluating the success of treatments.

The Life Extension Foundation's protocol for hepatitis C includes:

1) The standard dose of interferon is 3 million IU injected subcutaneously three

times a week for six months, prescribed by an infectious disease physician. Interferon is the FDA-approved therapy for treatment of hepatitis C. It only works in a minority of patients.

2) About 1,000 mg a day of ribavirin (taken in three doses) for six months. Ribavirin is an unapproved drug that increases the effectiveness of interferon therapy.

3) About 10 capsules of decaffeinated green tea extract capsules in three daily doses for a total of 1,000 mg a day of polyphenols. Green tea reduces serum iron levels.

4) The standard doses of Life Extension Mix and Life Extension Herbal Mix. Please note that some hepatitis C patients encounter liver enzyme elevations in response to the moderate doses of vitamin A, niacin and beta-carotene in Life Extension Mix. If your liver enzyme levels elevate after starting Life Extension Mix, then discontinue it and take most of the nutrients contained in Life Extension Mix separately. Beta-carotene possesses unique immune enhancing benefits that could help suppress the hepatitis C virus.

5) Reduce serum and liver iron levels to a minimum. Green tea, garlic and chelation therapy may facilitate this. Iron promotes hepatitis virus induced liver injury and precludes successful treatment with interferon. Verify that liver iron levels have been reduced before starting interferon therapy.

6) Other liver protecting nutrients and immune boosting therapies may be contemplated, including milk thistle extract, 150 mg three times a day, 500 mg of licorice extract three times a day, 2,000 mg a day of garlic, and vitamin C ranging from 5,000 to 20,000 mg a day.

Product availability: Green tea, licorice, silymarin, garlic, vitamin C, beta-carotene, Life Extension Mix and Life Extension Herbal Mix can be ordered by phoning 1-800-544-4440. Call for a list of offshore mail order companies that supply medications like ribavirin to Americans for personal use.

HIV Infection (AIDS)
(Opportunistic Infections)

Free radicals have been linked to much of the immune system destruction caused by the HIV (human immunodeficiency virus). Recent studies show that the HIV virus depletes cellular glutathione levels and is associated with free radical injury to critical immune system components. Scientific evidence shows that antioxidants can protect immune function, and that certain nutrients may prevent or slow the progression of HIV infection.

A major controversy has developed in the scientific community as to whether the HIV virus is the only agent responsible for the decline in immune function clinically defined as acquired immune deficiency syndrome (AIDS). In 1985, the Life Extension Foundation first proposed that the decline in immune function in HIV-positive individuals might be prevented or slowed by taking high-potency nutrient supplements. Since 1985, several hundred medical papers have provided evidence that the basic mechanisms involved in HIV-related immune system destruction are associated with deficiencies in vitamins, minerals and amino acids. Another conclusion that emerges from the scientific literature is that some people with healthy immune systems who are positive for the HIV virus may never develop immune suppression or AIDS. They remain perfectly healthy in spite of having antibodies to the HIV virus.

Antibody production occurs when the immune system is exposed to a foreign body such as a virus. Having HIV antibodies shows you have been infected by the HIV virus, but does not necessarily mean that you will develop AIDS. What this tells us is that most people should be on a nutrient-supplement program, not only to protect against AIDS but also to protect against cancer, the common cold, influenza, auto-immune diseases, hepatitis B and C, and other diseases.

The Foundation's HIV Treatment Protocol is comprised of the following three elements:

1) Nutritional immune support
2) Hormonal immune system support
3) European immune-boosting therapies

A critical part of our protocol is monthly blood monitoring to assess the effectiveness of whatever HIV treatment choice(s) you make. Since many FDA approved anti-viral drugs are toxic, regular blood tests can warn you against life-threatening organ damage by indicating toxicity before symptoms appear.

Among the nutrients that HIV patients should consider taking is the amino acid n-acetyl-cysteine (NAC). Much of the immunologic decline caused by the HIV virus involves depletion of cellular glutathione levels, resulting in massive free radical damage to immune system cells throughout the body. An effective way of boosting cellular glutathione levels is to take n-acetyl-cysteine. The suggested dose of NAC for those who are HIV positive is 600 mg three times a day. Two to 3 grams of vitamin C should be taken with each 600 mg dose of NAC.

For AIDS patients with severe liver impairment, NAC could become toxic if ingested over an extended period of time. We suggest that this small sub-group switch to 500 mg a day of pure glutathione instead of NAC.

Another glutathione precursor is the trace mineral selenium, which also counteracts potentially damaging free radicals and may inhibit chemicals that the HIV virus requires for reproduction. The minimum dose of selenium is 300 mcg daily, but HIV patients should consider taking 600 to 1,000 mcg daily. There are many inexpensive selenium supplements on the market, but none are better than Super Selenium Complex, which includes three forms of elemental selenium to provide different health benefits to the body.

A nutrient that is often overlooked by those who are HIV positive is the amino acid arginine, which enhances immune function via several different mechanisms, including stimulation of growth hormone secretion. Arginine has been shown to be an effective way of preventing AIDS-related wasting syndrome. The suggested dose for HIV patients is 6 to 15 grams of arginine a day on an empty stomach, preferably at bedtime.

Arginine is available as a powder, but the most convenient way of taking it is as arginine caplets. Each caplet contains 1,200 mg of arginine, which enables a person to consume high doses of the amino acid, without having to swallow a large number of capsules.

Another amino acid often overlooked by HIV-positive individuals is L-carnitine, which has been shown to boost immune function via several different mechanisms, to protect the heart against AZT-induced toxicity, and to enhance essential fatty acid and glucose uptake. High doses of L-carnitine have enhanced immunologic and metabolic functions in HIV patients who were deficient in L-carnitine. The suggested dose of L-carnitine for HIV patients is 2,400 mg a day in two divided doses on an empty stomach.

A popular supplement used by HIV-positive patients is coenzyme Q10. Studies indicate that coenzyme Q10 boosts immune function. In a pilot study in AIDS patients, coenzyme Q10 provided significant benefits to these patients. Coenzyme Q10 has been shown to be deficient in HIV-infected people. We suggest that HIV patients take at least 200 mg a day of coenzyme Q10.

Studies indicate that AIDS patients suffer from severe malabsorption of vitamin B12 and have a severe B12 deficiency. AIDS-related dementia has been reversed by the administration of vitamin B12. Some forms of AIDS dementia could be caused by a simple vitamin B12 deficiency. Vitamin B12 is not absorbed well when taken orally. We suggest that those who are HIV positive take B12 tablets that dissolve under the tongue. Three 500 mcg sublingual B12 tablets a day are suggested. If a blood test reveals a continuing B12 deficiency, weekly B12 injections should be considered.

In a study in the January-April 1995 issue of the *Yale Journal of Biology and Medicine*, AIDS patients were given 100,000 IU of beta-carotene a day. After four weeks of beta-carotene treatment, total lymphocyte counts rose by 66% and T-helper cells rose slightly. Six weeks after beta-carotene treatment, the immune cell measurements returned to pretreatment levels. While this study demonstrated no toxicity associated with high dose beta-carotene supplementation, the Life Extension Foundation recommends against high dose beta-carotene in AIDS patients who also have hepatitis. For some people with hepatitis, long-term use of beta-carotene could cause liver enzyme elevation, indicating potential liver damage. Many people infected with HIV also have been infected with hepatitis B or C. HIV/AIDS patients who do not have hepatitis or other liver damage should consider taking 25,000-to 100,000 IU a day of beta-carotene. Healthy people seeking to boost overall immune function should consider 25,000 IU a day of beta-carotene along with other complimentary antioxidants.

There are many other nutrients that appear to benefit those infected with HIV. Life Extension Mix contains potent doses of 52 different disease-preventing nutrients that can be taken in a convenient, economical form. HIV infected people should take three tablets of Life Extension Mix three times a day.

The immune-enhancing properties of certain herbal extracts are gaining considerable attention in the scientific literature. Herbal extracts are expensive because large quantities of bulk herbs have to be used to produce a relatively small amount of pharmaceutical herbal extract. In order to make the daily intake of disease-fighting herbs affordable, a powdered Life Extension Herbal Mix was designed, incorporating 27 different herbs into one drink mix. The suggested daily dose is one to two tablespoons taken first thing in the morning. Some of the herbal extracts contained in Life Extension Herbal Mix may produce anti-viral activity in addition to immune-boosting properties.

Hormones synchronize immune function. An immune system that is not precisely synchronized will not function optimally. The Foundation's HIV Treatment Protocol works best in HIV positive individuals with 500+ T-helper cells counts. HIV causes immune system destruction and desynchronization. Hormone-replacement therapies can protect and restore immune functions. Preliminary evidence suggests that HIV infection can be slowed by the nightly intake of melatonin.

Researchers now believe that the AIDS virus replicates at a furious pace from the time of infection, creating as many as 2 billion new viruses a day. The reason there appears to be such a long incubation period between the time of infection and the development of AIDS symptoms is because the immune system is creating new anti-viral cells as quickly as the AIDS virus replicates. At some point, however, the AIDS virus overwhelms the ability of the immune system to produce anti-viral cells and the patient succumbs to immune suppression, eventual immune system destruction and, finally, death.

The knowledge that the immune system responds aggressively to fight the AIDS virus means that therapies that enhance the immune system could be effective AIDS therapies. Melatonin enhances the production of T-helper cells, the very cells lost to HIV infection. Melatonin also enhances the production of other immune system components known to be affected by HIV infection, including natural killer cells (NK), interleukin-2, -4, and -10, gamma interferon, eosinophils, and red blood cells. In addition to enhancing the production of cells being killed by the AIDS virus, melatonin may also prevent HIV cellular destruction via its action as an antioxidant.

The latest evidence suggests that melatonin is even more effective than nutrient antioxidants in suppressing immune cell-killing free radicals generated by the HIV virus. One study, conducted by Dr. Russel Reiter of the University of Texas in Austin, indicated that melatonin may have a direct effect on HIV replication. For HIV to replicate, it needs a substance called nuclear factor kappa-B (NKF). Since the amount of NKF is reduced by 23% at night, Dr. Reiter sought to determine whether melatonin is responsible for the nightly decline in NKF. When Dr. Reiter injected rats with melatonin during the day, he observed a reduction of NKF binding activity of 43%. This finding suggests that melatonin may interfere in the division of HIV viruses by cutting off their supply of NKF.

Dr. George Maestroni, a pioneer in melatonin immunotherapy, conducted a pilot AIDS study in Italy where 11 HIV-infected people were given 20 mg of melatonin every night. After a month of treatment, the patients had a 35% increase in T-helper cells, a 57% increase in natural killer cells, and a 76% increase in lymphocyte production!

In spite of these remarkable findings, this line of research has not been pursued because melatonin is not a patentable drug that can generate billions of dollars of profits for the pharmaceutical giants.

Melatonin appears to benefit AIDS patients in many other ways, including protection against AZT toxicity and the wasting syndrome. We suggest that HIV patients obtain the book "Melatonin," by Dr. Russel Reiter and Jo Robinson. This book contains newly discovered findings about AIDS and melatonin.

The suggested dose of melatonin for HIV patients ranges from three to 30 mg nightly.

Studies have shown that HIV infection progresses only when serum levels of the hormone DHEA begin to decline. The speculation from these studies is that maintaining healthy blood levels of DHEA might prevent HIV infection from progressing to full blown AIDS. DHEA is now used widely by HIV patients. Its beneficial action may not be due to any direct anti-viral effect, but rather to DHEA's ability to protect immune functions against a wide array of insults.

The Life Extension Foundation recommends that all HIV infected patients and most people over 40 have their blood levels of DHEA tested, and then take DHEA supplements to restore their serum DHEA levels to that of a healthy 21-year-old. An appropriate dosage for men is 25 mg, three times a day. For those with liver disease, DHEA capsules should be opened and held under the tongue for 10 to 20 minutes and then swallowed. DHEA can possibly contribute to liver damage in people with hepatitis or cirrhosis. Before starting DHEA replacement therapy, refer to our DHEA Precautions.

For those who can afford it, growth hormone therapy could be very beneficial for HIV-infected and AIDS patients. Growth hormone boosts immune function, is a protease inhibitor, and promotes anabolic cell renewal and muscle building.

T-cells are produced and mature in response to hormones secreted by the thymus gland. Aging causes shrinkage of the thymus gland. The resulting reduction in the production of thymic hormones is a major cause of the progressive age-related decline in immune function. HIV infection adversely affects hormone secretion from the thymus gland.

As noted in an earlier protocol, Thymic Protein A has been shown in laboratory and animal experiments to cause the T-4 lymphocyte to mature, thereby initiating a specific cell-mediated immune response. This specific protein has been shown to be a stimulant in animal models for the production of interleukin-2. Interleukin-2 production by T-4 cells is the benchmark measurement for T-cell maturity and initiation of immune response.

The following is worth repeating verbatim:

A trial with 22 cats infected with feline immunodeficiency virus (FIV) concluded that this protein enhances immune response to infectious agents measured serologically, diminishes disease symptoms, lengthens survival and increases lymphocyte values.

A daily dose of four micrograms of this material may make a major difference in longevity by strengthening the immune system through its T-cell "programming" role. The more T-cells that are properly functioning, the more immune response may be mounted against metastasized cancer cells.

Initial reports from those undergoing chemotherapy indicate that Thymic Protein A has maintained their total white blood count at acceptable levels during the therapy. It is well-known among oncologists that chemotherapy and radiation will often induce a serious drop in white blood count to dangerous levels, which may dictate cessation of therapy. Healthy people can take one packet every day or every other day. Those with disease whose treatment is dependent on a strong immune system may need three packets a day for several months.

Thymex provides extracts of fresh, healthy tissue from the thymus and other glands that produce the disease-fighting cells of our immune system.

The primary ingredient in Thymex is immunologic tissue from the thymus gland. Also included in Thymex is tissue from the lymph nodes and spleen which produce the white blood cells that engage in life-or-death combat with invading organisms in our bloodstream under the "instruction" of the thymus gland.

Thymex is a synergistic formula that contains herbal activators and a full complement of natural homeopathic nutrients, in addition to fresh, healthy thymus, lymph and spleen tissues. Thymex is a professional formula normally dispensed through doctor's offices. Thymex has been extensively used to amplify the immune potentiating effect of DHEA replacement therapy. According to a physician most familiar with DHEA, thymus extract is required to obtain the immune system boosting benefit of DHEA.

Another therapy to boost thymus gland activity is isoprinosine. Isoprinosine is approved by almost every regulatory agency in the world except the U.S. Food and Drug Administration (FDA) In 1990, *The New England Journal Of Medicine* published findings that Isoprinosine slows the progression of HIV infection! This report is one of hundreds of studies showing that isoprinosine boosts immune function in cancer patients, HIV patients, and healthy people.

In 1985, the Life Extension Foundation recommends that HIV-infected people take isoprinosine to slow the decline in immune function that leads to full blown AIDS. Isoprinosine and other immune-boosting drugs work best when taken on an alternative dosing schedule, two months on, and two months off.

Here is an immune boosting program for healthy and immune-compromised patients to consider:

Isoprinosine Therapy — 2,000 to 3,000 mg daily for two months. Repeat every other two months.

After completing isoprinosine therapy, we suggest a two month regimen of:

Thymus Therapy — four Thymex capsules a day for two months, or one to three paks a day of Thymic Protein A. Thymus therapy can be used when isoprinosine is not used.

Once a year dosing of:

Biostim Therapy — Three month dosing schedule as follows: 2 tablets daily for eight days, then stop for three weeks; 1 tablet daily for eight days, then stop for three weeks; 1 tablet daily for eight days, then stop for nine months.

Proper levels of thyroid hormones are crucial for optimal immune function. Blood tests do not always accurately detect a thyroid hormone deficiency. One method of determining if you are thyroid deficient is to take your body temperature about 30 minutes before lunch. If your temperature is consistently below normal, you may want to take a thyroid hormone supplement. The TSH test (thyroid stimulating hormone) is extremely sensitive to both hypo- and hyper-thyroid conditions, often showing subclinical disorders.

Popular prescription thyroid replacement drugs are Synthroid (synthetic thyroid hormone), Armour, Forest Pharmaceuticals (natural thyroid hormone), and Cytomel (T3 thyroid fraction). You must be careful not to overdose on thyroid hormone, so the advice of a knowledgeable physician is important when considering thyroid hormone supplementation or replacement.

HIV infection causes excessive cortisol production from the adrenal glands that can decimate immune function. It is thus crucial to suppress excessive cortisol production. There are 17 European studies showing that HIV causes some of its destruction of the immune system by stimulating excessive cortisol production.

DHEA and melatonin may suppress cortisol levels. Two tablets of the European procaine drug, KH3, taken twice a day on an empty stomach, is suggested as the best way of suppressing elevated cortisol levels in cancer and AIDS patients. One or two tablets of KH3 can be taken first thing in the morning on an empty stomach, and then one or two KH3 tablets again an hour before dinner.

It is difficult to test cortisol levels in the blood because adrenal surges of cortisol can occur erratically throughout the day. That's one reason why this important cause of immune system destruction has been largely ignored by American doctors. However, a resting morning level of cortisol, taken before 9 a.m., may be quite significant in determining overall cortisol status in the body.

The FDA has approved four cytotoxic anti-viral drugs to slow the progression of HIV infection. These drugs are AZT, ddI, ddC, and 3TC. There are additional cytotoxic anti-viral drugs that will soon be approved. There is enthusiasm in some parts of the AIDS community that various combinations of these anti-viral drugs could enable those with HIV infection and clinically diagnosed AIDS to maintain long-term remissions.

Recent studies show that various combinations of these anti viral drugs are working better than AZT alone. Two studies indicate that a combination of AZT and 3TC, along with one of the new relatively non-toxic protease inhibitors may be the ideal combination to try first in AIDS patients.

In several studies published in 1994, AZT was compared to a placebo with no difference in overall survival rates. In some cases, AZT caused an *increase* in mortality. Recognizing that AZT monotherapy is clearly *not* the solution to AIDS, some of the AIDS support groups are suggesting that aggressive combinations of almost every anti-viral drug available be tried in AIDS patients. These combination therapies can, in the short-term, produce a significant reduction in the PCR (viral load testing) and even an increase in CD4 (T-helper cells). Regular blood tests would be needed to monitor the toxicity of these anti-viral drugs to determine when to switch from one toxic combination to another.

Our concern is that, if combination anti-viral therapy produces irreversible damage to the immune system, there could very well be no increase in survival, even though the therapy might kill a large number of HIV viruses and infected immune cells. It is interesting to note that, in two recent studies documenting that combination anti-viral drug therapy is better than AZT monotherapy, those who had never taken an anti-viral drug had higher survival rates than those who had previously taken AZT. One reason for the better effect on these "anti-viral virgins" was that not as much drug resistance to anti-viral drugs had developed in them. The use of AZT results in the development of drug-resistant strains of HIV within one to two years.

Another reason the "anti-viral virgins" did better is that their immune systems may not have been previously damaged by toxic drugs such as AZT and ddI. Since HIV is a slow progressing disease, and since blood tests enable you to monitor the efficacy of the Foundation's protocol, most HIV patients should consider following our non-toxic protocol first before resorting to anti-viral drug therapy.

Product availability: n-acetyl-cysteine, arginine, coenzyme Q10, Life Extension Mix, Life Extension Herbal Mix, melatonin, selenium, carnitine, vitamin B12, beta carotene, DHEA, Thymic Protein A and Thymex are available by calling 1-800-544-4440. For access to drugs like isoprinosine and Biostim, ask for a list of offshore suppliers who will mail-order these products to Americans for personal use. Growth hormone therapy is available from a few doctors in the U.S. and abroad. Call for a list of doctors who offer this therapy.

Hypertension
(High Blood Pressure)

There are many nutrients that may reduce or eliminate the need for anti-hypertensive medications. Nutrients do not work immediately to lower blood pressure the way drugs do, so it is important to carry through nutritional blood pressure-lowering therapy over a period of four to 12 weeks. Physician cooperation is crucial if you are to reduce your intake of blood pressure-lowering drugs safely. Regular blood pressure monitoring is mandatory in order to determine if the nutritional regimen you are following is controlling your blood pressure.

The two nutrients best documented to control hypertension are garlic and coenzyme Q10. The amount of standardized garlic extract needed to lower blood pressure is between 1,500 and 3,000 mg a day. The amount of coenzyme Q10 needed to lower blood pressure is between 200 and 300 mg a day. The coenzyme Q10 should be taken in a liquid oil capsule for optimal assimilation. After following this garlic/coenzyme Q10 regimen for four weeks, consult your physician about reducing the dosage of your anti-hypertensive medication. The objective is to be able to slowly reduce your intake of drugs as the natural anti-hypertensive effective of garlic/coenzyme Q10 begins to take effect. It is crucial to monitor your blood pressure closely, since the garlic/coenzyme Q10 combination does not work for everyone.

Some people have high blood pressure because they are deficient in certain minerals that keep blood pressure in balance. Anyone with elevated blood pressure should be taking between 500 and 2,000 mg of elemental magnesium a day. About 80% of Americans are magnesium deficient, and low levels of magnesium are associated with hypertension and arterial disease.

Even if magnesium fails to lower your blood pressure, it can reduce the risk of complications such as stroke. Among the most popular types of anti-hypertensive drugs are calcium channel blockers. These drugs are sold under trade names such as Norvasc and Procardia. Magnesium is nature's calcium-channel blocker. It inhibits excessive calcium infiltration into cells. Magnesium is safe to take, with the only adverse side effect being diarrhea when too much is taken.

In addition to magnesium, those with high blood pressure should consider taking 500 mg of potassium. A potassium deficiency can cause high blood pressure in some people. Unlike magnesium, which is very safe, too much potassium can be lethal. A blood test can reveal if you need additional potassium.

Supplemental calcium may help some women lower their high blood pressure. Before attempting to use magnesium and potassium to treat hypertension, please pay attention to the caution at the end of this protocol.

High doses of fish oil concentrates have lowered blood pressure in some people. It requires eight to 10 capsules of Mega-EPA capsules of fish oil to duplicate those studies. There are cardiovascular and other health benefits associated with taking fish oil, so if your GI tract can tolerate such a high daily dose of fish oils, then you may lower your blood pressure and gain other benefits.

Some other blood pressure-lowering nutrients include vitamin C in doses of 3,000 to 10,000 mg and the amino acid arginine in doses of 5,000 mg one to three times a day. Arginine can work synergistically with ACE-inhibiting anti-hypertensive drugs such as Vasotec and Capoten. This is important for those with chronic hypertension who fail to respond to conventional or alternative therapies.

An herbal extract that may reduce blood pressure is forskolin. Between 1981 and 1994, forskolin was tested in more than 5,000 *in vitro* studies to assess its cell regulating effects. Forskolin showed a wide range of cardiovascular benefits. It appears to lower blood pressure, improve arterial blood flow, strengthen heart contractions, and relieve angina (heart) pain.

Studies show that forskolin relaxes arteries. High blood pressure is often associated with a reduction in arterial elasticity. Forskolin has a vasodilating effect on arteries that is thought to be the mechanism by which it lowers blood pressure.

If you'd like to see if forskolin replaces your anti-hypertensive drugs, extreme caution is mandatory and physician cooperation essential. You should reduce the dosage of your anti-hypertensive drug very slowly while increasing your intake of forskolin. Monitor your blood pressure on a daily basis. If you do not exercise caution, an acute hypertensive event could occur, resulting in a stroke.

CAUTION: Do not use forskolin if you have prostate cancer.

Our general precaution is that, if you're going to attempt to use any of the nutrients the Foundation recommends to replace anti-hypertensive drugs, you must do so with the cooperation of your physician. You cannot assume that any nutrients will be able to replace a drug that is effectively controlling your blood pressure. Daily blood pressure monitoring is mandatory to insure that the nutrient regimen you are following is really keeping your blood pressure under control.

If nutrients fail to keep your blood pressure under control, our favorite class of anti-hypertensive drugs are the ACE inhibitors. ACE stands for angiotensin-converting-enzyme, which causes hypertension by constricting the arterial system. By blocking the angiotensin-converting enzyme, which is what ACE inhibitors do, the arterial system can be returned to a more youthful state of elasticity. Popular ACE Inhibiting drugs are Capoten and Vasotec. Nutrients such as arginine and forskolin also inhibit arterial constriction by improving arterial elasticity.

Those with hypertension often have artery disease. See the Atherosclerosis protocol for additional suggestions.

Product availability: Forskolin, coenzyme Q10, Mega-EPA, garlic, vitamin C, Life Extension

Mix, garlic, potassium, calcium, magnesium, and arginine are available by calling 1-800-544-4440. Capoten and Vasotec are prescription drugs that should be prescribed by a physician knowledgeable in treating hypertension.

Hypoglycemia

Low blood sugar caused by excessive release of insulin from the pancreas can cause fatigue, weakness, loss of consciousness, even death. In hypoglycemia attacks, there is too much insulin and not enough blood sugar. Insulin can be partially neutralized by taking the amino acid cysteine along with vitamin B1 and vitamin C.

Hypoglycemics should start out with doses of 500 mg of cysteine along with 250 mg of vitamin B1 and 1,500 mg of vitamin C, once a day. The second week, this dose should be administered twice a day and, by the third week, three times a day. The objective is to prevent hypoglycemic attacks by neutralizing excess insulin. Every hypoglycemic is slightly different, so the dosage ranges will vary from person to person.

Another possible cause of low blood sugar is the inability to release glycogen (stored sugar in the liver) secondary to vitamin B6 and chromium deficiency. Some hypoglycemics are helped by the administration of 100 to 250 mg of the vitamin B6 metabolite pyridoxal 5-phosphate and 200 mcg of chromium daily.

Product availability: The amino acid cysteine, vitamin B1, vitamin B6, vitamin C caps, pyridoxal 5-phosphate, and chromium picolinate are available by calling 1-800-544-4440.

Immune Enhancement

Free radicals have been linked to immune system damage caused by normal aging. A strong immune system is critical to the prevention of infection by viruses, fungi, and bacteria. Cancer cells are thought to form regularly, and a vigilant immune response is required to kill or inactivate these transformed cells before they become malignant tumors. Members of the Life Extension Foundation have long been encouraged to follow a daily antioxidant regimen that protects against immune-suppressing free radicals.

The incidence of cancer and new infectious diseases has been increasing every year in the U.S. Many dangerous bacteria have become resistant to antibiotics that once kept them in check, and they are now a threat to our lives. Scientific evidence shows that antioxidants can protect and enhance immune function.

The cornerstone of any program to boost immune function involves making sure that you are consuming every nutrient that has a role in maintaining a healthy immune system. The most convenient way of obtaining most of the nutrients needed for healthy immune function is to take three tablets, three times a day of the 52-ingredient Life Extension Mix. In addition, one capsule a day of Life Extension Booster provides added amounts of nutrients that protect immune system cells against damaging free radicals.

A powdered Life Extension Herbal Mix incorporates 27 different herbs into one daily drink. The suggested daily dose is one tablespoon, taken first thing in the morning.

Some other nutrients that have a positive effect on immune function include L-carnitine in doses of 1,800 to 2,400 mg a day, and coenzyme Q10 in doses of 100 mg to 300 mg a day.

The Foundation's Immune Enhancement protocol is designed to enhance immune function in people who are aging, are receiving cancer chemotherapy, or who have chronic viral or bacterial infections.

Aging, cancer chemotherapy and certain viruses and bacteria all cause immune system destruction and desynchronization. The most effective hormone therapy to protect and improve immune function is melatonin, which enhances the production of T-helper cells, which are necessary to identify cancer cells, viruses, fungi, and bacteria.

Melatonin also enhances the production of other immune components including natural killer cells, interleukin-2, interleukin-4 and interleukin-10, gamma interferon and eosinophils. The latest evidence suggests that melatonin is even more effective than nutrient antioxidants in suppressing immune cell-killing free radicals.

Studies have documented that DHEA has a beneficial role in maintaining healthy immune function. The Life Extension Foundation recommends that most people over 40 have their blood levels of DHEA tested, and then take supplemental DHEA accordingly to restore their serum DHEA levels to that of a healthy 21-year-old. This usually can be accomplished by taking 25 mg of DHEA, three times a day for men, and 15 mg three times a day for women.

T-cells mature in response to hormones secreted by the thymus gland. Aging causes a shrinkage of the thymus, and the resulting reduction in the production of thymic hormones is a major cause of the progressive decline in immune function that occurs with aging. By taking two to four capsules a day of the glandular extract formula Thymex, you can replace some of the thymic hormones lost to aging.

As noted in an earlier protocol, Thymic Protein A has been shown in laboratory and animal experiments to cause the T-4 lymphocyte to mature, thereby initiating a specific cell-mediated immune response. Because of its importance, and the fact that readers interested only in specific protocols might not have read this material previously, it is worth repeating here verbatim:

> Thymic Protein A has been shown to be a stimulant in animal models for the production of interleukin-2. Interleukin-2 production by T-4 cells is the benchmark measurement for T-cell maturity and initiation of immune response.
>
> A daily dose of four micrograms of this material may make a major difference in longevity by strengthening the immune system through its T-cell "programming" role. The more T-cells that are properly functioning, the more immune response may be mounted against metastasized cancer cells.

Initial reports from those undergoing chemotherapy indicate that Thymic Protein A has maintained their total white blood count at acceptable levels during the therapy. It is well-known among oncologists that chemotherapy and radiation will often induce a serious drop in white blood count to dangerous levels, which may dictate cessation of therapy. Healthy people can take one packet every day or every other day. Those with disease whose treatment is dependent on a strong immune system may need three packets a day for several months.

A less-expensive thymic enhancing product is Thymex. Thymex provides extracts of fresh, healthy tissue from the thymus and other glands that produce the disease-fighting cells of our immune system.

The primary ingredient in Thymex is immunologic tissue from the thymus gland. Also included in Thymex is tissue from the lymph nodes and spleen which produce the white blood cells that engage in life-or-death combat with invading organisms in our bloodstream under the "instruction" of the thymus gland.

Thymex is a synergistic formula that contains herbal activators and a full complement of natural homeopathic nutrients, in addition to fresh, healthy thymus, lymph and spleen tissues. Thymex is a professional formula normally dispensed through doctor's offices. Thymex has been extensively used to amplify the immune potentiating effect of DHEA replacement therapy. According to a physician most familiar with DHEA, thymus extract is required to obtain the immune system boosting benefit of DHEA.

Aging, cancer and AIDS often generate sub-optimal levels of thyroid hormone production. Proper levels of thyroid hormones are crucial for optimal immune function. Blood tests do not always detect a thyroid hormone deficiency. However, a TSH (thyroid stimulating hormone) test is recommended.

If your temperature 30 minutes before eating is consistently below normal, you may want to start taking a thyroid hormone supplement, directed by your physician.

Popular prescription thyroid replacement drugs are Synthroid (synthetic thyroid hormone, T4) and Cytomel (T3 thyroid hormone).

You must be careful not to overdose on thyroid hormones, so the advice of a knowledgeable physician is important when considering thyroid hormone therapy. Soy protein extract can boost thyroid output and eliminate the need for thyroid hormone replacement.

Aging, cancer and AIDS can stimulate excessive cortisol production from the adrenal glands, which decimates immune function. It is thus crucial to inhibit excessive cortisol production.

As has been noted in the HIV Infection (AIDS) Protocol, there are 17 European studies showing that HIV causes the destruction of the immune system by stimulating excessive cortisol production.

DHEA and melatonin may suppress cortisol levels. High doses of the European procaine drug KH3, taken at least twice a day, is suggested as the best way of suppressing elevated cortisol levels in cancer, AIDS, and stressed-out patients. One to two tablets of KH3 can be taken first thing in the morning on an empty stomach, and then one to two KH3 tablets can be taken again one hour before dinner on an empty stomach. It is difficult to test cortisol levels in the blood because adrenal surges of cortisol can occur erratically throughout the day. That's one reason why this important cause of immune system destruction has been largely ignored by American doctors.

Here is an immune-boosting regimen for immune-compromised patients:

- **Thymic Protein A:** One to two 4-microgram packets under the tongue.
- **Biostim therapy:** Three month dosing schedule as follows: 2 tablets daily for eight days, stop for three weeks; 1 tablet daily for eight days, stop for three weeks; 1 tablet daily for eight days, stop for nine months. Repeat Biostim therapy once a year.

Product availability: Life Extension Mix, Life Extension Booster, Thymex, coenzyme Q10, carnitine, melatonin, Soy Power, and DHEA are available by phoning 1-800-544-4440. Ask for a listing of offshore companies that sell Biostim and KH3.

Insomnia

Insomnia can be caused by a wide variety of factors, but for people over age 35 or 40, the most common cause of insomnia is deficiency of the pineal gland hormone melatonin. Melatonin is the hormone released by the pineal gland to induce drowsiness and to enable the body to enter the deep sleep patterns characteristic of youth.

Young people gradually release melatonin from their pineal gland in response to darkness in order to induce drowsiness. Young pineal glands then continue to secrete melatonin slowly for about five hours to enable the body to enter the various stages of deep sleep that enables them to feel revitalized and rejuvenated the next morning. The continuous secretion of melatonin throughout the night causes young people to stay asleep, thereby feeling completely refreshed when they wake up in the morning.

Melatonin has been shown in many scientific studies to be the safest and most effective sleep-enhancing therapy in the world. While most people find that taking one 3 mg capsule of melatonin before bedtime helps to solve their sleep problems, some people still wake up too frequently during the night and/or too early in the morning, even after taking melatonin.

In order to duplicate the mechanisms by which the young pineal gland induces youthful sleep patterns, a formula called Natural Sleep has been developed. This formula contains two different melatonin delivery systems that work together to generate the same kind of secretion of melatonin that occurs naturally in young people. Here is how Natural Sleep works. First, the Natural Sleep capsule bursts open in the stomach within five minutes after swallowing it to provide immediate-release melatonin to induce the drowsiness needed to get to sleep. Then Natural Sleep gradually introduces tiny beadlets of sustained-release melatonin into your digestive tract.

The sustained-release beadlets enable people to stay asleep to avoid the nocturnal tossing and turning characteristic of age-related sleep disturbances. Only pharmaceutical-grade melatonin is used in Natural Sleep. This is the identical form of melatonin used in the published studies documenting melatonin's insomnia-relieving properties.

Each capsule of Natural Sleep contains 2.5 mg of immediate-release melatonin plus 2.5 mg of sustained release melatonin for an average daily dose of 5 mg of melatonin. This is the average dose most people find effective to enable them to enjoy a complete night's rest every night.

Natural Sleep also contains pyridoxal-5-phosphate, an expensive, non-stimulating form of vitamin B6 that helps to convert the dietary amino acid tryptophan into serotonin, another brain chemical required to enter sleep patterns. Vitamin B12 is included in the formula because of studies showing that it can normalize circadian rhythms, thereby enabling people to enter sleep without stress or tension. Chromium picolinate and chromium polynicotinate are included in the new formula to help lower blood sugar levels that can inhibit the ability to fall asleep. Niacinamide ascorbate, magnesium, calcium, and inositol are included in Natural Sleep to help induce a state of relaxation.

Some people use the herb valerian to fall asleep. Valerian produces a drug-like hypnotic effect within the central nervous system similar to benzodiazepine drugs such as Valium and Halcion. Since valerian-containing products are often promoted as natural herbal remedies, the public mistakenly believes it is safe to take on a regular basis. Studies indicate, however that there is a significant toxicity risk when taking valerian over an extended period of time. Since a tolerance effect occurs with valerian, due to its Valium-like properties, people often need to take greater and greater amounts of it as time goes by in order to continue to obtain the desired hypnotic effect.

The chronic use of valerian could result in permanent liver damage along with potential central nervous system impairment. The Life Extension Foundation has thoroughly investigated the use of herbal insomnia remedies such as valerian, hops, and passion flower, and found that they have an unacceptable risk of toxicity with long-term use.

Natural Sleep does not contain any potentially toxic herbal extracts. Insomnia is often a life-long affliction, requiring the continuous need for nightly self-medication. The ingredients in Natural Sleep have been thoroughly investigated for long-term safety, and can be taken for an indefinite period of time without any risk of toxicity or tolerance.

Depression is often an underlying cause of insomnia. For alternative suggestions to FDA-approved antidepressant drugs, access the Foundation's Depression protocol.

Product availability: To order Natural Sleep or other melatonin products, call 1-800-544-4440.

Jet Lag

Crossing time zones can lead to jet lag. Jet lag is caused by disruption of the body's circadian rhythm cycle because of a rapid move to a new time zone. The body's circadian rhythm is controlled by the release of the pineal hormone melatonin.

The best way of using melatonin to alleviate jet lag is to take a 3 mg capsule of melatonin the night before you leave, and another 3 mg capsule on the first night you go to sleep in your new destination. The melatonin will adjust your circadian rhythm to the new time zone, and you should wake up feeling as if you were home. If you are able to sleep on the plane, taking melatonin at that time could enable you to arrive at your new destination fully refreshed.

Product availability: Pharmaceutical-grade melatonin supplements in a wide range of potencies are available by calling 1-800-544-4440.

Kidney Disease

The kidney is an extremely delicate organ and diseases of the kidney are difficult to treat. The kidney has a pivotal role in maintaining taurine balance. In a study in *Amino Acids* (11:1 1996), taurine was shown to concentrate in a unique pattern along the specialized cells of the kidneys (nephrons). Taurine was able to protect against experimentally induced lipid peroxidation of the renal tubular and glomerular cells. The beneficial effects of taurine were due to its antioxidant actions.

The researchers concluded that clinical trials are warranted to determine the usefulness of taurine as an adjunct therapy in the treatment of progressive glomerular disease and diabetic nephropathy>.

Suggested supplementation with taurine is 1,000 mg, two to three times a day.

For kidney stones, take about 2,000 mg of magnesium a day to inhibit calcium oxalate formation.

Refer to the Acetaminophen (Tylenol) Poisoning: Acute And Chronic protocol to learn about a common cause of kidney disease.

Refer to the Diabetes Type I protocol if you are diabetic.

Product availability: Taurine and magnesium are available by phoning 1-800-544-4440.

Learning Disorders

Refer to Attention Deficit Disorder (ADD) or Age-Associated Mental Impairment (Brain Aging).

Leukemia-Lymphoma (and Hodgkin's Disease)

Cancers of the blood-forming organs and lymph tissues respond better to conventional chemotherapy than most forms of cancer. The rate of cure of Hodgkin's lymphoma using chemotherapy is between 70% and 80%. Alternative cancer therapies should be used with caution when treating leukemia or lymphoma patients because most alternative therapies boost immune cell function, which could speed the proliferation of leukemia and lymphoma cancer cells.

There are some alternative therapies which can be effective in treating leukemia or lymphoma. A vitamin A analog has been approved for promyelocytic leukemia. This drug inhibits leukemia cell division and helps them to mature into normal cells. We recommend that leukemia and lymphoma patients ask their oncologists to prescribe this drug, which is called Vesanoid.

If your doctor will not prescribe Vesanoid because the FDA has not approved it for your type of cancer, we suggest that you use 100,000 to 300,000 IU a day of water-soluble vitamin A liquid. Monthly blood tests are needed to guard against the possibility of vitamin A liver toxicity.

Important: Refer to the Symptoms of Vitamin A Toxicity, in Appendix A.

Vitamin D3 and its analogs can induce leukemia and lymphoma cells to differentiate into normal cells. The Life Extension Foundation suggests that leukemia/lymphoma patients take 4,000 to 6,000 IU of vitamin D3 a day on an empty stomach. Monthly blood tests to monitor serum calcium and parathyroid hormone levels should be done to protect against vitamin D3 toxicity.

Soy extracts may inhibit leukemia/lymphoma cell proliferation by interfering with tyrosine kinase, the enzyme that cancer cells need for replication. Two heaping tablespoons a day of Super Soy Extract powder provide about 40 mg of genistein and 200 mg of isoflavones. Genistein, saponin, and other isoflavones are the ingredients in soy that scientists believe have cancer inhibiting properties. Super Soy Extract is also available in tablet form, but requires 20 tablets a day to obtain the amount contained in two heaping tablespoons of good-tasting powder.

Do not take soy extract when undergoing radiation therapy because the genistein in soy can interfere with the ability of the radiation to kill cancer cells. The Life Extension Foundation recommends that leukemia/lymphoma patients use these alternative therapies in addition to conventional therapy. If you don't want to use conventional therapy, call the Foundation at 1-800-544-4440 for a referral to an alternative cancer clinic.

Product availability: Water-soluble vitamin A liquid, vitamin D3 caps and Super Soy Extract are available phoning 1-800-544-4440. Vesanoid is a prescription drug that should be prescribed by your oncologist or hematologist.

Liver (Cirrhosis)

Liver degeneration can be caused by chronic alcohol (ethanol) intake, viral disease, FDA-approved drugs, malnutrition, congestive heart failure, and various hepatic toxins. Cirrhosis of the liver occurs when too many liver cells break down and become infiltrated with non-functioning fat cells.

It is possible to regenerate a degenerated liver if extraordinary therapies are followed and the underlying cause of the cirrhosis is eliminated. Nutritional therapies to help regenerate the liver include a daily regimen of 500 mg of vitamin B1, 75 mg of vitamin B2, 1,500 mg of vitamin B5, 200 mg of vitamin B6, 1,500 mg of choline, 1,600 mcg of folic acid, 3,000 mg of vitamin C, 800 IU of vitamin E, and 100 mg of coenzyme Q10.

Avoid niacin, vitamin A and beta-carotene, as these nutrients can be harmful to a severely damaged liver. Acetyl-L-carnitine should be taken in two daily doses of 1,000 mg each, and a daily dose of 600 mg a day of n-acetyl-cysteine should be taken. Green tea in a dose of four to 10 standardized 100 mg capsules a day can be used to lower toxic levels of iron that may be generating dangerous free radicals in the liver. If there is at least a 20% reserve capacity remaining, 5 to 10 grams of arginine can help to lower toxic ammonia levels in the blood caused by a defective liver, and can also help to facilitate liver regeneration.

An important therapy to help restore liver function involves the branched-chain amino acids. This includes twice-daily administration of 1,200 mg of leucine, 600 mg of isoleucine and 600 mg of valine. The flavonoid silymarin in doses of 300 mg a day may be helpful, along with 1,500 mg a day of the herbal extract curcumin.

CAUTION: Do not use curcumin if you have biliary tract obstruction because curcumin could eliminate the flow of bile excretion through the bile duct.

The European antidepressant drug S-adenosylmethionine (SAM) has potent liver regeneration properties. Suggested dose is four to eight 200 mg tablets of SAM throughout the day until normal liver function is restored. Regular liver function blood tests are required to assess the effectiveness of whatever therapy is being used. For specific anti-viral therapies to help eradicate hepatitis B or hepatitis C, refer to our Hepatitis C and Hepatitis B protocols.

Product availability: SAM, vitamin B1, vitamin B2, vitamin B5, vitamin B6, folic acid, choline, vitamin C, vitamin E, coenzyme Q10, acetyl-L-carnitine, n-acetyl-cysteine, green tea, arginine, curcumin, silymarin and the branched-chain amino acid complex can be ordered by phoning 1-800-544-4440. SAM can be ordered by overseas companies, for information call 1-800-544-4440.

Lupus

Lupus is thought to be caused by autoimmune reactions. Refer to the Life Extension Foundation's Autoimmune Disease protocol. Lupus patients should exercise extreme caution when attempting any new medical therapy as there is a chance the condition could be made worse.

Macular Degeneration (Dry)

Dry macular degeneration is characterized by a deficiency of blood flow to some parts of the eye, causing atrophy and a slow loss of vision.

Nutrients that may improve microcapillary circulation in the eye include ginkgo biloba at 120 mg a day, grape seed extract at 150 mg a day, and bilberry extract at 150 mg a day.

Hydergine in doses of 4 to 5 mg a day and higher has shown significant benefits for dry macular degeneration. Antioxidant nutrients such as selenium, 200 mcg a day, alpha lipoic acid, 500 mg a day, and glutathione, 500 mg a day should also be considered. The standard daily dose of Life Extension Mix, three tablets, three times a day, provides adequate levels of vitamin B-complex, zinc and other nutrients that are crucial for ocular function.

The daily application of the vitamin A-based VIVA Drops, can provide antioxidant protection to the lens of the eye. Wrap-around UV-blocking sunglasses provides significant protection against UV sun rays.

Studies suggest that a majority of patients with dry macular degeneration are at a high risk of developing more-dangerous wet macular degeneration of their eye. Therefore, anyone with dry macular degeneration should also refer to the Foundation's protocol on Wet Macular Degeneration.

Product availability: Ginkgo biloba extract, proanthocyanidins (grape seed extract), bilberry extract, selenium, alpha lipoic acid, glutathione, zinc, Life Extension Mix, VIVA Drops, and wrap-around sunglasses can be obtained by calling 1-800-544-4440.

Macular Degeneration (Wet)

Wet macular degeneration is characterized by an overgrowth of leaky blood vessels into the retina of the eye. When these blood vessels rupture, it causes severe visual loss, leading usually to blindness. Those who eat a large amount of spinach and collard greens have very low rates of wet macular degeneration.

The phytochemicals that protect against wet macular degeneration are lutein and zeaxanthin. Life Extension Mix and Chloroplex both contain lutein. Those with early-stage wet macular degeneration, should try Lutein Plus powder which provides potent concentrations of zeaxanthin and lutein. One tablespoon a day of Lutein Plus vegetable powder is suggested to prevent or slow the progress of wet macular degeneration.

Soy contains the phytochemical genistein, which has anti-angiogenesis properties. Those with wet macular degeneration may want to take two heaping tablespoons a day of Super Soy Extract so they can obtain enough genistein to possibly inhibit blood vessel growth in the eye. Super Soy Extract is available in tablet and powder form.

Free radical damage has been implicated in the development of wet macular degeneration. The daily dose of Life Extension Mix consisting of three tablets, three times a day will provide broad-spectrum antioxidant protection against free radical damage to the eye. An additional 30 mg of zinc should also be considered.

Product availability: Lutein powder, Super Soy Extract, Life Extension Mix, zinc, Lutein Plus and wrap-around UV blocking sunglasses are available by phoning 1-800-544-4440.

Medical Testing Protocols

The Life Extension Foundation has advocated regular medical testing since 1983 for the purpose of optimizing your personal life extension program. Regular blood testing enables you to detect:

1) Abnormalities that may predispose you to diseases that are treatable if caught at an early stage, e.g. cancer, diabetes, cardiovascular disease.

2) Toxicities that could be counteracted to prevent organ damage by adjusting your nutrient-drug intake, e.g. liver damage caused by hepatotoxic drugs, vitamin A, iron overload, etc.

3) Hormone imbalances that can accelerate your rate of aging if not corrected, e.g., DHEA deficiency or cortisol overload.

4) Other imbalances that could be adjusted to enable you to become healthier, more energetic, sexier and stronger.

Here are some of the important tests that can be used to assess your health and longevity, and the results you should strive to attain:

❖ **Glucose: Optimal level should be under 100.**

A consistent effect of calorie restriction is a reduction in serum glucose levels to within normal range. Calorie restriction is the only documented method of extending maximum life span. Calorie restricted people often have serum glucose levels between 70 and 80. When glucose levels are over 100, accelerated aging can occur via several mechanisms.

Glucose-lowering nutrients include 200 mcg of chromium picolinate with every meal, and/or 7.5 mg of vanadyl sulfate three times a day, and/or four decaffeinated green tea capsules with every meal, and/or fiber supplements. If your glucose level is too high, you should have your thyroid hormone level checked. If it is too low, you should consider low-dose thyroid hormone under a doctor's supervision. Another method of improving thyroid function is taking 6 to 30 grams of a highly concentrated soy extract, which can help to normalize your thyroid hormone levels.

❖ **Iron: Optimal level should be under 100.**

Iron is a catalyst for free radical activity that increases the risk of heart disease, Alzheimer's disease, cancer, and a host of degenerative diseases. Low iron levels have been shown to protect against cancer and heart disease in large human populations.

Iron-lowering nutrients include four decaffeinated green tea capsules and/or four Garlic/EDTA capsules with every meal, and/or undergoing a series of intravenous chelation treatments under the care of a physician, and/or donating a pint of blood to yourself for future use.

❖ **Cholesterol: Optimal LDL cholesterol level below 120. Optimal HDL cholesterol level above 50.**

Oxidized LDL cholesterol adheres to the inner linings of arteries, which contributes to atherosclerosis. It also promotes abnormal arterial clotting.

HDL cholesterol removes excess fat and other types of cholesterol from the arterial system.

Nutrients that favorably alter cholesterol levels, i.e., lower dangerous LDL cholesterol and elevate HDL cholesterol, include 200 mcg of chromium picolinate twice a day, 30 grams a day of soluble fiber, 1,000 to 3,000 mg a day of niacin with meals, and 2,000 mg a day and higher of vitamin C. Herbal extracts such as curcumin and gugulipid have dose-related cholesterol-lowering effects.

❖ **Triglycerides: Optimal triglyceride level is below 100.**

Triglycerides combine a fatty acid and glycerol. Elevated triglyceride levels predispose a person to atherosclerosis and abnormal platelet aggregation.

Nutrients that may lower elevated triglyceride levels include high doses of fish oil and garlic.

Why Blood Tests Are Not Used Regularly

The high cost and inconvenience of regular blood testing prevents many people from being tested as often as they should be.

Another problem with blood testing is that different labs often produce varying readings from the same blood specimen, making the results of regular testing difficult to interpret.

The Life Extension Foundation receives blood test results for evaluation from members who sometimes use different laboratories every time they're tested. In many cases the member is not even aware that different laboratories were used in testing.

Another problem is that commercial testing laboratories seldom perform the unique tests that Foundation members request, which means that a lab technician may be doing a DHEA serum test, for example, for the first time on your blood!

In order to standardize the methods used for all blood tests, the Life Extension Foundation has made an arrangement with a nationwide testing laboratory to perform all basic blood testing. For specialized tests to measure DHEA, growth hormone, and cortisol, the Foundation has contracted with an expert medical technologist who has been performing these unusual tests for 15 years.

Here is a description and discount prices for the most popular blood tests:

Complete Blood Chemistry/Blood Count

This testing panel includes LDL, HDL, total cholesterol, triglycerides, iron, glucose, liver and kidney function, and many more important tests.

These tests detect blood changes that may predispose you to a wide range of degenerative diseases. They also provide information to assess whether or not the drugs and nutrients you may be taking are causing liver, kidney or heart damage.

We suggest that this test battery be performed annually. If a serious abnormality is detected such as elevated glucose, cholesterol or iron, testing should be repeated more often to determine the efficacy of whatever therapy you are using to correct the potentially life-shortening abnormality.

Non-member price $55.00, member price $37.00.

Fibrinogen

Elevated levels of fibrinogen predispose you to arterial clotting that can cause a heart attack or a stroke. Elevated fibrinogen may be at least as great a risk factor for coronary artery disease as elevated LDL cholesterol. Optimal fibrinogen levels should be under 300.

Fibrinogen-lowering nutrients include bromelain in doses of 250 to 1,000 mg twice a day, and/or eight fish oil capsules a day, and/or beta-carotene in doses of 25,000 IU to 100,000 IU a day and/or vitamin C in doses exceeding 2,000 mg a day, and/or taking a European drug called Bezafibrate.

Non-member price $55.00, member price $37.00.

Prostate Specific Antigen (PSA)

The PSA test is more than 80% accurate in detecting prostate cancer and measuring the effectiveness of prostate cancer therapies.

The Life Extension Foundation believes that men over 40 should have a PSA test annually. And men over 60 should have this test every six months.

Individuals with prostate cancer should have a PSA test every 30 days in order to measure the efficacy of the prostate cancer therapy they are using.

Non-member price $60.00, member price $40.00.

Immune Cell Subset Tests

For people with cancer, HIV infection, chronic herpes outbreaks, hepatitis, autoimmune disorders or other diseases that suppress immune function, or who have declining immune function due to normal aging, the Immune Cell Subset Test shows your T-Helper to T-suppressor cell ratio, your total T-Helper cell count, and the activity of your Natural Killer Cells. This information can be used to help develop an immune system-boosting program that could put these diseases into long term remission.

The Immune Cell Subset Test should be repeated several months after the initiation of immune-boosting therapies such as isoprinosine, melatonin, gamma linolenic acid (GLA), and DHEA, with the objective of restoring your immune system to normal, healthy function.

Non-member price $315.00, member price $210.00.

Hormone And Cancer Profiles

If you are considering hormone replacement therapy, we suggest that you take one or more of the tests below. Low DHEA levels can be raised to youthful levels by taking DHEA or pregnenolone. We suggest that after you take your initial DHEA sulfate test to determine the dosage you need, further DHEA testing be done three weeks and six months after commencing DHEA and/or pregnenolone replacement therapy and every six months thereafter.

Men who take DHEA or pregnenolone should have a PSA test done because DHEA may elevate testosterone levels, which can cause existing prostate cancer cells to hyperproliferate. DHEA and pregnenolone are usually contraindicated in men with prostate cancer. However, some scientists favor its limited use in prostate cancer patients.

Men (and women to a lesser extent) should consider testing to determine if DHEA is elevating their testosterone levels, which could produce an anti-aging effect.

Women (and men to a lesser extent) should consider testing for Total Estrogen to see if DHEA is elevating their estrogen levels, which might reduce or eliminate their need for estrogen replacement therapy.

Ovarian and breast cancer patients should consider that DHEA supplementation may increase estrogen levels in some individuals, and that estrogen may be a contributing factor to these disorders. In this respect, the estrogen receptor blocking properties of melatonin may prevent estrogen from causing such a problem.

New findings indicate that growth hormone plays an important role in maintaining many functions of youth including the formation of new bone matrix and the maintenance of normal protein synthesis in brain cells.

Aging is associated with the excess secretion of cortisol from our adrenal glands. Cortisol is a glucocorticoid hormone that suppresses immune function, inhibits healthy brain cell metabolism, promotes atherosclerosis, and accelerates aging. The drawback of cortisol testing is that it needs to be done twice in the same day, before 9 a.m. and in the afternoon to obtain reliable results.

Cortisol-reducing therapies include:

  1) Vitamin C (at least 4 grams a day)
  2) Aspirin
  3) DHEA or pregnenolone replacement therapy
  4) Double doses of the procaine formulas KH3 or GH3

If you have elevated cortisol, we suggest trying several of the therapies below and then repeating the cortisol test monthly until you find the right combination of therapies to reduce your cortisol levels adequately.

	Member Price	Non-Member Price
DHEA Sulfate	$51.00	$77.00
Free Testosterone	$78.00	$112.00
(men and women)		
Estradiol	$68.00	$102.00
Total Progesterone	$68.00	$102.00
Ovarian Cancer Marker (CA 125)	$77.00	$115.00
Breast Cancer Marker (CA 27.29)	$77.00	$115.00
Gastric-Pancreatic Marker (CA 19-9)	$77.00	$115.00

Somatomedin C (IGF-1)	$159.00	$238.00
(Growth Hormone marker)		
Cortisol	$40.00	$60.00

Cancer Profile

Dr. Emil Schandl, a clinical biochemist and oncobiologist, with the Center for Metabolic Disorders and American Metabolic Testing Laboratories, has developed a battery of blood tests designed to predict your risk of developing cancer (CA) long before symptoms occur. This CA Profile includes the HCG and HCG-b hormones, PHI (phophohexose isomerase) and GGTP (g-glutamyl transpeptidase) enzymes, CEA (carcinoembrionic antigen), TSH (thyroid stimulating hormone), and DHEA-S (dehydroepiandrosterone, the "stress, immunity, and longevity hormone"). Dr. Schandl suggests a PTH (parathyroid hormone) test also to evaluate calcium status in the bones.

The CA Profile yields 90 positives out of 100 pathologically established malignancies. Because of its capacity to foretell the development of cancer years before a tumor is apparent, a positive finding is a serious warning sign of a developing cancer. The CA Profile tests can also be used to monitor the response of cancer patients' to various therapies. An increasing value of a tumor marker may indicate the benefits or futility of a therapy.

The CA Profile can be combined with specific cancer tests, such as the PSA, CA 27.29 (to detect breast cancer), and CA 125 (to detect ovarian cancer), to provide the most complete picture of your risk and/or the status of almost every cancer.

	Member Price	Non-Member Price
Cancer Profile	$233.00	$331.00
PTH (parathyroid hormone)	$84.00	$126.00

Cancer may actually be the number one killer of humans on this continent. Whereas there is no certain cure for cancer, it may be preventable. Fortunately in most cases, treatments and therapies can successfully extend life by many years. It is essential for cancer patients and their physicians to know how a person is responding to therapy. Biochemical testings are the quickest and most sensitive heralds in this respect.

Persons who appear to be healthy may be harboring growing, developing cancer cells without any physical signs or symptoms. In other words, no diagnosis can be made by X-rays or other established methods. The importance of early diagnosis, made possible by biochemical testings, cannot be over emphasized!

Dr. Schandl's biochemical Cancer Profile, done on blood, can monitor the progress of cancer therapy and can, as published in the *Journal of the National Cancer Institute,* foretell the development of malignancies more than two years prior to diagnosis.

The CA Profile, together with a chemistry profile (SMAC or similar), CBC with differential and platelet count, PTH for the evaluation of calcium metabolism, PSA for men over 40, or CA-125 and CA 27.29 for women, is the most comprehensive evaluation available for prevention, early detection and therapeutic monitoring of metabolic disorders.

Dr. Schandl has tested several thousand patients. The results of these tests not only indicate whether or not cancer is present but also measure the fluctuating conditions of the patient. Obviously this capacity is essential for assessing the effectiveness of the therapy instituted. The possible early diagnosis so afforded may add years of precious human life via prompt attention to the developing problem.

Even though our scientists consider the CA Profile to be the most comprehensive of its kind, a negative score does not entirely rule out the presence of cancer. It does, however, provide a reasonable degree of confidence.

The blood usually carries messages of ill health before such a condition could be detected by any other method. However, it should be mentioned that the final, definitive diagnosis for cancer is tissue/cell examination by a pathologist. The CA Profile is a very powerful tool as a part of a diagnostic work-up. A positive value may suggest, and sometimes strongly, the presence or the process of developing a cancer. The tests, in general, are not organ specific.

The CA Profile tests for the following:

HCG	May be elevated in cancer, stress related to cancer, a developing cancer, or pregnancy. Normal: less than one mIU/mL; gray up to 2.0.
PHI	May be elevated above 42 in cancer, developing cancer, active AIDS, other viral disease, or acute heart, liver or muscle disease. Normal: less than 42 U/L.
GGTP	May be elevated above 41 U/L in females and 53 U/L in males in diseases of the liver, pancreas, and the biliary system.
TSH	Thyroid stimulating hormone, for thyroid and oxygen metabolism. Normals: 0.4-3.1 mcIU/mL.
DHEA-S	Adrenal stress, immunity, and longevity hormone; low or zero in most cancer patients. Normal: F 35- 430 mcg/dL, M 80 - 560 mcg/dL. Results must be interpreted in reference to a person's age.
CEA	Carcinoembrionic antigen is elevated in just about all malignancies. Normals: less than 2.5 ng/mL.

Also Recommended:

PSA	For men over the age of 40 to detect prostate cancer. Normals: less than 4.0 ng/mL.
PTH	Parathyroid hormone, for the detection of calcium

	depletion from the bone, e.g., osteoporosis. Normals: 0 - 27 ng/dL.
CA-125	A sensitive marker for residual epithelial carcino mas of the ovary. Normals are less than 35 U/mL.
CA 27.29	A sensitive breast cancer marker. Normals: less than 32 U/mL.

Somatomedin-C (IGF-1) Human youth/longevity/growth hormone

To order the CA Profile, contact your physician. M.D., D.O., chiropractor, podiatrist, or dentist has to request the tests. For Medicare, the M.D. or D.O. must provide a UPIN number and diagnostic code number.

Clinical Biochemical Parameters in Cancer Diagnosis and Therapy

A clinical biochemical profile was constructed for early detection and therapy monitoring of malignancies. The profile was composed of HCG-B and CEA determinations by RIA and phosphohexose isomerase (PHI) and g-glutamyl transferase (GGT) by enzyme kinetic methods. When all four tests were used, 94% of diagnosed cancer patients, regardless of type or location of the malignancy, showed at least one elevated value. The omission of CEA resulted in 92% such success. HCG-B was elevated in 68% of the patients. PHI in 36%, GGT in 39%, and CEA in 51%. There were some differences noticed between male and female patients.

Elevated markers were observed in patients without diagnosed cancers: HCG-B 41%, PHI 16%, GGT 12%, and CEA 21%. Several patients in this category were cancer suspects, e.g., they had lumps in the breast or lymph gland enlargement, and were later diagnosed as having malignancies. Cancer patients were periodically tested using the Cancer Profile and it was possible to monitor favorable or unfavorable responses to therapies. The Cancer Profile was used as a diagnostic aid in the detection of malignancies and in the progress monitoring of patients.

A Letter From Dr. Schandl

"I designed the CA Profile while in the Nuclear Medicine department of a large hospital. My work was to inject people with radioactive substances for performance of various scans: brain, bone, liver, kidney, heart, lung, etc. I felt very uncomfortable making people radioactive for the tests, touching the radioactive materials, and having to be near the now-radiating people injected.

"The doses used were well within acceptable limits by all regulatory agencies. However, I have always maintained there is no such thing as safe radiation. So, having an excellent background in clinical chemistry, radiation biology, biochemistry, biology, genetics, and enzymology, I composed the CA Profile. It is made up of various tests. It is not invasive or radioactive. It requires no radioactive substances nor any X-rays, CAT scan radiation or even nuclear magnetic imaging (MRI). MRI involves speedy resonance of hydrogen atom protons due to an induced electromagnetic field, which is 3,000 to 25,000 times that of our Earth's own field.

"No surgical manipulations are used. Most commonly used diagnostic modalities can potentially cause cancer themselves. A recent issue concerning mammograms is an example. There also is considerable information on the carcinogenic effects of high-energy, high-frequency magnetic (or any) radiation.

"The CA Profile is simply composed of blood tests. The only invasiveness is the prick of a needle. To assure specimen stability, samples must be handled strictly as instructed. Tests are performed weekly and results reported on Mondays. Early detection and monitoring of cancers is thus reliably achieved.

"The CA Profile is being used by many doctors in the U.S. as well as in Europe, Canada, South America, the Philippines and the Atlantic island communities.

"Many years of experience show the predictive value can be as high as 92 percent. This means if there are 100 establish cases with active cancer, 92 will yield positive results. Do not forget, however, the absolute final diagnosis is a biopsied specimen, i.e. tissue pathology. A warning positive test result may warrant a complete change of lifestyle through metabolic therapy. An M.D., D.O., chiropractor, podiatrist, dentist or acupuncture physician can order the tests."

Sincerely yours in health,

Dr. Emil K. Schandl

How To Order Blood Tests

You can order blood tests by mail by calling 1-800-544-4440. All tests must be pre-paid unless the tests are covered by Medicare or other insurance.

As soon as you place your order, you will be sent a package to inform you of the location of the nearest blood drawing stations, as well as a pre-paid requisition, blood testing vials, and a postage-paid return envelope if you are ordering specialized tests. You should take the requisition to any of the blood-drawing stations in your area. A phlebotomist will draw the appropriate specimens of your blood, which should then be shipped to our laboratory for analysis.

You (or your physician) will then be mailed your test results. These results will show if you have any abnormalities. If the results show abnormalities, you should make sure you show these results to your personal physician, who can determine if you have any serious problems and what you can do about them.

If longevity risk factors such as glucose, iron, cholesterol, fibrinogen and CA Profile are abnormal, or even slightly elevated, you can take nutritional steps to reverse the trend, repeat the test in 45 to 60 days, and then chart your progress in improving your health and your chances of living longer in good health.

Important notes:

1) If you intend to bill your tests to an insurance company or Medicare, you need to submit a completely filled out insurance claim form, including your physician's UPIN number, an M.D. or DO's, name, address, phone, and the prescription for the tests. Other licensed practitioners of the healing arts who can order blood tests are chiropractors, podiatrists, dentists and acupuncturists. The Foundation cannot do mail-order blood testing paid by Medicare or other types of insurance without a health care practitioner first ordering the test.

2) Blood testing is an important and exacting science. Interpretations depend on the knowledge and expertise of trained clinical scientists. Therefore, it is recommended that you work closely with your physician or other qualified health professional for a satisfactory outcome.

Product availability: To order mail-order blood tests, phone 1-800-544-4440.

Meningitis

Meningitis is an acute, life-threatening inflammatory condition caused by a pathogen that requires immediate conventional medical care.

Depending on the pathogen involved, refer to either Bacterial Infections or Viral Infections.

Also see the Life Extension Foundation Immune Enhancement protocol and the HIV Infection protocol.

Menopause

Menopause, which involves the natural cessation of menstruation, is an event stemming from the lack of ovarian function and the subsequent curtailment of ovarian hormone secretion. During menopause, menstrual patterns change dramatically, estrogen levels fall and FSH (follicle-stimulating hormone) and LH (luteinizing hormone) levels increase. During this time, 65% of the requests for treatment are due to night sweats and 45% are due to psychological syndromes.

The average age for those seeking treatment for menopause is 44. Currently, the most prescribed hormone replacement therapy is Premarin, a form of estrogen, which alleviates some of the symptoms of menopause, and increases the risk of hormone-dependent cancers. The primary symptoms of menopause are:

❖ Vasomotor: Hot flashes, palpitations, spontaneous sweating, panic attacks and the inability to sleep.

❖ Psychological: Anxiety, mood swings, depression, poor memory and lack of concentration.

❖ Urogenital: Sexual organ atrophy, dysparenuria (pain during sex), trigonitis, frequent and urgent urination.

❖ Skeletal: Osteoporosis, vertebral crush fractures, and femoral neck fractures. Symptoms usually begin well into menopause.

❖ Cardiovascular: Ischemic heart disease and/or cerebrovascular disease. Symptoms usually begin well into menopause.

The Foundation's protocol for the treatment of menopause and post-menopause symptoms:

1) Safe estrogen and progesterone replacement therapy using pregnenolone, and/or DHEA. Pregnenolone is converted into both estrogen and progesterone in the body. DHEA can also convert to estrogen.

2) For some women, supplementation with TriEst (which contains 80% estriol, the safe form of estrogen) is needed.

3) High potency vitamin and mineral supplementation.

For further information on female hormone replacement therapy, refer to the Foundation's Estrogen Replacement protocol.

Product availability: Pregnenolone, Natural Estrogen, and progesterone cream are available by calling 1-800-544-4440. When calling the Foundation, ask for a listing of offshore companies that sell estriol and TriEst.

Menstrual Disorders
(Premenstrual Syndrome)

PMS is a woman's body telling her that something is not working properly. The causes may be nutritional, hormonal, or in some rare cases toxic metals. PMS is not another name for premenstrual cramps. PMS is a combination of symptoms that occur two to 14 days before the onset of menstruation. There are many symptoms and they vary from person to person. They increase in severity with age because of declining progesterone levels. Many factors contribute to the severity of PMS other than age, including heredity, diet, progesterone deficiency, stress, and very frequently the ingestion, intentional or otherwise, of synthetic hormones.

The symptoms of PMS can be alleviated by avoiding synthetic hormones either in the form of birth control pills or the even more dangerous hormones we get from dairy and meat. Cows bred for milk production are given large amounts of hormones and antibiotics to increase their milk production. The animals bred for their meat are injected with massive doses of hormones to increase their weight for sale. They are also fed diets with pesticide-laced grains.

Our own vegetable consumption is high in pesticides. However, vegetables are essential and there are ways to minimize our own pesticide consumption. Avoiding meats and dairy products would increase our health in numerous ways, including the alleviation of PMS and a reduced risk of reproductive cancers, particularly breast cancer.

Exercise enables bones to retain their youthful density by creating the bone-forming cells known as osteoblasts. Progesterone is also involved in the formation of bone-forming osteoblasts. Exercise also releases tension, increases endorphin levels, which lessen pain and increases our sense of well being. It also maximizes metabolism, and increases our energy and our ability to deal with stress.

Diet is a major player in reducing the symptoms of PMS. A low fat, high complex carbohydrate, high phyto-protein diet has been shown to enhance general health, ward off diseases, and significantly reduce the symptoms of PMS. Soy is the best source of protein, especially for women, because it gives us natural estrogens that are converted in our bodies into other hormones as needed. When we rely on animal meats for our protein, both the fat and the chemicals endanger our health.

We know that too much fat can endanger our lives, but the essential fatty acids (EFA) are essential in the natural production of hormones. EFAs help us to maintain healthy weight, improve cardiovascular health, improve skin, hair and nail appearance, as well as the elasticity and texture of the skin, thus improving our self-image. A poor or declining appearance can lead to depression, stress, anxiety, a decline in health — and the desire to do anything about it.

Nutritional supplements are very important. Even the medical community has recently, albeit grudgingly, admitted that we cannot get adequate nutrition. from diet alone. Women need more B vitamins, especially 200 to 300 mg of vitamin B6, starting two weeks before their periods. This should be combined with calcium and magnesium to improve the health of the bones, teeth, and cardiovascular system.

Udo's Choice Flax Oil provides the best combination of omega-3 and omega-6 essential fatty acids. One to two tablespoons a day is suggested. Mineral Formula For Women (4 to six capsules a day) provides an excellent source of the calcium and magnesium women need to ward off the symptoms of PMS.

Product availability: Vitamin B6, Mineral Formula For Women and Udo's Choice Flax Oil can be obtained by phoning 1-800-544-4440.

Migraine

Migraine headaches can be relieved in some people by taking 10 to 40 mg of the beta-blocking drug Propranolol. Those with very low blood pressure, congestive heart failure and asthma should avoid this class of drugs.

An herbal extract called feverfew has been used successfully in Europe to prevent migraine headaches. The recommended dose is one capsule daily containing a minimum 600 mcg of the active ingredient parthenolide.

Another European anti-migraine therapy is hyperforat, an extract from the herb St. John's Wort. The suggested dose of St. John's Wort is one tablet, twice a day.

The regular use of the hormone melatonin has been reported to reduce the incidence of migraine attacks and cluster headaches. The suggested dose is 3 to 10 mg a night for people over 40. Younger people may only need 500 mcg to one mg of melatonin every night.

Newly approved conventional drugs are now providing more migraine suffers with relief. The most effective of these drugs is Imitrex, an expensive drug available in oral and injectable forms, which can knock out an impending migraine headache before it can get going. Imitrex may have dangerous side effects in the elderly.

Product availability: Propranolol and Imitrex are drugs that need to be prescribed by your doctor. Mygracare (feverfew), St. John's Wort and melatonin can be ordered singly or in a Protocol Pak by phoning 1-800-544-4440.

Multiple Sclerosis (MS)

Multiple sclerosis (MS) is a debilitating disease caused by the loss of the protective, insulating myelin sheath covering the nerve fibers in the brain, spinal cord and peripheral nervous system. Muscle weakness, numbness, visual disturbances and multiple disabilities characterize this disease.

There are several theories to explain what causes the destruction of the myelin sheath in MS patients. Some doctors believe it is an autoimmune attack. Others believe a virus may be involved in myelin sheath destruction. Dr. Emil Schandl published a paper in the *American Journal of Clinical Nutrition* that presented a strong correlation between MS and exposure to carbon monoxide from automobile exhaust, fossil-fuel-utilizing heating devices and cigarette smoking, as well as vitamin B6 deficiency. A smoker has little hope of recovering from MS because of the constant high level of carbon monoxide that cigarette smoking produces. This means that MS patients should avoid second-hand cigarette smoke and carbon monoxide exposure whenever possible.

The Life Extension Foundation's protocol for MS is based partially on the work of Dr. Hans Neiper of Germany, who has used high-potency nutrient supplements to treat multiple sclerosis for many years. The FDA has banned the importation of Dr. Neiper's MS nutrient formulas, but the Foundation has attempted to follow his recommendations.

To help correct autoimmune disorders and protect against free radical injury to the myelin sheath, the 52-ingredient Life Extension Mix should be taken in doses of four tablets, three times a day. One capsule of Life Extension Booster should be taken daily, along with four capsules of Mineral Formula For Men and four capsules of Mineral Formula For Women. These formulas contain important minerals that have helped both men and women MS patients. To protect the myelin sheath against a deficiency of essential fatty acids, eight capsules a day of Mega-EPA fish oil, and four capsules a day of Mega-GLA borage oil should be taken. These oils help to suppress autoimmune reactions and provide the building blocks to help rebuild the myelin sheath.

Hydergine (five to 20 mg a day) and/or acetyl-L-carnitine (1,000 mg, twice a day) and/or alpha lipoic acid (400 mg, twice a day) should be taken to provide myelin sheath protection and energy enhancement to the nerve fibers. Coenzyme Q10 in doses of 100 mg three times a day can be especially important for MS patients. Coenzyme Q10 should be taken in oil-filled capsules for maximum assimilation. The addition of 100-250 mg of vitamin B6 in the form of pyridoxal phosphate, and 1,000 mcg of sublingual (to be taken under the tongue) vitamin B12 could be extremely beneficial.

Product availability: Life Extension Mix, Life Extension Booster, Mineral Formula For Men, Mineral Formula For Women, Mega-EPA, Mega-GLA, acetyl-L-carnitine, alpha lipoic acid, coenzyme Q10, pyridoxal 5-phosphate and vitamin B12 are available by phoning 1-800-544-4440. Call for a list of overseas pharmacies that sell high-potency hydergine to Americans for personal use.

Muscle Building

Aging causes a progressive catabolic (breaking down) effect on muscle tissue that results in muscle atrophy and a general weakening of the entire body. The underlying causes of muscle wasting are well-documented in the scientific literature. One cause of muscle atrophy is the age-associated breakdown of carbohydrate metabolism that precludes the efficient use of insulin and glucose to rebuild muscle mass.

Therapies that can restore youthful carbohydrate metabolism include 200 mcg of chromium picolinate with every meal, 5 to 15 grams of the amino acid arginine on an empty stomach, and thyroid and DHEA hormones.

The age-associated decline in cellular energy production is another cause of muscle atrophy. A cell-energy enhancing program would include the daily intake of 1,000 to 2,000 mg of acetyl-L-carnitine, 100 to 300 mg of coenzyme Q10, one tablespoon of Udo's Choice flax oil, and the standard dose of the 52-ingredient multi-nutrient Life Extension Mix.

Many body builders take a large number of supplements to generate an anabolic effect in order to build muscle mass. The most efficient way of taking most of the nutrients used by body builders is to take three heaping scoops of Optifuel powder by Twinlab. Optifuel provides the full range of amino acids and other anabolic nutrients. It should be used in conjunction with an exercise program for maximum results.

Woman should refer to the Life Extension Foundation's Estrogen Replacement Therapy protocol. Estrogen is an important anabolic hormone in women. For those who can afford human growth hormone therapy, a marked anabolic effect on muscle mass can occur in older people. For a referral to a physician with expertise in administering growth hormone replacement therapy, call the Life Extension Foundation at 1-800-544-4440.

Product availability: Chromium picolinate, Life Extension Mix, Optifuel, acetyl-L-carnitine, coenzyme Q10, DHEA, arginine and Udo's Choice Blend Oil can be ordered by phoning 1-800-544-4440. Thyroid hormone and growth hormone replacement therapy should be prescribed by your doctor.

Muscular Dystrophy

Muscular dystrophy is a group of diseases characterized by weakness and wasting of skeletal muscle tissue, without the breakdown of nerve tissue. Each type of muscular dystrophy is different with regard to the group of muscles affected and the rate of progression of the disease.

A recent study showed significant benefits when muscular dystrophy patients were given high doses of coenzyme Q10. The recommended dose of coenzyme Q10 is one 100 mg oil-filled coenzyme Q10 capsule, three times a day.

Vitamin E and selenium deficiencies may play important roles in the development of this disease. The suggested doses are 400 IU of vitamin E three times daily, and 200 mcg of selenium three times daily. Muscular dystrophy patients should refer to the Life Extension Foundation's Muscle Building and Catabolic Wasting protocols for additional suggestions.

Product availability: Coenzyme Q10, vitamin E, and selenium are available singly or in a Protocol Pak by calling 1-800-544-4440.

Myasthenia Gravis

Myasthenia gravis occurs because of a defect in the transmission of nerve signals from nerve fibers to muscles. The result is severe long-term muscle weakness. Mainstream scientists have not yet conducted studies to explore the relationship between nutrition, nutritional therapies and myasthenia gravis. There are nutritional therapies that appear to play an important role in the functioning and maintenance of muscle tissue.

Essential fatty acids are crucial for maintaining the myelin sheath that contains nerve fibers and is often damaged during the course of the disease. Therefore, patients should consider taking eight capsules a day of Mega-EPA, a fish oil concentrate that provides a potent dose of the omega-3 fatty acids. Two capsules a day of Mega-GLA provides the critical omega-6 fatty acid gammalinolenic acid (GLA).

The lipotropic agents choline and inositol are required to utilize the fatty acids; 1,000-2,000 mg a day of each could be helpful. To boost the levels of the neurotransmitter acetylcholine and to boost neurological cellular energy levels, five capsules a day of Cognitex (which includes choline and synergistic co-factors) is suggested. Free radical damage should be reduced by taking three tablets, three times a day, of Life Extension Mix.

To improve the transmission of nerve signals, 400 mg of alpha lipoic acid should be taken twice a day. Vitamin D3 at a dose of 1,000 IU a day could help with calcium ion exchange, which is needed for nerve conduction. Hydergine can be prescribed by your physician in the range of 5 to 20 mg a day, and deprenyl at a dose of 5 mg taken twice a week.

Product availability: The essential fatty acids Mega-EPA and Mega-GLA along with alpha lipoic acid, vitamin D3, vitamin E, choline, inositol, Cognitex, vitamin D3 and Life Extension Mix can be ordered by calling 1-800-544-4440. Your doctor can prescribe hydergine and deprenyl. If you want to order these products by mail from low-cost offshore pharmacies, call 1-800-544-4440 to ask for a list of companies that ship medicines to Americans for personal use only.

Nails

Nails are composed of a protein called keratin, woven together by the sulfur-containing amino acid cysteine. When nails don't grow properly or have other abnormalities, it is often caused by a nutritional deficiency:

1) A lack of vitamin A and calcium causes dryness and brittleness.

2) A vitamin B deficiency causes fragility with horizontal and vertical ridges.

3) A vitamin B12 deficiency leads to rounded and curved nails.

4) A lack of protein, folic acid and vitamin C causes hangnails.

5) A lack of "friendly bacteria" (lactobacillus) leads to fungus under and around the nails.

6) A deficiency in hydrochloric acid contributes to splitting nails.

7) Low iron can cause "spoon" nails and/or vertical ridges.

We suggest the following:

✔ Life Extension Mix — Three tablets, three times a day, with food.

✔ Biosil — six drops orally per day.

✔ Designer Protein — two servings per day.

✔ L-cysteine — 1,000 mg per day.

✔ Biotin — 2,000 mcg a day

Product availability: Life Extension Mix, biosil, designer protein, l-cysteine and biotin can be ordered singly or in a Protocol Pak by calling 1-800-544-4440.

Neuropathy

Neuropathies involve inflammation and wasting of the nerves, often manifested in severe chronic pain and weakness. Neuropathies can be caused by diabetes, poisoning, FDA-approved drugs, viruses, bacteria and other factors.

Nutrients used to treat neuropathies are acetyl-L-carnitine at a dose of 1,000 mg twice a day and alpha lipoic acid at a dose of 400 mg twice a day.

Essential fatty acids are recommended at a dose of five to eight capsules a day of Mega-EPA fish oil concentrate and four to five capsules a day of Mega-GLA borage oil concentrate.

To suppress free radical injury to nerve fibers, take the 52-ingredient Life Extension Mix at a dose of three tablets, three times a day.

DHEA may be of help in some cases of neuropathy. Refer to DHEA Precautions and dosage suggestions before using DHEA.

Product availability: Acetyl-L-carnitine, alpha lipoic acid, Mega-EPA, Mega-GLA, DHEA and Life Extension Mix can be ordered by calling 1-800-544-4440.

Obesity (Weight Loss)

The Life Extension Foundation does not have a permanent cure for obesity, but we offer several innovative therapies that can make the success of various drugs, psychiatric care, and other obesity therapies more effective. Refer to the Foundation's Weight Loss protocols to find therapies that enhance the efficacy of an anti-obesity program.

Organic Brain Syndrome

Refer to the Life Extension Foundation's protocols for Alzheimer's Disease.

Osteoporosis

Osteoporosis is characterized by the loss of bone density to the point that small holes appear in the bones. It can cause pain, especially in the lower back, fractured bones, loss of body height and bone deformity.

Osteoporosis occurs because of hormonal imbalances that interfere with bone forming cells, called osteoblasts, which pull calcium, magnesium and phosphorous from the blood in order to build bone mass. Osteoblasts require the hormone progesterone. The other hormones that promote bone-forming osteoblasts are DHEA, melatonin, growth hormone and vitamin D3.

To maintain youthful bone-forming capability during and after menopause, women should be on progesterone replacement therapy. The most effective progesterone therapy may be a topical natural progesterone cream. Pre-menopausal women should use ¼ to ½ teaspoon daily starting at day-15 of their menstrual cycle, until the end of the menstrual cycle. Post-menopausal women should use ¼ to ½ teaspoon of topical progesterone cream once daily. Those with severe osteoporosis should use ½ teaspoon morning and night for the first jar of natural progesterone cream, then ¼ teaspoon morning and night for the second jar.

Natural progesterone cream should be applied to different areas of the skin with each application to prevent saturation of the fat cells in any one area of the body. It should be rubbed on the wrists, the face, the breasts, the underarms and thighs.

Pregnenolone is a hormone that breaks down into DHEA, progesterone, estrogen and testosterone. Women may be able to get some or all of the combined benefits of topically applied progesterone cream and estrogen/DHEA/testosterone replacement by taking 50 to 200 mg a day of pregnenolone.

DHEA can stimulate osteoblast activity and boost estrogen levels to help prevent bone loss.

Most women use 15 mg of DHEA, three times a day. Refer to DHEA Precautions before using DHEA or pregnenolone.

Estrogen is beneficial for bones because it promotes the action of osteoclasts, which remove dead portions of demineralized bone. DHEA may produce enough estrogen to maintain youthful osteoclast activity.

Women over the age of 35 or 40 should consider taking melatonin in the range of 500 mcg to 6 mg every night to help prevent osteoporosis and reduce the carcinogenic risks associated with estrogen replacement therapy. Refer to the Life Extension Foundation's protocol on Estrogen Replacement Therapy for more information.

Blood tests can help to determine optimal individual dosing of these hormone replacement therapies. As can be seen from our hormone replacement recommendations, calcium supplementation is only part of our osteoporosis prevention and treatment program. The Life Extension Foundation recommends that women take between 1,000 and 1,500 mg of elemental calcium along with 600 to 1,000 mg of elemental magnesium every day, plus about 1,000 IU of vitamin D3 to insure optimal calcium absorption. A woman can obtain these high doses of elemental minerals as well as vitamin D3 by taking the standard dose of Life Extension Mix every day along with six capsules of the Mineral Formula For Women. Life Extension Mix also provides other vitamins and minerals required to maintain youthful bone density.

A number of women take calcium tablets, but calcium is a strong binding agent that is often difficult to break down in the digestive tract. Calcium capsules, however, burst open in the stomach within five minutes for quick absorption into the bloodstream.

For those with severe osteoporosis, higher amounts of calcium and vitamin D3 may be required, along with a 6-month regimen of growth hormone replacement therapy. A parathyroid hormone (PTH) test must be performed to see if calcium is leaving the bones, i.e., the process of demineralization is occurring. An elevated PTH level indicates the possibility of osteoporosis, secondary to calcium deficiency. You can order blood tests by mail by calling 1-800-544-4440.

Effective alternatives to estrogen drugs are natural estrogens derived from plants. Refer to the Estrogen Replacement protocols for more information.

Product availability: Progesterone cream, DHEA, pregnenolone, Natural Estrogen, Mineral Formula For Women, vitamin D3, Life Extension Mix and melatonin can be obtained by calling 1-800-544-4440. If you need growth hormone replacement therapy, ask for doctors who have expertise in this area. Call the Life Extension Foundation at 1-800-544-4440 for information on blood testing.

Pain

The Life Extension Foundation's fundamental protocol for pain management is to eradicate the underlying cause of chronic pain. You should, therefore, first consider the specific condition causing your pain, such as arthritis, and refer to the protocol for this condition.

For general pain relief, some people find that boosting brain levels of the endorphins can provide natural pain suppression. This approach isn't an effective way of dealing with acute pain, but is the safest method of alleviating chronic pain.

By taking 500 mg of the nutrient amino acids dl-phenylalanine or 500 mg of tyrosine two to three times a day, you can raise your brain endorphin levels to reduce, and perhaps eliminate, chronic pain of almost any type.

CAUTION: Before starting on such a pain-management program, refer to our Phenylalanine Precautions.

Recent studies have shown that the pineal gland hormone melatonin has natural pain suppressing properties. For nighttime pain relief, 3 to 10 mg of melatonin should be taken before bedtime. Melatonin should only be used at night before bedtime, not during the day.

Refer to the Migraine Protocol for more information on melatonin's pain-relieving properties.

Product availability: Dl-phenylalanine, melatonin and tyrosine are available singly or in a Protocol Pak by calling 1-800-544-4440.

Parathyroid (Hyperparathyroidism)

Too much parathyroid hormone is clinically defined as hyperparathyroidism. The excess parathyroid hormone pulls calcium from the bones, which overloads the blood system with excessive amounts of calcium. Many long-term degenerative diseases have been linked to this type of calcium imbalance.

A standard blood-chemistry test can reveal elevated calcium levels caused by hyperparathyroid disease. Only a PTH (parathyroid hormone) blood test can effectively diagnose hyperparathyroidism. People who do not have regular blood tests usually find out they have hyperparathyroidism when a bone suddenly breaks, a kidney stone develops, or when their kidneys fail altogether.

Surgery is necessary when there is a parathyroid tumor that causes the overproduction of parathyroid hormone. There are diagnostic procedures (MRI, CT scan, sonography) to determine if the excess parathyroid hormone is caused by a tumor or by a vitamin D3/calcium deficiency. If your blood test is high in calcium and parathyroid hormone, that also may be an indication of hyperparathyroidism.

The first step in countering parathyroidism is to take 4,000 IU of vitamin D3 every day along with 2,000 mg of elemental calcium. This much calcium and vitamin D3 will act as a signal to your parathyroid glands to stop producing so much parathyroid hormone. When your bloodstream is loaded with calcium, your parathyroid glands will no longer have to pull it from your bones to guarantee proper calcium metabolism. Many people undergo surgery to remove one or more parathyroid glands when all they need do is to take calcium and vitamin D3.

Product availability: Vitamin D3 and an encapsulated calcium-mineral formula called Mineral Formula For Women can be ordered by phoning 1-800-544-4440.

Parkinson's Disease

For every decade we live past age 40, we lose on average of about 10% of our dopamine-producing brain cells. Once 80% of these brain cells have died, Parkinson's disease is often diagnosed. Parkinson's disease is characterized by uncontrolled muscle tremors, rigidity, depression, weakness and an unsteady gait.

Studies have shown that if healthy people take antioxidants throughout most of their lives, their risk of acquiring Parkinson's disease is reduced considerably. However, when Parkinson's patients are given vitamin E by itself there is no slowdown in disease progression. Since Parkinson's patients have already sustained massive damage to crucial brain cells, aggressive multiple therapies are required to have a chance of significantly slowing the natural progression of the disease.

The Life Extension Foundation's protocol for Parkinson's disease is based on studies showing that low doses of several drugs work better than high doses of a single drug. The Foundation receives updates from its members about the efficacy or lack of efficacy of the therapies it recommends. We would appreciate hearing from as many Parkinson's patients, their families or doctors about the effects of our Parkinson's disease protocol. The 14 components that comprise this protocol are suggested because of evidence of their safety and efficacy in treating the multiple underlying neurological disorders linked to the disease.

1) Bromocriptine — Lowest effective dose to begin with. Usually 1.25 mg a day. May be withheld until later in the disease phase.

2) Sinemet (controlled release) and/or Sinemet (L-dopa plus a dopa decarboxylase inhibitor) — Lowest effective dose to begin with. Some doctors withhold Sinemet until later in the progression of the disease in order to give the Parkinson's patient more time to benefit from Sinemet before its effects wear off.

3) Amantadine — Lowest effective dose to begin with. Usually 300 mg a day.

4) Deprenyl — Lowest effective dose to begin with. Between 1.25 and 5 mg a day. Deprenyl dosing has been significantly reduced based on studies showing that high doses of deprenyl may be detrimental to Parkinson's patients.

5) Hydergine — 10 to 20 mg every day.

6) Acetyl-L-carnitine — 1,000 mg, twice a day.

7) Phosphatidylserine — 200 mg, twice a day.

8) NADH — 5 to 10 mg, twice a day.

9) DHEA — 100 mg three times a day and/or pregnenolone, 50 mg, three times a day. Pregnenolone is a DHEA precursor.

10) Coenzyme Q10 — 100 mg, three times a day.

11) Life Extension Mix — three tablets, three times a day. Avoid if taking Sinemet because the vitamin B6 in Life Extension Mix can prevent L-dopa from reaching the brain. Take other antioxidants in place of Life Extension Mix that do not contain vitamin B6.

12) Melatonin — 3 to 10 mg, every night at bedtime.

13) Life Extension Booster — one capsule, twice a day.

14) Human growth hormone — two IU daily, by injection

This protocol attempts to cover the many neurological problems, neurochemical imbalances, and hormonal deficiencies associated with Parkinson's disease. While the drug and some of the hormone therapies in this protocol have to be carefully monitored, the nutrient therapies can be used safely on a regular basis to help protect and improve overall neurological functions.

Product availability: DHEA, melatonin, pregnenolone, acetyl-L-carnitine, Life Extension Mix, Life Extension Booster, NADH, Cognitex, LECI-PS (phosphatidylserine) and coenzyme Q10 can be ordered by phoning 1-800-544-4440. A neurologist should carefully prescribe the other medications. Call 1-800-544-4440 if you need a referral to a physician knowledgeable in the use of growth hormone therapy.

Phenylalanine and Tyrosine Precautions

There are some people who cannot use the amino acid phenylalanine. This includes those born with a genetic deficiency that prevents them from metabolizing phenylalanine (Phenylketonuria or PKU), those with high blood pressure, and people with cancer. Phenylalanine and tyrosine can promote cancer cell division, especially malignant melanoma.

Phobias

Phobias are common. Surveys have shown that more than half of those surveyed admit to having one or more phobias. People become phobic when the adrenal glands release large amounts of adrenaline and the brain releases its own form of adrenaline, norepinephrine, an excitatory neurotransmitter that stimulates cells in the brain and other parts of the body. Epinephrine initiates its effects by binding to beta-adrenergic sites on the cell membrane.

By taking a beta-blocking drug before a phobia-inducing event, such as public speaking, the excess adrenaline and norepinephrine will not create the anxiety, shaking, heart palpitations, sweating and queasy stomach that characterize a phobia. The first beta-blocking drug was propranolol, and it has more than 30 years of clinical use to document its safety.

Propranolol is available in low-cost generic form. The suggested dose is 10 to 40 mg of propranolol before a phobia-inducing event such as flying in an airplane or meeting new people. People with very low blood pressure, certain forms of congestive heart failure, and asthma should not take propranolol or other beta-blocking drugs. Nutritionally, vitamin B3 (niacin) and calcium may be beneficial.

Product availability: Propranolol is a prescription drug. For a listing of knowledgeable physicians in your area who will prescribe propranolol to treat phobia, call 1-800-544-4440. Vitamin B3 (niacin) is available by calling 1-800-544-4440.

Pregnenolone Precautions

Since pregnenolone is converted into DHEA within the body, some of our precautions for DHEA may apply to pregnenolone. For some people, pregnenolone may raise DHEA serum levels to reduce the need for DHEA supplementation.

Women may experience an increase in progesterone after taking pregnenolone, which may eliminate the need for natural progesterone cream and progestin drugs. Proper blood testings of various hormones will reveal the likely metabolic pathway in each individual. Refer to DHEA Precautions for more information.

Premenstrual Syndrome

Refer to the Menstrual Disorders-Premenstrual Syndrome (PMS) protocol.

Prevention Protocols

If you are healthy now and want to stay that way, the Life Extension Foundation has designed protocols that incorporate the most scientifically substantiated disease-preventing nutritional formulas.

The Foundation's Prevention Protocols consist of the Top 11 most important supplements for the average person to take every day to reduce their risk of contracting the degenerative diseases of aging. Remember, Prevention Protocols are for healthy people. Those seeking to treat an existing disease can refer to the other protocols in this book.

The following Prevention Protocols are listed *in order of importance*:

Recommendation No. 1: Life Extension Mix

Life Extension Mix is a super-potent formula containing 52 different vegetable extracts, vitamins, minerals, amino acids, herbal extracts and other unique antioxidants that cannot be found in any other multi-nutrient product.

Life Extension Mix saves people time and money by combining the most popular nutrient supplements into one product, thus enabling most people to eliminate the need to take many separate bottles of B-complex, vitamins C and E, mineral supplements, etc.

The Life Extension Foundation mandates that the ingredients in Life Extension Mix come only from pharmaceutical-grade suppliers such as Roche and Indena. These premium companies charge a lot more for their vitamin C, grape-seed extract, etc., but the pharmaceutical purity of these nutrients greatly exceeds the lower-cost generic versions that are so prevalent in the vitamin industry.

Life Extension Mix is the cornerstone of a comprehensive supplement program because it provides so many different disease-preventing nutrients. If you are on a budget, Life Extension Mix will provide you with more disease-preventing nutrients per dollar spent than any other product on earth.

Dosage: Three tablets at breakfast, three tablets at lunch and three tablets at dinner.

Recommendation No. 2: Life Extension Booster

Some nutrients are so well-documented to prevent disease that many people want to take even higher amounts than are contained in Life Extension Mix. The Life Extension Booster contains many important nutrients that cannot fit into the tightly packed Life Extension Mix formula.

Life Extension Booster is designed to be a convenient, low-cost method of obtaining the most important disease-preventing nutrients in just one capsule. The cost of these pharmaceutical-grade ingredients if bought separately would be much higher than what members pay for Life Extension Booster.

Dosage: One capsule a day with a meal.

Recommendation No. 3: Coenzyme Q10

One of the most researched disease-preventing nutrients is coenzyme Q10. The Life Extension Foundation was the first organization to introduce coenzyme Q10 to the American public, and since then hundreds of new studies have appeared in the scientific literature documenting the multiple life extension benefits of this versatile nutrient.

Coenzyme Q10 absorbs into the bloodstream much better when it is in an oil base. For this reason, we suggest that coenzyme Q10 be taken as a separate oil-based supplement. Most dry powder coenzyme Q10 supplements only absorb into the bloodstream at about half the rate of oil-based coenzyme Q10. Since coenzyme Q10 is a relatively expensive product, it makes sense to take it in an oil base.

Dosage: 30 to 100 mg daily with meals.

Recommendation No. 4: Melatonin

For people over age 40, melatonin may be the most-effective overall disease-preventing agent available, yet it costs virtually nothing.

Melatonin has been shown in hundreds of published studies to reduce the risk of numerous degenerative diseases, boost immune function, inhibit cancer-cell proliferation and slow aging. Many people take an average of 3 mg a night of melatonin to sleep better. If you are over 40 and sleep fine, we suggest taking only a 500 microgram (mcg) capsule of melatonin at bedtime. People over age 50 may consider higher doses of melatonin for disease prevention.

Dosage: 500 mcg to 3 mg at bedtime.

Recommendation No. 5: Trimethylglycine (TMG)

Trimethylglycine, or TMG, provides unique biological effects that make it a critical component of a disease-prevention program. TMG facilitates youthful methylation metabolism. Published research shows three specific benefits of enhancing methylation:

1) Methylation lowers dangerous homocysteine levels, thus lowering the risk of heart disease and stroke. Methylation is the primary process by which homocysteine is transformed into non-toxic compounds such as S-adenosylmethionine (SAM).

2) Methylation produces SAM, which may have potent anti-aging effects, and has been shown to alleviate depression, remylenate nerve cells, improve

Alzheimer's and Parkinson's disease patients, and protect against alcohol-induced liver injury.

3) Methylation protects DNA. Protecting DNA may slow cellular aging.

Enhancing methylation improves health and slows premature aging, and perhaps normal aging as well. Published research shows that methylation is related to a variety of disease states, including cardiovascular disease, cancer, liver disease, and neurological disorders.

Trimethylglycine is the most effect methylation-enhancing agent known.

Dosage: One to three tablets daily with meals.

Recommendation No. 6: Cognitex, Ginkgo And Other Neurological Enhancing Nutrients

Brain aging is a leading cause of disease, disability and death in the elderly. Healthy people seeking to slow down brain aging often notice cognitive-enhancing effects in response to Cognitex and ginkgo.

Slowing brain aging is the reason most people contact the Life Extension Foundation. While the antioxidants found in Life Extension Mix and Life Extension Booster protect against free radical damage to brain cells, there are other mechanisms of brain cell aging that may be prevented by nutrients such as phosphatidylserine, choline, pregnenolone and other components of the Cognitex formula.

If you take Life Extension Mix, you automatically receive ginkgo extract, so you do not need to take this expensive encapsulated nutrient separately.

Dosage: Five Cognitex capsules early in the day. One 120 mg ginkgo cap early in the day.

Recommendation No. 7: Saw Palmetto for Men, Mineral Formula for Women

Prostate enlargement is an inevitable consequence of aging for most men. An extract from the saw palmetto berry may prevent benign prostatic hypertrophy and possibly reduce the risk of prostate cancer.

Dosage: One capsule in the morning, one capsule in the afternoon or evening.

For women, osteoporosis is a common consequence of aging. In order to prevent bone loss, calcium supplements are often used. The problem is that most doctors don't know that osteoporosis is caused by a wide range of nutrient deficiencies, including deficiencies in magnesium, vitamin D3, and the hormones DHEA and progesterone. For calcium to prevent bone loss, adequate amounts of vitamin D3 and progesterone have to be available so that calcium, magnesium and phosphorous will be incorporated into the bone matrix.

Calcium tablets often fail to break down in the digestive tract, which is why the Mineral

Formula for Women is in capsule form. The capsules burst open within five minutes of swallowing, making the minerals and vitamin D3 immediately available for absorption into the bloodstream for incorporation into the bone.

Mineral Formula for Women contains the forms of calcium that have been shown to help prevent bone loss, compared to inexpensive calcium carbonate.

Dosage: five to nine capsules, preferably before bedtime.

Recommendation No. 8: Soy Extract

When Asians move to the United States and reduce their intake of soy, their risks of many forms of cancer increase substantially, even when other risk factors, such as higher fat diets, are taken into account. Soy consumption has been linked to significant decreases in cancer incidence, osteoporosis, menopausal discomfort and a host of other diseases that are prevalent in the Western world.

It is difficult for Americans to include enough soy in their daily diets to prevent disease. A product called Soy Power contains a standardized extract of isoflavones such as genistein, along with a wide range of anti-cancer phytochemicals such as saponin and lignan. Soy Power also provides essential fatty acids that are required for optimal health.

The standardized isolavones in Soy Power have natural estrogenic properties that enable some women to decrease or eliminate estrogen prescription drugs. Unlike FDA-approved estrogen drugs that have been shown to increase breast, ovarian and uterine cancer risks, natural estrogens have been shown to protect against reproductive cancers.

Dosage: Five tablets or one teaspoon a day.

Recommendation No. 9: Life Extension Herbal Mix

Numerous published studies show that specific herbal extracts can prevent a wide range of degenerative diseases and boost cognitive function. Life Extension Herbal Mix contains some of the best-documented herbals including green tea extract, gingko extract, grape-seed extract, bilberry extract, licorice extract and ginseng extract, along with 21 other disease-fighting phytochemicals such as chlorella and soy.

Herbal extracts are expensive because a large quantity of organic plant has to be used to produce a minute quantity of the pharmaceutical extract. Some members take only Life Extension Herbal Mix several times a week in order to reduce the monthly cost.

Dosage: One tablespoon early in the day, with or without food.

Recommendation No. 10: Garlic

Garlic is one of the better documented disease-preventing nutrients. Published studies have shown that garlic prevents cancer, boosts immune function and protects against many forms of cardiovascular disease. Garlic is left out of Life Extension Herbal Mix because it would adversely affect the taste of the product.

Dosage: Dependent on strength of particular brands.

Recommendation No. 11: Aspirin

The greatest cause of death and disability is an abnormal clot that develops inside an artery to cause a heart attack or a thrombotic stroke. While many of the nutrients included in the Prevention Protocols will reduce the risk of an abnormal blood clot forming inside a blood vessel, there is still a disease-preventing benefit for most people taking just one-quarter of one regular aspirin tablet every day with a heavy meal.

Low-dose aspirin prevents blood clots from forming inside arteries by a unique mechanism that is will-documented in the scientific literature.

Product availability: Life Extension Mix, Life Extension Booster, coenzyme Q10, melatonin, Trimethylglycine (TMG), Cognitex, ginkgo biloba, saw palmetto extract, Mineral Formula for Women, Soy Power, Life Extension Herbal Mix, garlic products and ¼ aspirin tablets (Healthprin) can be ordered by phoning 1-800-544-4440.

Prostate Cancer (Early Stage)

Unlike most forms of cancer, early-stage prostate cancer is almost completely controllable with complete hormone-blocking therapy. The drugs used to contain early-stage prostate cancer are FDA-approved, yet a recent survey showed that only 13% of urologists are using hormone-blocking therapy properly in early-stage prostate cancer patients.

If your PSA level is less than 11, the odds are that the cancer is confined to the prostate sack. Even if your PSA is over 11, there is still a good chance that the combination of FDA-approved hormone blocking therapy along with our innovative cancer treatment protocols can result in long-term remission. You should institute a three- to nine-month course of complete hormone blockade by using the FDA-approved drug Casodex and then receiving a pellet implant of FDA-approved Lupron a week later. This combination therapy should reduce your PSA level to less than 1 after only a few months. Casodex is taken every day and the Lupron pellets re-administered every three months.

When taking Casodex, it should first be taken orally for one week prior to an injection of Lupron that will last for three months. Many urologists do not know that Lupron causes a temporary prostate cancer cell flare up if Casodex (or Flutamide) is not first given one week prior to Lupron's administration.

For many years, the Foundation has advocated that prostate cancer patients first try three to nine months of complete hormone blockade before considering any permanent therapies.

The rationale is to shrink the prostate cancer volume by inhibiting testosterone production and blocking testosterone receptor sites on prostate cells. Testosterone is responsible for most prostate cancer cell proliferation. Blocking testosterone will cause an elevated PSA blood reading to drop to virtually zero within two months. The reduced PSA is indicative of a significant drop in prostate cancer cell activity. The PSA (Prostate Specific Antigen) test is an extremely accurate measure of prostate cancer cell activity. Peer-reviewed studies show that hormone blocking therapy instituted before aggressive therapy significantly increases your chances of a "cure!"

Studies have shown that prolactin may also be involved in prostate growth, and a rising serum level of prolactin indicates progression in patients with advanced prostate cancer.

The presence of prolactin receptors in prostate cancer cells may facilitate the entry of testosterone into prostate cells. Since testosterone-blocking therapies do not completely eliminate testosterone from the blood, it is conceivable that prolactin could carry a small amount of residual testosterone into the prostate cells and cause cancer growth. Suppressing prolactin secretion with relatively safe prescription drugs thus appears to be another method of slowing the progression of prostate cancer.

In a study in the *European Journal of Cancer* (Vol 31A, No. 6, 1995), the use of a pro-lactin suppressing drug (bromocriptine) with flutamide and orchiectomy (surgical removal of the testes) resulted in a 61-percent suppression of primary prostate growth, compared with only a 48-percent reduction with orchiectomy and flutamide only. After 36 months, only 40 percent of the group receiving bromocriptine and orchiectomy/flutamide experienced disease progression, compared to 60 percent in the orchiectomy/flutamide-only group. Most prostate cancer patients, understandably, prefer taking the drug Lupron instead of undergoing orchiectomy. Lupron may be more effective than orchiectomy.

Prostate cancer patients should have their prolactin levels checked via a blood test. If your prolactin levels are elevated, you should consider one of the following prescription drug regimens prescribed by a physician:

- ✔ Bromocriptine, 5 mg one to two times a day; or
- ✔ Pergolide, 0.25 mg to 0.5 mg twice a day; or
- ✔ Dostinex, 0.5 mg twice a week

Check your prolactin levels again in 30 days to make sure the drug you choose is, in fact, suppressing prolactin release from the pituitary gland into your blood.

Dostinex is the newest and cleanest drug to use. Dostinex has fewer side effects than the older drugs, is more effective in suppressing prolactin than the older drugs, and requires dosing only twice a week.

If a person continuously stays on hormone blocking therapy, after four years the prostate cancer cells will mutate to a new form of cancer cell that will not need testosterone to proliferate. Once the cancer cells become "androgen-independent," the prostate cancer is usually out of control and will freely metastasize throughout the body.

The Foundation has been recommending only a three- to nine-month course of Casodex and Lupron therapy. Prolactin suppression therapy may be continued longer. During this period, it is suggested that innovative cancer control therapies be incorporated to see if long-term remission can be achieved. Prostate cancer patients usually take two tablespoons a day of Super Soy Extract powder along with about 4,000 IU of vitamin D3, four saw palmetto extract capsules and as much as the Foundation's published Cancer Treatment protocol as possible. The Foundation especially recommends that prostate cancer patients take four to ten decaffeinated green tea extract capsules each day.

Before and after hormone-blocking therapy is discontinued, prostate cancer patients should take a PSA test every 30 days to see if the innovative cancer therapies are keeping the prostate cancer under control. Serum calcium and parathyroid hormone blood tests also are suggested to make sure that the relatively high daily doses of vitamin D3 are not causing toxicity.

In many cases, the PSA stays low after hormone-blocking therapy has been discontinued. If the PSA level does increase again to more than 4, the prostate cancer patient is then encouraged either to go on another three to nine month hormone-blocking regimen and alter their innovative cancer control regimen, or seek out a permanent solution such as enhanced radioactive seed implantation or cryoablation therapy. When a permanent remission is being sought, it is critical the prostate cancer patient have undetectable levels of PSA by previously being on a three- to nine-month hormone blocking therapy regimen.

In a study published in the *Journal of Steroid Biochemistry and Molecular Biology* (May 1996), prostate cancer was treated in mice with either continuous hormone-blocking therapy or the intermittent-hormone blocking regimen recommended by the Life Extension Foundation. The results showed that five to six cycles of intermittent hormone blockade were possible before the prostate cancer cells mutated to a form that did not need testosterone to proliferate. There was an initial 66% greater time period of prostate cancer cell control in the intermittent group compared with the group receiving continuous hormone blockade. In the late term of the study, the mice on intermittent hormone-blocking therapy had an astounding 3.78-fold reduction in their PSA levels compared to the mice receiving continuous hormone-blocking therapy.

This study showed that continuous hormone blocking therapy accelerates the rate at which prostate cancer cells become resistant to testosterone blocking therapy and that intermittent hormone blockade significantly increases the length of effectiveness of hormone blocking therapy in the long-term treatment of prostate cancer.

There are many prostate cancer patients following the Foundation's protocols with success. Individuals have personal decisions to make, based on a wide range of factors, regarding how they are going to deal with their prostate cancer in the long run. *Every* prostate cancer patient should consider three to nine months of complete hormone blockade before attempting any form of permanent therapy, such as surgery, radiation, cryoablation, radioactive seeds, etc.

Product availability: Super Soy extract, Soy Power, green tea extract, vitamin D3 capsules and saw palmetto extract can be ordered singly or in a Protocol Pak by phoning 1-800-544-4440.

Prostate Cancer
(Metastasized/Late Stage)

Refer to the Life Extension Foundation Cancer Treatment protocol. Follow hormone blocking therapies listed in the early-stage Prostate Cancer protocol if the prostate cancer cells have not become refractory to hormone blockade. Initiate prolactin suppression drug therapy if prolactin levels in the blood are even slightly elevated.

Prostate Enlargement
(Benign Prostatic Hypertrophy)

The benign enlargement of the prostate gland affects most men over the age of 60. The enlarged prostate blocks the flow of urine from the bladder which can produce mild to severe urinary obstruction. The inability to completely evacuate the bladder is especially troublesome at night. Men with prostate enlargement often complain about having to get up multiple times throughout the night to urinate. Benign prostate disease can mean a higher risk of prostate cancer in the future. The Life Extension Foundation's protocol to shrink enlarged benign prostate glands also is designed to reduce the future risk of prostate cancer.

One cause of prostate enlargement is overproduction of a hormone metabolite called dihydrotestosterone (DHT), which is considered a prime culprit in the development of benign prostate enlargement and, possibly, prostate cancer. The stimulating nature of dihydrotestosterone in the development of prostate disease is well-documented, since castration before age 40 prevents prostate enlargement and prostate cancer. Additionally, castration is a proven therapy to reverse both benign and malignant prostate disease. These findings suggest strongly that strategies to reduce DHT levels would prevent many forms of prostate disease.

The evidence that DHT is a cause of prostate disease came from observations in 1974 that men with low blood levels of DHT maintain normal muscle mass, libido and a small prostate compared to men with average DHT levels who suffer from enlarged prostates, frontal hair recession, diffuse beard growth and acne. It appears that DHT is responsible for many of life's undesirable ills affecting males. Testosterone is converted into DHT by the enzyme 5 alpha reductase, which increases as men grow older, causing elevated DHT production, decreased serum testosterone and enlargement of the prostate gland. When the action of 5 alpha reductase is blocked, dramatic reductions in DHT levels occur.

The reduction in DHT production via inhibition of 5 alpha reductase produces normalization of prostate volume and improvements in urinary and sexual function in men suffering from benign prostatic hypertrophy. Additionally, a decline in DHT could impact favorably on hairline recession, acne and excess facial hair. In females, testosterone is produced in the adrenal glands, and blocking dihydrotestosterone could be especially effective in ridding the patient of unwanted facial hair.

For many years, the Foundation has recommended the European drug Permixon as an effective therapy for benign prostatic hypertrophy. Permixon is a standardized extract from the saw palmetto berry. Permixon was used in Europe almost 20 years before the FDA approved an expensive drug called Proscar that can cause serious side effects in some men.

Permixon works via two primary mechanisms:

1) It blocks the enzyme 5 alpha reductase, thereby inhibiting the serum conversion of testosterone to dihydrotestosterone.

2) It blocks receptor sites on cell membranes that are required for the prostate cells to absorb DHT and testosterone.

By reducing serum DHT levels and displacing DHT and testosterone from prostate cells, the proliferation of prostate cells is inhibited, resulting in a reduction in prostate volume and in most cases, relief from the symptoms of prostate enlargement.

Studies have shown that saw palmetto produces significant improvement in those with prostate enlargement resulting in the following clinical benefits:

❖ Reduction of nocturnal urinary urgency
❖ Increased urinary flow rate
❖ Reduced residual volume in the bladder
❖ Reduction in uncomfortable urination symptoms

A paper in *Current Therapies, Research, Clinical Experience* reports on a Belgian study involving 505 men with benign prostate disease. The results showed that saw palmetto improved urinary flow, reduced residual urinary volume and prostate size, and improved quality of life after only 45 days of treatment. After 90 days, 88% of the patients and treating physicians considered the treatment effective. In addition, the study showed for the first time that saw palmetto does not mask the PSA score as Proscar has been shown to do. The researchers concluded by stating, "The extract of saw palmetto appears to be an effective and well-tolerated pharmacologic agent in treating urinary problems accompanying benign prostatic hypertrophy."

For most men, two saw palmetto extract capsules a day will shrink an enlarged prostate gland to provide relief from benign prostate disease. If this is not successful, a combination of saw palmetto extract and another European prostate medication called pygeum will provide relief in almost 90% of cases. Pygeum inhibits DHT and produces an anti-edema effect that can shrink enlarged prostate glands significantly.

For the 10% to 20% of men who do not obtain sufficient benefit from the saw palmetto and pygeum extracts, the addition of the prescription drug Hytrin has proven benefit. For those in whom all nutrient and drug therapies fail, temporary testosterone blockade of prostate cell receptor sites with the drug Casodex for three months may provide significant prostate gland shrinkage. Casodex is not approved by the FDA to treat benign prostatic hypertrophy, but your doctor can legally prescribe it.

Avoid the surgical procedure known as a transurethral resection. It involves the insertion of a device into the urethra, and the grinding away of part of the prostate gland. Many painful side effects can occur as a result of this procedure. There is a microwave procedure that appears to benefit those with severe benign prostatic hypertrophy. This newly approved procedure should be available soon in most cities.

Soy extract contain potent concentrations of phytoestrogens that counteract the effects of DHT. Men with enlarged prostate glands should take two heaping tablespoons a day of good-tasting soy extract powder.

Product availability: Saw palmetto extract, soy extract and saw-palmetto/pygeum extract are available by calling 1-800-544-4440. Hytrin, Lupron, and Casodex are drugs that should be prescribed by your doctor.

Pulmonary Insufficiencies

Refer to the Emphysema and Chronic Obstructive Pulmonary Disease protocols.

Retinopathy

Diseases of the eye, diagnosed as retinopathies, are often caused by nutrient deficiencies. Diabetic retinopathy, for example, has been shown to be caused by a deficiency of vitamin B6. In order to rule out a nutritional deficiency as a cause of retinopathy, it is suggested that three tablets, three times a day, of Life Extension Mix be taken for 10 weeks. Life Extension Mix contains 52 different high-potency nutrients, including the complete B-complex vitamins that are often deficient in retinopathies.

Product availability: Life Extension Mix can be ordered by calling 1-800-544-4440.

Seasonal Affective Disorder (SAD)

Research is being conducted to understand a depressive state that occurs when the days get shorter. The early loss of sunlight appears to induce chemical changes in the brain that bring on depression.

In some people, melatonin makes the symptoms of seasonal affective disorder worse. These people should stop melatonin or reduce its dosage during the times of the year when darkness appears early in the day.

Some people take prescription antidepressants, such as Prozac, only during the time of the year they are affected by seasonal affective disorder.

Refer to the Foundation's protocol for Depression. People who are afflicted with SAD should consider the Foundation's natural protocol before resorting to conventional antidepressant drugs.

Skin Aging

The most important thing to do to prevent skin aging is to protect your skin from exposure to ultraviolet (UV) light. That means wearing a sunscreen every time you go outdoors. If you look at the skin in areas of your body not exposed to the sun, you'll see that it is far more youthful than your face and hands which are chronically bombarded with UV light.

The oral intake of antioxidants, especially the proanthocyanidin flavonoid found in grape seed extract, can boost the production of collagen and elastin. Grape seed extract also provides broad-spectrum protection against damaging free radicals that cause proteins in the skin to crosslink and form wrinkles.

Vitamin C taken orally and applied topically enhances collagen production and protects against free radicals. The average dose of grape seed extract to protect against skin aging is 200 mg a day along with several thousand milligrams of vitamin C. The grape seed extract we recommend contains 50 mg of pharmaceutical-grade extract along with 250 mg of vitamin C from buffered calcium ascorbate.

The skin plays an important role in immune function. Boosting the health of the skin increases the natural rate of cell renewal and repair. Epidermal growth factors encourage young cells to replace old cells in the upper layers of the skin. The stimulation of epidermal growth factors is one of the mechanisms responsible for the anti-aging effects of the prescription drug Retin-A.

Aging causes the skin to lose moisturizing components such as NaPCA, lactic acid and hyaluronic acid, required for skin cells to retain moisture. Replacing these natural moisturizing factors topically can produce a youthful, moistening effect in dry, aged skin. Skin damaging free radicals can be suppressed by the topical application of antioxidants such as vitamin E, vitamin C and EDTA.

A well-documented mechanism of skin aging is the accumulation of dead cells at the surface of the skin. Young skin rapidly produces fresh skin cells that move to the surface to replace old, damaged cells, but aged skin forms a natural glue that binds to dead skin cells and prevents them from sloughing off.

The topical application of alpha-hydroxy fruit acids can gently remove dead cells at the surface of aged skin and more quickly expose the young cells underneath. The effects of the daily application of alpha-hydroxy fruit acids are to reduce the appearance of fine lines and enlarged pores, and expose more youthful appearing skin cells. The topical application of RNA and yeast cell wall extracts can stimulate greater production of youthful skin cells, thus potentiating the appearance-enhancing effect of the alpha-hydroxy acids.

You can purchase five or 10 different commercial products at very high prices that can provide these well-documented anti-aging factors, or you can obtain all of them in a product called Rejuvenex, which includes alpha-hydroxy fruit acids, the complete moisturizing complex, cell-renewing nutrients such as retinyl palmitate, RNA, and a special yeast cell-wall extract, topical antioxidant vitamins, epidermal growth factors, and a light sunscreen to protect against daily indoor and outdoor ultraviolet light exposure.

For those seeking a highly potent alpha-hydroxy skin product, a formula designed by Durk Pearson and Sandy Shaw called Look & Feel provides high concentrations of all the alpha-hydroxy fruit acids that have shown an anti-wrinkling effect.

Product availability: Rejuvenex, proanthocyanidins (grape seed extract), vitamin C and Look & Feel can be ordered by phoning 1-800-544-4440.

Stress

Refer to the Life Extension Foundation's Anxiety protocol.

Stroke (Hemorrhagic)

Twenty percent of strokes are caused by a rupture in an artery of the brain. Blood flow is disrupted to the area of the brain normally served by the ruptured artery, which usually results in paralysis or death. Hemorrhagic stroke can be caused by high blood pressure, an aneurysm in a brain artery or an overdose of blood thinning medication.

The acute treatment for hemorrhagic stroke is different from the treatment for stroke caused by a blood clot. That is why a CAT scan has to be done in a hospital setting to determine whether an apparent stroke has been caused by a ruptured artery or an arterial blood clot.

When a hemorrhagic stroke occurs, blood thinning agents like aspirin and ginkgo biloba have to be avoided. A hemorrhagic stroke not only deprives a portion of the brain of blood, but also causes massive free radical injury from the iron-rich blood that saturates brain cells.

The emergency room doctor should immediately administer 10 mg of hydergine sublingually and 10 mg of hydergine orally. Liquid hydergine should be avoided in treating hemorrhagic stroke because of its high alcohol content. Hydergine is a powerful antioxidant that helps to protect brain cells from free radical injury and death. More importantly, hydergine protects brain cells from oxygen deprivation and improves their ability to utilize oxygen, something that is critical when there a disruption of blood supply to an area of the brain.

In Europe, hydergine is administered on an acute-care basis to prevent permanent brain damage due to stroke. Since the FDA has not approved hydergine for acute stroke, most emergency room doctors are reluctant to prescribe it. You (or your medical surrogate) should insist on hydergine being administered when symptoms of an acute stroke are present. Hydergine should be readily available from the hospital pharmacy.

What will not be available from the hospital pharmacy is the European medication piracetam, which can protect brain cells against injury and death after interruption of blood. The administration of 4,800 mg of piracetam orally can provide considerable protection against permanent neurologic injury.

To learn about therapies that may strengthen the arteries in the brain to prevent hemorrhagic stroke, refer to the Life Extension Foundation's protocols on treating Cerebral Vascular Disease.

To learn about therapies that might help to restore neurological function lost to a hemorrhagic stroke, refer to the Life Extension Foundation's protocol for Age-Associated Mental Impairment (Brain Aging).

Product availability: You can order high-potency hydergine tablets and piracetam from offshore suppliers who ship to Americans for personal use. Some people keep hydergine in their medicine cabinet for emergency administration in case of a heart attack, stroke or accident. Many people take hydergine and piracetam every day to help prevent neurological aging. For a list of offshore sources for these drugs, phone 1-800-544-4440.

Stroke (Thrombotic)
(also Transient Ischemic Attack)

Eighty percent of strokes are caused by a blood clot that forms in an artery in the brain. The blood clot blocks the flow of blood to a portion of the brain resulting in paralysis or death. A stroke caused by a blood clot is called a thrombotic stroke, as opposed to stroke caused by a breakage in a cerebral artery, which is called a hemorrhagic stroke.

Underlying risk factors for thrombotic stroke are cerebral atherosclerosis, hypertension, excessive blood clotting factors such as fibrinogen and LDL cholesterol, heart valve defects, diabetes and aging. More than 400,000 Americans suffer a thrombotic stroke yearly. When a thrombotic stroke occurs, it is crucial to dissolve the blood clot blocking an artery in the brain.

The FDA has approved a clot-busting drug called TPA. You should insist that the emergency room doctor administer the drug TPA (sold under the brand name Activase) immediately in order to bust open the clot that is preventing blood from reaching a portion of your brain. TPA stands for tissue plasminogen activator. It is a natural clot-dissolving substance produced by your body.

TPA has saved the lives of hundreds of thousands of heart attack victims. However, the FDA took eight years to approve TPA as a treatment for thrombotic stroke. TPA has been used in progressive emergency rooms in the U.S. as an unapproved drug to treat thrombotic stroke. Patients may encounter severe resistance from emergency room doctors who are reluctant to administer it, even if a patient's life at stake. In the latest study, 30% more stroke victims were able to regain full use of their faculties after receiving TPA.

While TPA can bust open the blood clot that causes blood vessel blockage, there are other complications that occur during a thrombotic stroke that have to be addressed if permanent brain damage is to be prevented. Any interruption in blood flow causes an oxygen imbalance that results in massive free radical damage. It is critically important to have antioxidants in your bloodstream when TPA is administered to reduce the free radical damage that will occur when blood flow is restored.

The most potent antioxidant that hospital pharmacies normally stock is hydergine. You should insist that the emergency room doctor administer 10 mg of hydergine sublingually, and another 10 mg of hydergine orally in liquid form. Hydergine is a powerful antioxidant that reduces free radical damage. Hydergine will increase the amount of oxygen delivered to the brain, enhance the energy metabolism of brain cells, and protect brain cells against both the low and high oxygen environments that thrombotic stroke victims often encounter.

Hydergine is used routinely in Europe as a treatment for stroke, but most emergency room doctors in the U.S. are reluctant to prescribe it because the FDA does not recognize its value in preventing brain cell death. Paralyzed stroke victims consume billions of health care dollars every year. The reason that most thrombotic stroke victims are permanently paralyzed is that the FDA had stopped patients from being treated with medications to prevent brain cell death.

If you have access to the European drug piracetam when stroke symptoms occur, brain cell damage can be prevented or at least mitigated. Recommended dose is 4,800 mg of piracetam administered immediately. If you know a thrombotic stroke is occurring, large quantities of antioxidant vitamins and herbs such as ginkgo biloba would be of benefit.

The problem is, if it's a brain hemorrhage (hemorrhagic stroke) instead of a blood clot (thrombotic stroke), these nutrients could cause additional cerebral bleeding. Magnesium in an oral dose of 1,500 mg is a safe nutrient to relieve arterial spasm, a common problem in thrombotic stroke. If you take high-potency antioxidant nutrients at least three times a day, your chances of fully recovering from a thrombotic stroke would be vastly improved.

If you already suffer from brain-cell damage caused by a previous thrombotic stroke, please refer to the Life Extension Foundation's protocol on treating Age-Associated Mental Impairment (Brain Aging).

To learn how to prevent a stroke or transient ischemia attacks (TIAs), refer to the Atherosclerosis protocol .

Product availability: If you want to keep hydergine and piracetam in your medicine cabinet for emergency use during a heart attack, stroke or accident, phone 1-800-544-4440 for a list of offshore pharmacies that will ship these products by mail to Americans for personal use. Many people take hydergine and piracetam every day to prevent brain-cell injury due to normal aging.

Surgical Precautions

Refer to the Life Extension Foundation's Anesthesia And Surgery Precautions protocol.

Thyroid Deficiency

Many people over age 40 are thyroid deficient, but blood tests fail to detect this subtle hormonal deficit that can be a cause of weight gain, fatigue, immune impairment, adult onset diabetes and premature aging.

One way of detecting thyroid deficiency is to take your temperature about 30 minutes before lunch for seven days. If your temperature is consistently below 98.6 degrees F, you may be thyroid deficient. Drugs that can be prescribed to treat severe thyroid deficiency include Cytomel, Synthroid and Armour.

Natural therapies that may correct underlying thyroid deficiency include 1 mg a day of iodine, 500 to 1,000 mg of the amino acid tyrosine, 3 mg of melatonin at bedtime, 10 grams a day of soy extract (which provides at least 40 mg of genistein), and DHEA replacement therapy. An appropriate dose for men is 25 mg of DHEA, three times a day; an appropriate dose for women is 15 mg of DHEA, three times a day. Refer to DHEA Precautions before beginning DHEA therapy.

Correcting a thyroid deficiency can slow down some of the degenerative diseases associated with normal aging and help you lose weight. Natural therapies boost youthful levels of thyroxine, which is safer than replacing it with drugs such as Synthroid.

Product availability: Melatonin, tyrosine, Super Soy Extract powder or tablets and DHEA are available singly or in a Protocol Pak by calling 1-800-544-4440. Thyroid medication should be prescribed by a knowledgeable physician.

Tinnitus

Chronic ringing in the ears is a frequent complaint of the elderly that is clinically diagnosed as tinnitus. Some studies have shown that 120 to 240 mg a day of pharmaceutical-grade ginkgo biloba can alleviate tinnitus. Other studies fail to show benefits for ginkgo in treating this condition.

If ginkgo does not work, 10 to 15 mg a day of hydergine should be considered or 20 to 40 mg a day of vinpocetin, as there is some evidence that these neurologic-enhancing therapies can alleviate tinnitus in some people.

Product availability: To order pharmaceutical ginkgo biloba extract, phone 1-800-544-4440. Ask for a list of offshore suppliers who will ship high-potency hydergine and vinpocetin to Americans for personal use.

Trauma

Permanent injury or death due to trauma is often caused by free radicals generated when the tissues of the body are physically disrupted. This is well documented in spinal cord injury cases where the free radical damage that occurs immediately after the injury is what causes permanent paralysis.

Antioxidants should be immediately administered to most victims of trauma to protect against free radical injury. Trauma that involves massive bleeding may preclude the use of antioxidants such as ginkgo that could accelerate hemorrhaging.

To protect brain cells against oxygen deprivation or permanent damage from direct trauma to the head, 10 mg of sublingual hydergine should be immediately administered along with 10 mg of hydergine LC capsules. If piracetam is available, 4,800 mg of piracetam should be administered to further protect against brain damage.

In laboratory studies where two groups of animals were exposed to the same traumatic force, animals given high doses of vitamin C died less frequently than animals not given vitamin C. Antioxidants appear to protect against many forms of permanent damage inflicted by trauma.

The hormone pregnenolone has been shown to protect against paralysis from spinal cord injury in laboratory animals. The immediate administration of 400 mg of pregnenolone along with 800 IU of vitamin E to a spinal injury patient might be advisable. Vitamin E could speed the bleeding process, so do not use vitamin E if excessive bleeding is occurring.

Product availability: vitamin C, vitamin E and pregnenolone can be ordered by calling 1-800-544-4440. Call for a list of offshore companies that sell high-dose hydergine and piracetam to Americans for personal use.

Urinary Tract Infections

Chronic urinary tract infections cause discomfort to many people, especially women. The over-prescribing of antibiotics to treat recurring urinary tract infections often results in chronic yeast infections. The urinary tract is vulnerable to chronic bacterial infection because of the ability of bacteria to bind to the wall of the bladder and urethra.

Studies document that drinking eight glasses of cranberry juice twice a day can eradicate most urinary tract infections. As long as the cranberry juice is continued, the infections are not likely to return. Cranberry juice works by preventing bacteria from adhering to the linings of the urinary tract. Most people find it difficult to drink sixteen 8-ounce glasses of cranberry juice a day, but a there is a dietary supplement called Cranex Cranberry Juice Concentrate that provides the equivalent of eight 8-ounce glasses of cranberry juice in just one capsule. That means that people predisposed to urinary tract infections only need to take two capsules to consume the active ingredients in 16 glasses of cranberry juice.

Product availability: You can order Cranex Cranberry Juice Concentrate by calling 1-800-544-4440.

Valvular Insufficiency/Heart Valve Defects

There are many causes of heart valve defects and degeneration, ranging from congenital defects to age-associated calcification. Since heart-valve diseases are anatomical in nature, it is difficult to address the problem from a nutritional standpoint.

Leaky heart valves put a strain on the heart because blood is not being pumped efficiently through the chambers of the heart. To alleviate the burden placed on the heart by a defective valve, we suggest you follow the Congestive Heart Failure/Cardiomyopathy protocol.

Vertigo

Vertigo involves feelings of dizziness, faintness, and the inability to maintain normal balance in a sitting or standing position. There are many causes of vertigo, including ear infection, ear surgery or accidental injury to the ear.

If conventional medicine is unable to diagnose and treat vertigo, you may want to consider taking medications that can correct a neurological deficit that may be causing your vertigo. Some people have found that 5 to 10 mg a day of hydergine can be an effective therapy for vertigo. Other people have successfully used 2,400 to 4,800 mg of piracetam a day for this condition. A third option is to take 20 to 40 mg of vinpocetin a day.

Product availability: To obtain high-potency hydergine, piracetam, or vinpocetin, phone 1-800-544-4440 for a list of offshore suppliers who ship these products to Americans for personal use.

Weight Loss

Weight gain associated with aging is one of the most significant health problems in the Western world.

Obesity is an underlying risk factor for hypertension, adult-onset diabetes, heart disease, and stroke, and is a major cause of the overall loss of energy experienced by so many people.

People over age 30 often become overweight from a metabolic disorder, which makes it extremely difficult for them to slim down by dieting. The reason diets don't work is that dieting interferes with the ability of the body to burn sugar, and that blood sugar which is not used to generate energy is stored as body fat.

We tend to put on weight as we grow older in part because aging impairs our ability to metabolize carbohydrates. Since most food is eventually broken down into glucose (blood sugar), the age-related decline in our ability to metabolize glucose is a significant cause of degenerative disease and excessive weight gain associated with aging.

A cause of impaired carbohydrate metabolism is subclinical thyroid deficiency. Blood tests are not always reliable in diagnosing this condition. A study found that 18% of elderly people who were initially diagnosed as having normal thyroid levels were later found to have significant thyroid deficiency after undergoing extensive testing. Many physicians believe that most people over 40 suffer from a subclinical thyroid deficiency that contributes to their weight gain.

People start getting fat over the age of 30 for reasons that are just now beginning to be understood by the scientific community. Based upon newly emerging evidence, the Life Extension Foundation has developed a unique new fat loss strategy.

The thyroid gland secretes hormones involved in cellular energy expenditure. When you go on a diet, there is a decrease in thyroid hormone secretion that causes your body's metabolic rate to slow down. This decrease occurs because your thyroid gland thinks you are starving and tries to conserve energy until you find more food to eat.

Everyone who has ever dieted knows about the rebound effect. How your body resists losing weight while you "starve yourself," but then puts the weight back on with devastating quickness after you eat a little more. This is why dieting is such a miserable way to try to lose weight. Now you know why! It's because your thyroid gland fights you all the way by reducing your energy efficiency in order to keep you from losing weight!

This biological mechanism involving the thyroid gland, which evolved to counter the very real risk of starvation for hundreds of thousands of years, is what sabotages you in today's world of plenty when you deliberately eat less in an attempt to lose weight!

To give you an idea how your thyroid gland dictates how much you weigh, consider the fact that, when the thyroid produces too much thyroid hormone, the most common clinical symptom is the significant loss of weight! The name for the disease caused by an overactive thyroid gland is hyperthyroidism, and in 76% to 83% of cases, the patient's first complaint to their doctor is about how much weight they've been losing!

Clinical studies have consistently shown that dieting produces a decline in thyroid output resulting in a severe reduction in resting energy expenditure. This reduced metabolic rate prevents cells from burning calories to produce energy. If the cells do not take up glucose to produce energy, the sugar is stored as fat within the body. The *only* way dieting can produce significant long-term weight loss is for the cells to take up glucose for conversion into energy rather than into body fat!

One way of boosting thyroid function in order to lose weight and fight fatigue is to take supplemental thyroid hormone. People who have serious thyroid hormone deficiency should take it under the care of a doctor, but for most people the adverse side effects of supplementation with thyroid hormone outweigh the benefits.

While there are studies showing that thyroid supplementation promotes weight loss in some people, it can also kill you! Excessive thyroid hormone can cause rapid heart rate and atrial fibrillation that could lead to a heart attack or stroke. The problem is not thyroid deficiency per se, but that people become thyroid deficient in response to dieting. In short, thyroid supplementation doesn't always work and can be dangerous!

Later in this protocol, we're going to reveal a safe and effective natural way of losing weight by boosting your thyroid function without having to take thyroid hormone!

There are several reasons why thyroid hormone supplementation hasn't consistently produced weight loss in clinical studies:

1) Commercially available thyroid supplements may not provide all the thyroid hormones needed to restore optimal carbohydrate metabolism. When safe doses of thyroid supplements are given to dieters, their resting energy expenditure still does not approach their pre-diet level, even though measurable serum levels of thyroid hormone are up to 130% higher than pre-diet levels.

2) The thyroid supplements currently on the market have only been tested by themselves in clinical studies. When only one therapy is tested at a time without producing dramatic results, the therapy is considered useless. Thyroid deficiency is only one factor that works against successful weight loss in response to dieting.

3) Normal diets do not provide optimal levels of minerals. Dieting can cause severe deficiencies of chromium and magnesium. These deficiencies cause insulin resistance, which is a major factor in carbohydrate metabolic disorders. Chromium and magnesium must be present if thyroid hormone is to work synergistically with insulin to drive glucose into cells for energy production.

4) There are other hormones such as DHEA and pregnenolone that boost the effect of thyroid hormone on carbohydrate metabolism.

The scientific evidence shows that dieting induces a thyroid-deficient state which slows the body's metabolic rate. If body weight is to be controlled by diet, something must be done to safely boost thyroid hormone to near pre-diet levels.

There is more than 80 years of scientific research to document the ability of soy protein to lower blood fat levels. A study in the Aug. 3, 1995, issue of *The New England Journal of Medicine* showed that soy protein lowered LDL cholesterol by 12.9% and triglycerides by 10.5%.

One mechanism by which soy reduces blood fats is by boosting thyroid hormone levels. Studies show that thyroid hormone literally burns up LDL cholesterol globules in the blood!

Because of the many documented health benefits from soy intake, the Life Extension Foundation suggests that anyone seeking to lose weight safely through dieting take between 6 to 30 grams a day of soy protein concentrate. Soy protein not only boosts thyroid hormone levels to burn sugar calories, but also contains an amino acid complex that helps to spare the body's protein stores, which are often broken down in response to dieting. The phytoestrogens and essential fatty acids in soy further help to promote weight loss.

The Life Extension Foundation has recommended soy protein concentrates to cancer patients for many years. A highly concentrated soy extract has been introduced for the specific purpose of preventing cancer. This super-concentrated soy extract is quite expensive.

The Foundation has found a new soy product that is only slightly less concentrated than the expensive soy extract we've recommended for adjutant cancer treatment. This new soy extract, which is called Soy Power, costs 40% less than soy extract for cancer.

Soy Power provides eight to 10 times more of the active ingredients of soy than conventional soy extracts. Some of these ingredients are the phytoestrogens genistein and the newly identified anti-cancer agent saponin.

Soy Power comes in powder or tablets. The powder has a light, pleasant-tasting nutty flavor. If you consume 6 to 30 grams of Soy Power in water, you may be able to skip a meal because the soy protein, essential fatty acids and the natural soy fiber have a satiating effect.

Soy Power tablets contain 1,200 mg of soy extract. The suggested dose is at least six Soy Power tablets a day.

Soy intake is associated with significant reductions in the risk of many forms of cancer and in blood fat levels. Many Foundation members are already taking supplemental soy to reduce their risk of cancer, especially breast and prostate cancer. Now that soy extract prices are 40% lower, more people can use soy every day for weight loss purposes.

While thyroid hormone plays a definite role in weight management, the scientific literature makes it clear that both magnesium and chromium are required to break down the cellular insulin resistance that causes higher-than-normal blood sugar levels.

Overweight people usually suffer from insulin impairment that prevents the proper cell uptake of carbohydrates (sugars). Excessive serum glucose is converted into body fat unless this insulin resistance is broken down and the cells are able to regain youthful carbohydrate metabolism.

Chromium has received widespread publicity for its ability to lower serum glucose levels by potentiating insulin sensitivity. Studies have shown that chromium supplementation results in a slight reduction in body fat and an increase in lean body mass.

New studies indicate that niacin improves the metabolic enhancing effect of chromium picolinate. In response to this research, 30 mg of niacin has been added to the 200 mcg chromium picolinate capsules. This small amount of niacin does not usually cause a niacin flush, but does increase the effects of chromium picolinate.

To improve the fat-reducing effects of dieting, the Foundation now suggests that one capsule of this new chromium picolinate be taken with every meal to facilitate youthful carbohydrate metabolism. The importance of taking a chromium capsule with each meal is illustrated in animal studies in which chromium was given throughout the day in order to lower serum glucose levels. When you consume food, your serum glucose levels rise significantly unless your cells are sensitized to insulin. Chromium will help sensitize your cells to insulin by helping to lower your blood sugar levels.

You shouldn't take more than three chromium capsules a day, and should always take antioxidant supplements when you take chromium to protect against free radical activity.

While chromium has received the most media attention, the scientific literature shows that magnesium plays an even more important role in regulating carbohydrate metabolism. Magnesium is involved in a number of enzymatic reactions required for cells to uptake and metabolize glucose. Magnesium deficiency causes insulin resistance and elevated blood sugar levels.

About 80% of Americans are magnesium deficient. When they go on a diet, they become severely deficient in magnesium, which causes the insulin resistance that contributes to the failure of the diet. Life Extension Mix contains high amounts of magnesium. For those going on a calorie-restricted diet, it is suggested that at least one 500 mg magnesium capsule a day be taken in addition to the full dose Life Extension Mix.

When animals are given supplemental DHEA, they eat as much as they want and stay thin. Unfortunately, DHEA by itself does not produce the same dramatic weight loss in humans as it does in animals.

DHEA is an important anabolic hormone that works with thyroid hormone, chromium and magnesium to improve carbohydrate metabolism. For people over 35 years of age, DHEA replacement therapy is suggested as part of an overall weight management program.

The average dose of DHEA for men should be 25 mg of DHEA, three times a day. Women only need 15 mg of DHEA, three times a day. Many people now use pregnenolone in place of (or in addition to) DHEA because pregnenolone naturally breaks down into DHEA and other weight-regulating hormones in the body. The suggested dose for pregnenolone is 50 mg in three daily doses.

A New Diet

Based upon the evidence showing why diets don't work, the Foundation now recommends a program to help dieters achieve safe, long-lasting weight loss. Most of the foods we eat are broken down into glucose (blood sugar) in your bloodstream. In response to the buildup of serum glucose, a healthy pancreas secretes insulin to tell our cells to absorb glucose from our blood. These cells take up glucose from the bloodstream to produce energy. Most of the glucose that is not taken up by the cells for energy production is stored as fat. While glucose can be stored for future use in the liver and muscles, people who overeat overload their glucose storage capacity. Glucose is converted into excess body fat if the cells become resistant to insulin and are unable to utilize glucose.

Aging seldom affects the ability of the pancreas to secrete insulin, but it does cause cells to resist insulin's instructions to take up glucose. This age-related cellular disorder is called "insulin resistance." It occurs when cells fail to absorb glucose, even in the presence of high insulin levels.

Remember, diets fail because thyroid-hormone levels fall, causing the body to conserve calories rather than burning them as energy. Diets also fail because of chromium and magnesium deficiencies that preclude proper carbohydrate metabolism. Aging causes a decline in DHEA production, making weight loss even more difficult in people over 40. Thyroid and DHEA hormone replacement, along with chromium and magnesium supplementation are the missing links that prevent moderate calorie restriction from producing long-term weight loss.

If you seek to lose weight, the following program should help you accelerate fat loss and then help to maintain your desired weight level:

- ✔ Soy Power — To boost thyroid hormone; 6 to 30 grams a day powder or tablets.
- ✔ Chromium Picolinate — To enhance glucose update; one capsule with each meal consisting of 200 mcg chromium/30 mg niacin.
- ✔ Magnesium — To break down insulin resistance. At least one capsule a day, consisting of 500 mg elemental magnesium.
- ✔ DHEA and/or Pregnenolone — To build lean body mass and reduce body fat. Refer to DHEA Protocol.

If you reduce your food intake moderately, and follow this program, you'll reach your desired weight level, improve your overall health, and never have to starve yourself again to lose weight.

Additional Weight-Loss Products

A nutrient that can block the enzyme ATP citrate lyase, which is required to convert blood sugar into body fat, is hydroxycitric acid (HCA). The suggested dose of HCA is 250 mg with every meal along with 200 mcg of chromium to help drive the sugar not being converted into body fat into the cells.

An herbal extract called Gymnea sylvestri can help suppress cravings for carbohydrates. If you take 50 mg of Gymnea sylvestri extract three times a day, you may be able to increase your will power to avoid body fat-inducing sugars in your diet. For some people, excess blood sugar is not the reason they are overweight. The problem is that they eat too much dietary fat. This fat is readily absorbed into the bloodstream and is converted into body fat.

Fiber can block the absorption of dietary fat into the bloodstream. The newest fat absorbing fiber is chitosan, which is composed of the exoskeletons of shellfish and insects. Chitosan has an electrical charge that specifically binds to fat molecules, inhibiting their absorption into the blood. It is suggested that people who eat fatty meals take four to eight 250 mg chitosan capsules just before eating to help absorb fat.

Other fat absorbing fibers are guar gum, pectin and psyllium seed husks. A multi-ingredient formula, called the All-In-One Weight Loss Formula, has been developed to contain the proper amounts of chromium, hydroxycitric acid, Gymnea sylvestri and a fat-absorbing fiber complex of pharmaceutical-grade chitosan and fat-absorbing psyllium seed husk, guar gum and pectin.

The suggested dose is four to eight capsules of All-In-One Weight-Loss Formula with every meal. Nutritionists have designed super low-calorie meal replacement cookies and powders to help you avoid high-fat meals.

Product availability: Chromium picolinate with niacin, soy Power, magnesium, chitosan, DHEA and All-In-One Weight-Loss Formula can be ordered by phoning 1-800-544-4440.

Wound-Healing
(Surgical Wounds, Trauma, Burns)

There is strong evidence that at least two nutrients and one juice — the amino acid arginine, the trace metal zinc, and the juice from the aloe vera plant — can enhance wound-healing significantly. The typical western diet contains about 5 grams a day of arginine, mainly from meat, fish, poultry and dairy products. Under normal physiologic conditions, arginine is a substrate for protein synthesis, creatine synthesis and polyamine synthesis which is involved in the control of cell division. Arginine also is involved in a metabolic pathway in which it is converted into nitric oxide.

It is well-documented that, following traumatic injury, there is a significantly increased need for arginine for a variety of metabolic functions. Animal studies have demonstrated that, following surgical trauma, dietary supplementation with arginine results in an increase in nitrogen retention and increased body weight, both of which are essential for successful recovery from traumatic injury.

Studies in patients undergoing gall bladder surgery have shown that taking 15 grams per day of arginine for three days significantly reduces nitrogen excretion, compared to patients receiving conventional nutritional support. In patients with gastrointestinal malignancies undergoing surgery, 25 grams a day of arginine (for seven days) improved their nitrogen balance five to seven days after surgery.

In a study published in *Surgery*, 85 patients with gastrointestinal malignances receiving dietary supplementation with arginine, omega-3 fatty acids and RNA showed major improvement in nitrogen balance compared to patients receiving a standard nutritional regimen. Patients in the arginine group recovered more rapidly and were discharged sooner from the hospital.

Animal studies have shown that arginine speeds wound-healing via several different mechanisms.

In a clinical study, in the August 1990 of *Surgery*, scientists recruited 36 healthy volunteers from medical and non-medical hospital personnel. None of the subjects suffered from diabetes, smoked, or took drugs known to impair wound healing. The 36 subjects were randomly placed into three groups of equal size. Group I received 100 ml/day of an aromatic syrup as a placebo. Group II received 30 grams of arginine aspartate in 100 ml of aromatic syrup (the equivalent of 17 grams/day of free arginine). Group III received 30 grams of arginine hydrochloride in 100 ml of aromatic syrup (the equivalent of 24.8 grams/day of free arginine). All supplements were taken throughout the day for two weeks. On days zero, seven and 14, peripheral blood was drawn for analysis after an overnight fast.

On the first day of the study, all the subjects underwent the creation of a "standard wound" (5 cm long, one mm in diameter) after receiving a local anesthetic with a 12-gauge needle. A catheter was inserted into the wound with one end sutured and left protruding from the skin. The wound was then covered with an occlusive, transparent dressing which was changed during the study as needed.

The primary finding of the study was that in both arginine groups, there was a significant increase in the amount of reparative collagen synthesized at the site of the wound. The scientists concluded, "To our knowledge, this is the first instance in which collagen synthesis has been shown to be enhanced to 'supranormal' levels."

In the same study, there was also marked enhancement in the activity and effectiveness of peripheral T lymphocytes in the bloodstream. Other studies in animals have shown that dietary supplementation with arginine increases the weight of the thymus which is the master gland of immunity, and reduces shrinkage of the thymus after trauma and in normally aging animals. The benefits of arginine for thymic function have also been demonstrated by its ability to restore thymic endocrine function by increasing blood levels of thymulin, one of the hormones secreted by the thymus gland.

Growth hormone plays a critical role in modulating the action of the immune system, and is essential for muscle growth and development. One of the primary reasons that the functioning of the immune system *and* muscular strength both decline dramatically as we grow older is the progressive, precipitous decline in growth hormone secretion with advancing age! There is strong evidence that arginine's ability to improve both wound-healing and immune-system function are related to its ability to stimulate the release of growth hormone.

The role of copper in healing was first observed by a German physician (Dr. Rademacher) who noted that broken bones seemed to heal faster when patients were given a copper salt during convalescence. Since then, the need for copper in the biosynthesis of bone and connective tissues has been established. The Life Extension Foundation does not recommend copper as a dietary supplement because of the preponderance of evidence that long-term excessive copper intake generates too much free radical activity throughout the body. The evidence makes it clear that, while copper is important for health and wound healing, it is potentially harmful if its intake is excessive. On the other hand, the therapeutic, short-term use of copper to enhance wound healing in localized injury sites is both reasonable and appropriate.

To accelerate wound-healing, the Foundation recommends 10 to 22 grams of supplemental arginine a day along with 90 mg of zinc and 8 mg of copper. Extra amounts of vitamin C is also very important for proper functioning of enzyme protocollagen hydroxylase, which is essential for wound-healing. Supplemental nutrients obtained by taking three tablets of Life Extension Mix three times a day can also aid in wound-healing.

Product availability: You can obtain premium-grade arginine powders, tablets and capsules, zinc, Aloe vera, copper, vitamin C and Life Extension Mix singly or in a Protocol Pak by phoning 1-800-544-4440.

Yeast Infections

For suggestions on treating chronic yeast infections, refer to the Life Extension Foundation's protocol on Candida Infection.

Avoiding Vitamin A Toxicity

Based upon hundreds of published studies, The Life Extension Foundation has recommended vitamin A analogs to cancer patients. For the many cancer patients who cannot gain access to vitamin A analogs because the FDA classifies them as "unapproved new drugs," the Foundation has recommended the use of **water-soluble vitamin A liquid drops**.

The dosage range of vitamin A lipid drops that cancer patients have been using is between 100,000 and 200,000 IUs a day. The Foundation has cautioned that these high doses could produce toxicity if taken over extended periods of time, yet cancer patients are often forced to risk some degree of toxicity to obtain an effective dose of vitamin A.

Anyone taking very high doses of vitamin A for cancer or any other reason should do so under the care of a physician, and should be on the lookout for symptoms of vitamin A toxicity. The following are common symptoms of vitamin A overdose that should be watched for in cancer patients taking high doses of any vitamin A product:

1) **Headache**
2) **Dizziness**
3) **Blurred vision**
4) **Joint pain**
5) **Dry lips**
6) **Scaly-dry skin**
7) **Excessive hair loss**

Blood tests showing elevated liver enzymes may be a sign of a vitamin A overdose. If any of these symptoms appear, please discontinue using vitamin A until the symptoms disappear and then resume vitamin A therapy at a much lower dosage. The cancer patient faces a dilemma in attempting to use the maximum dose of vitamin A to fight their cancer, while trying to avoid vitamin A toxicity.

Those with thyroid cancer should avoid vitamin A.

Therapy Caveats

Remember that the information contained in this book is not intended to replace the attention or advice of a physician or other health care professional. Anyone who wishes to embark on any dietary, drug, exercise, or other lifestyle change intended to prevent or treat a specific disease or condition should first consult with and seek clearance from a qualified health care professional.

There are a number of caveats individuals should be aware of when considering undergoing certain therapies, or when they are suffering from specific problems. They include, but are not limited to, the following:

Acetaminophen. The most popular form of acetaminophen is Tylenol, which can cause permanent kidney damage when taken over extended periods of time. This damage can be lethal to those with underlying kidney disease. There are no nutrient supplements known to protect against acetaminophen-induced kidney damage, although the amino acid taurine (1,000 mg 2 to 3 times a day) and some forms of dietary fiber might be helpful.

Adrenal diseases. Some adrenal diseases such as Addison's Disease involve under production of cortisol. This is a potentially acute life-threatening condition that requires expert physician intervention.

Arginine. For a minority of Type II diabetics, arginine can elevate their blood sugar by neutralizing insulin. Therefore, any diabetic contemplating using arginine or Powermaker II (Sugar-Free) should check their blood sugar with a glucometer every time they take an arginine supplement during the first three weeks they use arginine.

Bee products. When using any bee products for children, they should not be administered to children under the age of three.

Beta-carotene. When suffering from a damaged liver, avoid niacin, vitamin A and beta-carotene, as these nutrients can be harmful. Also, the Life Extension Foundation recommends against high dose beta-carotene in AIDS patients who also have hepatitis.

Biliary tract obstruction. Do not use curcumin if you have biliary tract obstruction because curcumin could eliminate the flow of bile excretion through the bile duct.

Caffeine. Those with cardiac arrhythmias should avoid caffeine, heavy alcohol intake, and dietary saturated fats.

Curcumin. Do not use curcumin if you have biliary tract obstruction because curcumin could eliminate the flow of bile excretion through the bile duct. High doses of curcumin on an empty stomach can cause stomach ulceration.

Depression. Anyone suffering from clinical depression of any type should be under the care of a physician.

DHEA. Those with prostate cancer should avoid DHEA. Generally, it is a good idea to use any hormone with caution under the direction of a competent physician.

Forskolin. Do not use forskolin if you have prostate cancer or low blood pressure. If you are going to attempt to use forskolin or any other alternative therapy to replace drugs that strengthen heart muscle contraction, then extreme caution is mandatory and physician cooperation essential. Tests should be conducted to make sure forskolin and other nutrients are maintaining sufficient cardiac output.

Forskolin and anti-hypertensive drugs. If you'd like to see if forskolin replace your anti-hypertensive drugs, extreme caution is mandatory and physician cooperation essential. You should reduce the dosage of your anti-hypertensive drug very slowly, while increasing your intake of forskolin and monitoring your blood pressure on a daily basis. If you do not exercise caution, an acute hypertensive event could occur resulting in a stroke.

Genistein. Do not take soy extract when undergoing radiation therapy because the genistein in soy can interfere with the ability of the radiation to kill cancer cells.

Hops. See valerian.

Hypertension. Our general precaution is that, if you're going to attempt to use any of the nutrients we recommend to replace anti-hypertensive drugs, you **must** do so with the cooperation of your physician. You cannot assume that any nutrients will be able to replace a drug that is effectively controlling your blood pressure. Daily blood pressure monitoring is mandatory to insure that the nutrient regimen you are following is really keeping your blood pressure under control.

Interleukin-2. While melatonin is strongly recommended for breast cancer patients, interleukin-2, which is often combined with melatonin, should be avoided by breast cancer patients. Interleukin-2 may promote breast cancer cell division.

Leukemia. Alternative cancer therapies should be used with caution when treating leukemia or lymphoma patients because most alternative therapies boost immune cell function, which could speed the proliferation of leukemia and lymphoma cancer cells.

Lupus. Lupus patients should exercise extreme caution when attempting any new medical therapy as there is a chance the condition could be made worse.

Lymphoma. Alternative cancer therapies should be used with caution when treating leukemia or lymphoma patients because most alternative therapies boost immune cell function, which could speed the proliferation of leukemia and lymphoma cancer cells.

KH3. People allergic to procaine (the active ingredient in KH3) or on sulfa drugs should not take KH3.

Niacin. When suffering from a several damaged liver, avoid niacin, vitamin A and beta-carotene, as these nutrients can be harmful.

Pain. Before starting on a pain management program, please refer to the Phenylalanine Precautions in this book.

Passion flower. See valerian.

Phenylalanine or tyrosine. There are some people who are genetically sensitive to phenylalanine and cannot take it. Hypertensive people should use phenylalanine with caution because it can elevate blood pressure in people who already have high blood pressure. Cancer patients should avoid taking extra phenylalanine and tyrosine because these amino acids can contribute to cancer cell proliferation.

Pregnenolone. See DHEA-Pregnenolone Precautions in this book.

Procaine. People allergic to procaine (the active ingredient in KH3) or on sulfa drugs should not take KH3.

Propranolol. People with very low blood pressure, certain forms of congestive heart failure, and asthma should not take propranolol or other beta-blocking drugs.

Shark liver oil. Do not take shark liver oil for more than 30 days because it may cause the overproduction of blood platelets.

Soy extract. Do not take soy extract when undergoing radiation therapy because the genistein in soy can interfere with the ability of the radiation to kill cancer cells.

Sulfa drugs. People allergic to procaine (the active ingredient in KH3) or on sulfa drugs should not take KH3.

Thyroid hormone therapy. You must be careful not to overdose on thyroid hormones, so the advice of a knowledgeable physician is important when considering thyroid hormone therapy.

Tyrosine. See Phenylalanine or tyrosine.

Appendix

Valerian. Some people use the herb valerian to fall asleep. Valerian produces a drug-like hypnotic effect within the central nervous system similar to benzodiazepine drugs such as Valium and Halcion. Since valerian-containing products are often promoted as natural herbal remedies, the public mistakenly believes it is safe to take on a regular basis. Studies indicate, however that there is a significant toxicity risk when taking valerian over an extended period of time. Since a tolerance effect occurs with valerian, due to its Valium-like properties, people often need to take greater and greater amounts of it as time goes by in order to continue to obtain the desired hypnotic effect. The chronic use of valerian could result in permanent liver damage along with potential central nervous system impairment. The Life Extension Foundation has thoroughly investigated the use of herbal insomnia remedies such as valerian, hops, and passion flower, and found that they have an unacceptable risk of toxicity with long term use.

Vitamin A lipid drops. The dosage range of vitamin A lipid drops that cancer patients have been using is between 100,000 and 200,000 I.U.s. a day. The Foundation has cautioned that these high doses could produce toxicity if taken over extended periods of time. Cancer patients are often forced to risk some degree of toxicity to obtain an effective dose of vitamin A.

Vitamin B6. Since high doses of B-6 have peripheral nerve toxicity, high doses (500 mg of B6 a day and higher) should only be used when a blood test documents the failure of folic acid, vitamin B12 and TMG to lower homocysteine levels.

Vitamin D3. Monthly blood tests to monitor serum calcium and parathyroid hormone levels should be done to protect against vitamin D3 toxicity.

Vitamin D3. Underlying kidney disease precludes high-dose vitamin D3 supplementation.

Acetaminophen (Tylenol) Poisoning
Acute And Chronic

Acute renal failure due to acetaminophen ingestion: a case report and review of the literature. J Am Soc Nephrol (UNITED STATES) Jul 1995

Acute hepatic and renal toxicity from low doses of acetaminophen in the absence of alcohol abuse or malnutrition: evidence for increased susceptibility to drug toxicity due to cardiopulmonary and renal insufficiency. Hepatology (UNITED STATES) May 1994

Protective effect of oral acetylcysteine against the hepatorenal toxicity of carbon tetrachloride potentiated by ethyl alcohol. Alcohol Clin Exp Res (UNITED STATES) Aug 1992

Cholestyramine as an antidote against paracetamol-induced hepato- and nephrotoxicity in the rat. Toxicol Lett (NETHERLANDS) May 1989

Relation of analgesic use to renal cancer: population-based findings. Natl Cancer Inst Monogr (UNITED STATES) Dec 1985

Acetaminophen-induced depletion of glutathione and cysteine in the aging mouse kidney. Biochem Pharmacol (ENGLAND) Jul 7 1992

Cysteine isopropylester protects against paracetamol-induced toxicity. Biochem Pharmacol (ENGLAND) Feb 4 1992

Fatal acetaminophen poisoning with evidence of subendocardial necrosis of the heart. J Forensic Sci (UNITED STATES) May 1991

Intrinsic susceptibility of the kidney to acetaminophen toxicity in middle-aged rats. Toxicol Lett (NETHERLANDS) Jun 1990

Glutathione enhancement in various mouse organs and protection by glutathione isopropyl ester against liver injury. Biochem Pharmacol (ENGLAND) Jun 15 1990

A comparison of the protective effects of N-acetyl-cysteine and S- carboxymethylcysteine against paracetamol (acetaminophen)-induced hepatotoxicity. Toxicology (NETHERLANDS) Nov 1983

Acetaminophen hepatotoxicity. An alternative mechanism. Biochem Pharmacol (ENGLAND) Jul 1 1983, 32 (13) p2053-9

Glutathione Metabolism and Its Role in Hepatotoxicity. Pharmacologic Therapy, 1991;52:287-305

Overdose of Extended-Release Acetaminophen. New England Journal of Medicine, July 20, 1995;196

Adrenal Disease

Adrenocortical insufficiency. Clinical Enocrinology Metab (ENGLAND) Nov 1995, 14 (4) p947-76

Changes in serum concentrations of conjugated and unconjugated steroids. J Clin Endocrinol Metab (UNITED STATES) Oct 1994, 79 (4) p1086-90

Ovarian suppression with triptorelin and adrenal stimulation with adrenocorticotropin in functional hyperadrogenism: role of adrenal and ovarian cytochrome P450c17 alpha. Fertil Steril (UNITED STATES) Sep 1994, 62 (3) p521-30

Pattern of plasma dehydroepiandrosterone sulfate levels in humans from birth to adulthood: evidence for testicular production. J Clin Endocrinol Metab (UNITED STATES) Sep 1978, 47 (3) p572-7

Adrenal function and ascorbic acid concentrations in elderly women. Gerontology (SWITZER-LAND) 1978, 24 (6) p473-6

Age-Associated Mental Impairment
(Brain Aging)

Piracetam. An overview of its pharmacological properties and a review of its therapeutic use in senile cognitive disorders. Drugs Aging (NEW ZEALAND) Jan 1991, 1 (1) p17-35

Memory-enhancing effects in male mice of pregnenolone and steroids metabolically derived from it. Proc Natl Acad Sci U S A (UNITED STATES) Mar 1 1992, 89 (5) p1567-71

Piracetam elevates muscarinic cholinergic receptor density in the frontal cortex of aged but not of young mice. Psychopharmacology (Berl) (GERMANY, WEST) 1988, 94 (1) p74-8

Habituation of exploratory activity in mice: effects of combinations of piracetam and choline on memory processes. Pharmacol Biochem Behav (UNITED STATES) Aug 1984, 21 (2) p209-12

Profound effects of combining choline and piracetam on memory enhancement and cholinergic function in aged rats. Neurobiol Aging (UNITED STATES) Summer 1981, 2 (2) p105-11

Interaction between psychological and pharmacological treatment in cognitive impairment. Life Sci (ENGLAND) 1994, 55 (25-26) p2057-66

Impairment of learning and memory in shuttle box-trained rats neonatally injected with 6-hydroxydopamine. Effects of nootropic drugs. Acta Physiol Pharmacol Bulg (BULGARIA) 1993, 19 (3) p77-82

Latency of memory consolidation induced in mice by piracetam, a nootropic agent. Indian J Exp Biol (INDIA) Nov 1993, 31 (11) p898-901

References

Elevated corticosteroid levels block the memory-improving effects of nootropics and cholinomimetics. Psychopharmacology (Berl) (GERMANY) 1992, 108 (1-2) p11-5

A trial of piracetam in two subgroups of students with dyslexia enrolled in summer tutoring. J Learn Disabil (UNITED STATES) Nov 1991, 24 (9) p542-9

Aldosterone receptors are involved in the mediation of the memory-enhancing effects of piracetam. Brain Res (NETHERLANDS) Aug 6 1990, 524 (2) p203-7

Pharmacological restoration of scopolamine-impaired memory. Acta Physiol Pharmacol Bulg (BULGARIA) 1985, 11 (3) p37-43

Gerontopsychological studies using NAI ('Nurnberger Alters-Inventar') on patients with organic psychosyndrome (DSM III, Category 1) treated with centrophenoxine in a double blind, comparative, randomized clinical trial. Arch Gerontol Geriatr (NETHERLANDS) Jul 1989, 9 (1) p17-30

[Characteristics of the action of psychostimulants on learning and memory in rats] Biull Eksp Biol Med (USSR) Aug 1988, 106 (8) p161-3

Centrophenoxine: effects on aging mammalian brain. J Am Geriatr Soc (UNITED STATES) Feb 1978, 26 (2) p74-81

Centrophenoxine activates acetylcholinesterase activity in hippocampus of aged rats. Indian J Exp Biol (INDIA) May 1995, 33 (5) p365-8

On the role of intracellular physicochemistry in quantitative gene expression during aging and the effect of centrophenoxine. A review. Arch Gerontol Geriatr (NETHERLANDS) Nov-Dec 1989, 9 (3) p215-29

Neuronal lipopigment: a marker for cognitive impairment and long- term effects of psychotropic drugs [see comments] Br J Psychiatry (ENGLAND) Jul 1989, 155 p1-11

Age-related change in the multiple unit activity of the rat brain parietal cortex and the effect of centrophenoxine. Exp Gerontol (ENGLAND) 1988, 23 (3) p161-74

[Effect of centrophenoxine, piracetam and aniracetam on the monoamine oxidase activity in different brain structures of rats] Farmakol Toksikol (USSR) May-Jun 1988, 51 (3) p16-8

[Comparative neurophysiological study of the nootropic drugs piracetam and centrophenoxine] Farmakol Toksikol (USSR) Nov-Dec 1987, 50 (6) p17-20

Fluidizing effects of centrophenoxine in vitro on brain and liver membranes from different age groups of mice. Life Sci (ENGLAND) Dec 1 1986, 39 (22) p2089-95

Studies on the effect of iron overload on rat cortex synaptosomal membranes. Biochim Biophys Acta (NETHERLANDS) Nov 7 1985, 820 (2) p216-22

Alterations of the intracellular water and ion concentrations in brain and liver cells during aging as revealed by energy dispersive X- ray microanalysis of bulk specimens. Scan Electron Microsc (UNITED STATES) 1985, (Pt 1) p323-37

References

Alterations in the molecular weight distribution of proteins in rat brain synaptosomes during aging and centrophenoxine treatment of old rats. Mech Ageing Dev (SWITZERLAND) Dec 1984, 28 (2-3) p171-6

Study on the anti-hypoxic effect of some drugs used in the pharmacotherapy of cerebrovascular disease. Methods Find Exp Clin Pharmacol (SPAIN) Nov 1983, 5 (9) p607-12

Inability to deactivate the sympathetic nervous system in patients with brainstem infarction; correction of the disorder by centrophenoxine administration. Neurol Psychiatr (Bucur) (ROMANIA) Oct-Dec 1983, 21 (4) p425-39

Participation of adrenergic mechanisms in brain acetylcholine release produced by centrophenoxine. Acta Physiol Pharmacol Bulg (BULGARIA) 1979, 5 (4) p21-6

Acetyl-L-Carnitine: chronic treatment improves spatial acquisition in a new environment in aged rats. J Gerontol A Biol Sci Med Sci (UNITED STATES) Jul 1995, 50 (4) pB232-36

[Effects of L-acetylcarnitine on mental deterioration in the aged: initial results] Clin Ter (ITALY) Mar 31 1990, 132 (6 Suppl) p479-510

Effect of acetyl-L-carnitine on conditioned reflex learning rate and retention in laboratory animals. Drugs Exp Clin Res (SWITZERLAND) 1986, 12 (11) p911-6

The effects of acetyl-l-carnitine on experimental models of learning and memory deficits in the old rat. Funct Neurol (ITALY) Oct-Dec 1989, 4 (4) p387-90

Alzheimer dementia and reduced nicotinamide adenine dinucleotide (NADH)- diaphorase activity in senile plaques and the basal forebrain. Neurosci Lett (NETHERLANDS) Jan 7 1985, 53 (1) p39-44

Effects of phosphatidylserine in Alzheimer's disease. Psychopharmacol Bull (UNITED STATES) 1992, 28 (1) p61-6

Nootropic drugs and brain cholinergic mechanisms. Prog Neuropsychopharmacol Biol Psychiatry (ENGLAND) 1989, 13 Suppl pS77-88

Effects of phosphatidylserine in age-associated memory impairment. Neurology (UNITED STATES) May 1991, 41 (5) p644-9

Memory effects of standardized extracts of Panax ginseng (G115), Ginkgo biloba (GK 501) and their combination Gincosan (PHL-00701). Planta Med (GERMANY) Apr 1993, 59 (2) p106-14

[Activity of Ginkgo biloba extract on short-term memory] Presse Med (FRANCE) Sep 25 1986, 15 (31) p1592-4

References

Alcohol-Induced Hangover: Prevention

Protective action of ascorbic acid and sulfur compounds against acetaldehyde toxicity: implications in alcoholism and smoking. Agents Actions (SWITZERLAND) May 1975, 5 (2) p164-73

Sulfur amino acid metabolism in hepatobiliary disorders. Scand J Gastroenterol (NORWAY) May 1992, 27 (5) p405-11

[Severe somatic complications of acute alcoholic intoxication] Rev Prat (FRANCE) Oct 15 1993, 43 (16) p2047-51

[The therapeutic approach in optic neuropathy due to methyl alcohol] Oftalmologia (ROMANIA) Jan-Mar 1991, 35 (1) p39-42

Alcohol and brain damage. Hum Toxicol (ENGLAND) Sep 1988, 7 (5) p455-63

Acute ethanol poisoning and the ethanol withdrawal syndrome. Med Toxicol Adverse Drug Exp (NEW ZEALAND) May-Jun 1988, 3 (3) p172-96

Clinical signs in the Wernicke-Korsakoff complex: a retrospective analysis of 131 cases diagnosed at necropsy. J Neurol Neurosurg Psychiatry (ENGLAND) Apr 1986, 49 (4) p341-5

Thiamine status of institutionalised and non-institutionalised aged. Int J Vitam Nutr Res (SWITZERLAND) 1977, 47 (4) p325-35

[Vitamin B 1 deficiency in chronic alcoholics and its clinical correlation] Schweiz Med Wochenschr (SWITZERLAND) Oct 23 1976, 106 (43) p1466-70

Effect of S-adenosyl-L-methionine administration on red blood cell cysteine and glutathione levels in alcoholic patients with and without liver disease. Alcohol Alcohol (ENGLAND) Sep 1994, 29 (5) p597-604

Glutathione prevents ethanol induced gastric mucosal damage and depletion of sulfhydryl compounds in humans. Gut (ENGLAND) Feb 1993, 34 (2) p161-5

Effects of amino acids on acute alcohol intoxication in mice—concentrations of ethanol, acetaldehyde, acetate and acetone in blood and tissues. Arukoru Kenkyuto Yakubutsu Ison (JAPAN) Oct 1990, 25 (5) p429-40

A possible protective role for sulphydryl compounds in acute alcoholic liver injury. Biochem Pharmacol (UNITED STATES) Aug 15 1977, 26 (16) p1529-31

Protection against toxic effects of formaldehyde in vitro, and of methanol or formaldehyde in vivo, by subsequent administration of SH reagents. Physiol Chem Phys (UNITED STATES) 1976, 8 (6) p543-50

N-Acetylcysteine for Lung Cancer Prevention. Nico Chest May 1995;107(5):1437-1441.

S-Adenosylmethionine and the Liver. The Liver: Biology and Pathobiology, 3rd Edition, 1994; 27:461-470

Allergies

The effect of gamma-linolenic acid on clinical status, red cell fatty acid composition and membrane microviscosity in infants with atopic dermatitis. Drugs Exp Clin Res. 1994. 20(2). P 77-84

Fatty acid compositions of plasma lipids in atopic dermatitis/asthma patients. Arerugi. 1994 Jan. 43(1). P 37-43

Autoimmune disease and allergy are controlled by vitamin C treatment. IN VIVO (Greece), 1994, 8/2 (251-258)

Immune senescence and adrenal steroids: Immune dysregulation and the action of dehydroepiandrosterone (DHEA) in old animals. EUR. J. CLIN. PHARMACOL. (Germany), 1993, 45/SUPPL. 1 (S21-S23)

Omega-3 fatty acids in respiratory diseases: A review. J. AM. COLL. NUTR. (USA), 1995, 14/1 (18-23)

Vitamin C and the genesis of autoimmune disease and allergy (Review). In Vivo (Greece), 1995, 9/3 (231-238)

Is Linus Pauling, a vitamin C advocate, just making much ado about nothing? IN VIVO (Greece), 1994, 8/3 (391-400)

Asthma and vitamin C. ANN. ALLERGY (USA), 1994, 73/2 (89-99)

The effect of vitamin C infusion treatment on immune disorders: An invitation to a trial in AIDS patients (Review). INT. J. ONCOL. (Greece), 1994, 4/4 (831-838)

Chromium dermatitis and ascorbic acid. CONTACT DERMATITIS (DENMARK), 1984, 10/4 (252-253)

Colds and vitamin C. IRISH MED.J. (IRELAND), 1975, 68/20 (511-516)

Vitamin C metabolism and atopic allergy. CLIN.ALLERGY (ENGLAND), 1975, 5/3 (317-324)

Alzheimer's Disease

Isolated cerebral and cerebellar mitochondria produce free radicals when exposed to elevated CA2+ and Na+: implications for neurodegeneration. J Neurochem (UNITED STATES) Aug 1994, 63 (2)

Isoprenoids (coQ10) in aging and neurodegeneration. Neurochem Int (ENGLAND) Jul 1994, 25 (1) p35-8

Therapy for Alzheimer's disease. Symptomatic or neuroprotective? Mol Neurobiol (UNITED STATES) Aug-Dec 1994, 9 (1-3)

The mystery of Alzheimer's disease and its prevention by melatonin. Med Hypotheses (ENGLAND) Oct 1995, 45 (4) p339-40

References

Advances in the pharmacotherapy of Alzheimer's disease. Eur Arch Psychiatry Clin Neurosci (GERMANY) 1994, 244 (5)

Chrono-neuroendocrinological aspects of physiological aging and senile dementia. Chronobiologia (ITALY) Jan-Jun 1994, 21 (1-2) p121-6

Overview of clinical trials of hydergine in dementia. ARCH. NEUROL. (USA), 1994, 51/8 (787-798)

Combined cholinergic precursor treatment and dihydroergotoxine mesylate in Alzheimer's disease. IRCS MED. SCI. (ENGLAND), 1983, 11/12 (1048-1049)

Hydergine treatment and brain functioning (CNV rebound) in Alzheimer's patients: Preliminary findings. PSYCHOPHARMACOL. BULL. (USA), 1981, 17/3 (202-206)

Single-case study of clinical response to high-dose ergot alkaloid treatment for dementia. Preliminary report. GERONTOLOGY (SWITZERLAND), 1981, 27/1-2 (76-78)

Isoprenoids (coQ10) in aging and neurodegeneration. NEUROCHEM. INT. (United Kingdom), 1994, 25/1 (35-38)

Analyses of energy metabolism and mitochondrial genome in post-mortem brain from patients with Alzheimer's disease. J. NEUROL. (Germany), 1993, 240/6 (377-380)

Muscle biopsy in Alzheimer's disease: Morphological and biochemical findings. CLIN. NEUROPATHOL. (Germany), 1991, 10/4 (171-176)

Growth hormone secretion in Alzheimer's disease: Studies with growth hormone- releasing hormone alone and combined with pyridostigmine or arginine. DEMENTIA (Switzerland), 1993, 4/6 (315-320)

Selegiline: A review of its clinical efficacy in Parkinson's disease and its clinical potential in Alzheimer's disease. CNS Drugs (New Zealand), 1995, 4/3 (230-246)

Age-related memory decline and longevity under treatment with selegiline. LIFE SCI. (USA), 1994, 55/25-26

Long-term effects of phosphatidylserine, pyritinol, and cognitive training in Alzheimer's disease. A neuropsychological, EEG, and PET investigation. DEMENTIA (Switzerland), 1994, 5/2 (88-98)

Abnormalities of energy metabolism in Alzheimer's disease studied with PET. ANN. NEW YORK ACAD. SCI. (USA), 1991, 640/- (65-71)

Effects of phosphatidylserine in Alzheimer's disease. USA PSYCHOPHARMACOL. BULL. (USA), 1992, 28/1 (61-66)

Effect of phosphatidylserine on cerebral glucose metabolism in Alzheimer's disease. DEMENTIA (Switzerland), 1990, (197-201)

Decreased methionine adenosyltransferase activity in erythrocytes of patients with dementia disorders. Sweden European Neuropsychopharmacology (Netherlands), 1995, 5/2 (107-114)

References

Folate, vitamin B12 and cognitive impairment in patients with Alzheimer's disease. ACTA PSYCHIATR. SCAND. (Denmark), 1992, 86/4 (301-305)

Alzheimer's Disease: A 'cobalaminergic' hypothesis. MED. HYPOTHESES (United Kingdom), 1992, 37/3 (161-165)

Vitamin B12 and folate concentrations in serum and cerebrospinal fluid of neurological patients with special reference to multiple sclerosis and dementia J. NEUROL. NEUROSURG. PSYCHIATRY (United Kingdom), 1990, 53/11 (951-954)

Vitamin B12 levels in serum and cerebrospinal fluid of people with Alzheimer's disease. ACTA PSYCHIATR. SCAND. (Denmark), 1990, 82/4 (327-329)

Alzheimers disease/alcohol dementia: Association with zinc deficiency and cerebral vitamin B12 deficiency. J. ORTHOMOL. PSYCHIATRY (CANADA), 1984, 13/2 (97-104)

Carnitine and acetyl-L-carnitine content of human hippocampus and erythrocytes in Alzheimer's disease. Journal of Nutritional and Environmental Medicine (United Kingdom), 1995, 5/1 (35-39)

Advances in the pharmacotherapy of Alzheimer's disease. EUR. ARCH. PSYCHIATRY CLIN. NEUROSCI. (Germany), 1994, 244/5 (261-271)

Clinical and neurochemical effects of acetyl-L-carnitine in Alzheimer's disease. NEUROBIOL. AGING (USA), 1995, 16/1 (1-4)

Neuroprotective activity of acetyl-L-carnitine: Studies in vitro. NEUROSCI. RES. (USA), 1994, 37/1 (92-96)

Acetyl-L-carnitine and Alzheimer's disease: Pharmacological beyond the cholinergic sphere. ANN. NEW YORK ACAD. SCI. (USA), 1993, 695/- (324-326)

Acetyl-L-carnitine: A drug able to slow the progress of Alzheimer's disease? ANN. NEW YORK ACAD. SCI. (USA), 1991, 640/- (228-232)

Pharmacokinetics of IV and oral acetyl-L-carnitine in a multiple dose regimen in patients with senile dementia of Alzheimer Type. EUR. J. CLIN. PHARMACOL. (Germany), 1992, 42/1 (89-93)

Double-blind, placebo-controlled study of acetyl-l-carnitine in patients with Alzheimer's disease. CURR. MED. RES. OPIN. (United Kingdom), 1989, 11/10 (638-647)

The pharmacotherapy of Alzheimer's disease based on the cholinergic hypothesis: An update. Neurodegeneration United Kingdom),1995, 4/4 (349-356)

Aniracetam: A new nootropic drug with excellent tolerance for mild to moderate cognitive impairment in elderly people. DRUGS TODAY (Spain), 1994, 30/1 (9-24)

Auditory and visual event-related potentials in patients suffering from Alzheimer's dementia and multiinfarct dementia, before and after treatment with piracetam. FUNCT. NEUROL. (Italy), 1993, 8/5 (335-345)

Amnesia

[Antagonism of piracetam with proline in relation to amnestic effects]. Biull Eksp Biol Med (USSR) Mar 1985, 99 (3) p311-4

[Effect of mental stimulants on electroconvulsive shock-induced retrograde amnesia]. Pharmazie (GERMANY, EAST) Dec 1983, 38 (12) p869-71,

Hypoxia-induced amnesia in one-trial learning and pharmacological protection by piracetam. Psychopharmacologia (GERMANY, WEST) 1972, 25 (1) p32-40

Pre-clinical evaluation of cognition enhancing drugs. Prog Neuropsychopharmacol Biol Psychiatry (ENGLAND) 1989, 13 Suppl pS99-115

Nootropic drugs and brain cholinergic mechanisms. Prog Neuropsychopharmacol Biol Psychiatry (ENGLAND) 1989, 13 Suppl pS77-88

Specificity of piracetam's anti-amnesic activity in three models of amnesia in the mouse. Pharmacol Biochem Behav (UNITED STATES) Mar 1988, 29 (3) p625-9

[Effects of piracetam during prolonged use in an experiment] Effekty piratsetama pri dlitel'nom primenenii v eksperimente. Farmakol Toksikol (USSR) Jul-Aug 1985, 48 (4) p42-6

Amyotrophic Lateral Sclerosis (ALS)
(Lou Gehrig's Disease)

Free Radicals Appear to Fuel Lou Gehrig's Disease. Family Practice News, Rockville, MD

In vivo generation of hydroxyl radicals and MPTP-induced dopaminergic toxicity in the basal ganglia. Ann N Y Acad Sci (UNITED STATES) Nov 17, 1994, 738 p25-36

Detection of point mutations in codon 331 of mitochondrial NADH dehydrogenase subunit 2 in Alzheimer's brains. Biochem Biophys Res Commun (UNITED STATES) Jan 15 1992, 182 (1) p238-46

Deprenyl enhances neurite outgrowth in cultured rat spinal ventral horn neurons. J Neurol Sci (NETHERLANDS) Aug 1994, 125 (1) p11-3

Therapeutic trial with N-acetylcysteine in amyotrophic lateral sclerosis. Adv Exp Med Biol (UNITED STATES) 1987, 209 p281-4

Attempted treatment of motor neuron disease with N-acetylcysteine and dithiothreitol. Adv Exp Med Biol (UNITED STATES) 1987, 209 p277-80

Anti-Glutamate Therapy in Amyotrophic Lateral Sclerosis: A Trial Using Lamotrigine. Canadian Journal of Neurological Sciences, 1993; 20:297-301

A Controlled Trial of Riluzole in Amyotrophic Lateral Sclerosis. New England Journal of Medicine, March 3, 1994; 330(9):585-591

Aluminum Deposition in Central Nervous System of Patients with Amyotrophic Lateral Sclerosis From the Kii Peninsula of Japan. Neurotoxicology, 1991; 615-620

Free Radicals and Neuroprotection. By B, J. Wilder, M. D., Professor Emeritus of Neurology University of Florida College of Medicine and Consultant in Neurology Department of Veterans Affairs Medical Center

Anemia-Thrombocytopenia-Leukopenia

Folic acid supplementation improves erythropoietin response. Nephron (SWITZERLAND) 1995, 71 (4) p395-400

Partial amelioration of AZT-induced macrocytic anemia in the mouse by folic acid. Stem Cells (Dayt) (UNITED STATES) Sep 1993, 11 (5) p393-7

Megaloblastic anemia in patients receiving total parenteral nutrition without folic acid or vitamin B12 supplementation. Can Med Assoc J (CANADA) Jul 23 1977, 117 (2) p144-6

Modulation of tumor necrosis factor-alpha (TNF-alpha) toxicity by the pineal hormone melatonin (MLT) in metastatic solid tumor patients. Annals of the New York Academy of Sciences (USA), 1995, 768 (334-336)

[Anemias due to disorder of folate, vitamin B12 and transcobalamin metabolism]. Rev Prat (FRANCE) Jun 1 1993, 43 (11) p1358-63

[Is it necessary to supplement with folic acid patients in chronic dialysis treated with erythropoietin?]. Rev Med Chil (CHILE) Jan 1993, 121 (1) p30-5

Ineffective hematopoiesis in folate-deficient mice. Blood (UNITED STATES) May 1 1992, 79 (9) p2273-80

[Primary prophylaxis against cerebral toxoplasmosis. Efficacy of folinic acid in the prevention of hematologic toxicity of pyrimethamine]. Presse Med (FRANCE) Apr 2 1994, 23 (13) p613-5

Nutritional status of an institutionalized aged population. J Am Coll Nutr (UNITED STATES) 1984, 3 (1) p13-25

[Acquired, vitamin B6-responsive, primary sideroblastic anemia, an enzyme deficiency in heme synthesis]. Schweiz Med Wochenschr (SWITZERLAND) Oct 10 1981, 111 (41) p1533-5

Intakes of vitamins and minerals by pregnant women with selected clinical symptoms. J Am Diet Assoc (UNITED STATES) May 1981, 78 (5) p477-82

[Anemia with hypersideroblastosis during anti-tuberculosis therapy. Cure with vitamin therapy]. Nouv Rev Fr Hematol (FRANCE) Apr 14 1978, 20 (1) p99-110

[Myelopathy and macrocytic anemia associated with a folate deficiency. Cure by folic acid]. Ann Med Interne (Paris) (FRANCE) May 1975, 126 (5) p339-48

References

[Vitamin B 6 deficiency anemia]. Schweiz Med Wochenschr (SWITZERLAND) Oct 11 1975, 105 (41) p1319-24

Premature infants require additional folate and vitamin B-12 to reduce the severity of the anemia of prematurity. Am J Clin Nutr (UNITED STATES) Dec 1994, 60 (6) p930-5

Apoptosis mediates and thymidine prevents erythroblast destruction in folate deficiency anemia. Proc Natl Acad Sci U S A (UNITED STATES) Apr 26 1994, 91 (9) p4067-71

Acute folate deficiency associated with intravenous nutrition with aminoacid- sorbitol-ethanol: prophylaxis with intravenous folic acid. Br J Haematol (ENGLAND) Dec 1977, 37 (4) p521-6

Interactions between folate and ascorbic acid in the guinea pig. J Nutr (UNITED STATES) Apr 1982, 112 (4) p673-80

Modulation of human lymphoblastoid interferon activity by melatonin in metastatic renal cell carcinoma. A phase II study. Cancer (UNITED STATES) Jun 15 1994, 73 (12) p3015-9

A biological study on the efficacy of low-dose subcutaneous interleukin-2 plus melatonin in the treatment of cancer-related thrombocytopenia. Oncology (SWITZERLAND) Sep-Oct 1995, 52 (5) p360-2

A new class of antihypertensive neutral lipid: 1-alkyl-2-acetyl-sn-glycerols, a precursor of platelet activating factor. BIOCHEM. BIOPHYS. RES. COMMUN. (USA), 1984, 118/1 (344-350)

Metabolism of 1-O-alkyl-2-acetyl-sn-glycerol by washed rabbit platelets: Formation of platelet activating factor. ARCH. BIOCHEM. BIOPHYS. (USA), 1984, 234/1 (318-321)

Conversion of 1-alkyl-2-acetyl-sn-glycerols to platelet activating factor and related phospholipids by rabbit platelets. BIOCHEM. BIOPHYS. RES. COMMUN. (USA), 1984, 124/1 (156-163)

Anti-neoplastic action of peritoneal macrophages after oral admin. of ether analogues of lysophospholipids. EUR. J. CANCER PART A GEN. TOP. 1992, 28/10 (1637-1642)

Anesthesia and Surgery Precautions

Myocardial preservation by therapy with coenzyme Q10 during heart surgery. USA CLIN. INVEST. SUPPL. (Germany), 1993, 71/8 (S 155-S 161)

Effect of CoQ10 on myocardial ischemia/reperfusion injury in the isolated rat heart. Journal of the Japanese Association for Thoracic Surgery (Japan), 1995, 43/4 (466-472)

Free radical reaction products and antioxidant capacity in arterial plasma during coronary artery bypass grafting. J. THORAC. CARDIOVASC. SURG. (USA) 1994, 108/1 (140-147)

Oxygen radicals in cerebral vascular injury. CIRC. R RES. (USA), 1985, 57/4 (508-516)

Postischemic tissue injury by iron-mediated free radical lipid peroxidation. ANN. EMERG.

MED. (USA), 1985, 14/8 (804-809)

Oxygen free radical-induced histamine release during intestinal ischemia and reperfusion. EUR. SURG. RES. (Switzerland), 1989, 21/6 (297-304)

Role of iron ions in the genesis of reperfusion injury following successful cardiopulmonary resuscitation: Preliminary data and a biochemical hypothesis. ANN. EMERG. MED. (USA), 1985, 14/8 (777-783)

The biological significance of zinc. ANAESTHESIST (BERL.) (GERMANY, WEST), 1975, 24/8 (329-342)

Cortical pOsub 2 distribution during oligemic hypotension and its pharmacological modifications (Hydergine). SWITZERLAND ARZNEIM.-FORSCH. (GERMANY, WEST), 1978, 28/5 (768-770)

The use of piracetam (Nootrop) in post-anesthetic recovery of elderly patients. (A preliminary study). GREECE ACTA ANAESTHESIOL. HELL. (GREECE), 1981, 15/1-2 (76-80)

Free radical reaction products and antioxidant capacity in arterial plasma during coronary artery bypass grafting. J. THORAC. CARDIOVASC. SURG. (USA), 1994, 108/1 (140-147)

Free radical trapping agents in myocardial protection in cardiac surgery. FRANCE ANN. CARDIOL. ANGEIOL. (FRANCE), 1986, 35/7 BIS (447-452)

Biochemical studies of cerebral ischemia in the rat - Changes in cerebral free amino acids, catecholamines and uric acid. JAPAN BRAIN NERVE (JAPAN), 1986, 38/3 (253-258)

Glutathione status in human blood during surgery. CLIN. CHEM. ENZYMOL. COMMUN. (United Kingdom), 1988, 1/2 (71-76)

Effect of supplemental vitamin A on colon anastomotic healing in rats given preoperative irradiation. AM. J. SURG. (USA), 1987, 153/2 (153-156)

Effect of reduced glutathione on endocrine and renal functions following halothane anesthesia and surgery in man. JPN. J. ANESTHESIOL. (JAPAN), 1982, 31/8 (830-839)

Intraocular irrigating solutions and lens clarity. AMER.J.OPHTHAL. (USA), 1976, 82/4 (594-597)

Intraocular irrigating solutions. Their effect on the corneal endothelium. ARCH.OPHTHAL. (USA), 1975, 93/8 (648-657)

Anxiety and Stress

Nutritional management of the metabolically stressed patient. CRIT. CARE NURS. Q. (USA), 1995, 17/4 (79-90)

Propranolol in psychiatry. Therapeutic uses and side effects. Neuropsychobiology (SWITZERLAND) 1986, 15 (1) p20-7

References

Propranolol in experimentally induced stress. Br J Psychiatry Dec 1981, 139 p545-9

Modulation of the immunologic response to acute stress in humans by beta- blockade or benzodiazepines. FASEB J (UNITED STATES) Mar 1996, 10 (4) p517-24

Beta-adrenergic receptors are involved in stress-related behavioral changes. Pharmacol Biochem Behav (UNITED STATES) May 1993, 45 (1) p1-7

The effect of beta blockade on stress-induced cognitive dysfunction in adolescents. Clin Pediatr (Phila) (UNITED STATES) Jul 1991, 30 (7) p441-5

Modulation of baseline behavior in rats by putative serotonergic agents in three ethoexperimental paradigms. Behav Neural Biol (UNITED STATES) Nov 1990, 54 (3) p234-53

Effects of propranolol, atenolol, and chlordesmethyldiazepam on response to mental stress in patients with recent myocardial infarction. Clin Cardiol (UNITED STATES) Jun 1987, 10 (6) p293-302

Clinical Trials For Chronic Fatigue and Anxiety. Life Extension Update-February 1996. A study was conducted on 20 patients who had been ill with various forms of chronic fatigue from one-to-three months. Patients were registered and information collected in accordance with the protocol of the European Fatigue Study Group, which includes scales to measure anxiety, depression, muscle fatigue, mental fatigue, sleep disorders, and headache. Four placebo capsules were given to these patients daily during the first two weeks of the study. Then four capsules of garum extract were given daily for the next two weeks of the study. After two weeks on placebo, fatigue symptoms were reduced by an average of 14% and overall symptoms of anxiety, depression, and insomnia were reduced by 4%. After two weeks of taking garum extract, on the other hand, fatigue symptoms were reduced by 51% and overall symptoms by 65%. Two weeks after discontinuing garum extract therapy, fatigue symptoms increased 15% and overall symptoms increased 7%. These results show the broad-spectrum benefits of garum extract for people suffering from chronic stress and fatigue. It is interesting to note that the beneficial effects of garum extract persisted even after the treatment was stopped. Another study involved 40 patients who had been suffering from various forms of chronic fatigue for one-to-three months. Four capsules of garum extract per day was prescribed for two weeks. The results, based on the Fatigue Study Group criteria, showed conclusive average benefit of 50% for the ten functions that most accurately measure fatigue and depression. In a study of 60 patients taking garum extract, only three mild reactions were noted without the necessity of interrupting the treatment. The reactions were: one case of nervous irritation, one case of heartburn, and one case of diarrhea. No emotional tension or insomnia was reported and it was concluded that garum extract is extremely well tolerated and is without contraindications. In a soon to be published study on the treatment of anxiety in college students, garum extract was shown to be safe and effective in reducing anxiety in otherwise healthy subjects. Other studies are showing that, when garum extract reduces anxiety, it results in improved learning, including enhanced EEG (Electroencephalogram) brain wave activity.

Summary: Garum extract benefits 90% of patients with chronic stress and fatigue compared to only 30% of patients on placebo. An analysis of all the human clinical studies of garum extract to date shows overall positive results in the treatment of the symptoms of chronic stress, including fatigue, anxiety and depression.

Additional References:
See Garum. 1 0-volume edition of Dictionnaire Larousse.
Dr. J. BORY, Journees de Biochimie medicale de l'Ouest, Brest, 1981.
Ph. DARCET et al (Ann. Nutr. Alim., 1980, 34 277.901.
G. DURANT, G. PASCAL N. VODOVAR, H. GOUNELLE DE PONTANEL (Med. et Nutr., 1978, vol. XIV, 1 95-204).
GROWFORD and SINCLAIR, 1972 (J. Nutrition, 102-1315).
M. HENRY, researcher, Personal contribution.
LAMPTEY and WALTER, 1976 lJ. Nutrition, 106-86).
Professor P METAIS (Cahiers de Nutrition et Dietetique, 1980, vol. XV, n 3, 227
Prostaglandines et physiologic de la reproduction, International INSERM Symposium (Revue francaise des laboratoires-January 1980, n 77 4-5-6)

Arrhythmia (Cardiac)

Fish oil and other nutritional adjuvants for treatment of congestive heart failure. Medical Hypotheses (United Kingdom), 1996, 46/4 (400-406)

Evidence on the participation of the 3',5'-cyclic AMP pathway in the non-genomic action of 1,25-dihydroxy-vitamin D3 in cardiac muscle. Mol Cell Endocrinol (NETHERLANDS) Dec 1991, 82 (2-3) p229-35

1,25(OH)2 vitamin D3, and retinoic acid antagonize endothelin-stimulated hypertrophy of neonatal rat cardiac myocytes. J Clin Invest Apr 1 1996, 97 (7) p1577-88

[Effect of vitamin E deficiency on the development of cardiac arrhythmias as affected by acute ischemia]. Biull Eksp Biol Med (USSR) Nov 1986, 102 (11) p530-2

Antioxidant protection against adrenaline-induced arrhythmias in rats with chronic heart hypertrophy. Can J Cardiol (CANADA) Mar 1990, 6 (2) p71-4

The antiarrhythmic effects of taurine alone and in combination with magnesium sulfate on ischemia/reperfusion arrhythmia. Chinese Pharmacological Bulletin (China), 1994, 10/5 (358-362)

Prophylactic effects of taurine and diltiazem, alone or combined, on reperfusion arrhythmias in rats. Acta Pharmacologica Sinica (China), 1996, 17/2

The effects of antioxidants on reperfusion dysrhythmias. Ceska a Slovenska Farmacie (Czech Republic), 1995, 44/5 (257-260)

Protective effects of all-trans-retinoic acid against cardiac arrhythmias induced by isopro-

References

terenol, lysophosphatidylcholine or ischemia and reperfusion. Journal of Cardiovascular Pharmacology (USA), 1995, 26/6

Effects of dietary supplementation with alpha-tocopherol on myocardial infarct size and ventricular arrhythmias in a dog model of ischemia-reperfusion. J. AM. COLL. CARDIOL. (USA), 1994, 24/6 (1580-1585)

Magnesium flux during and after open heart operations in children. Ann Thorac Surg (UNITED STATES) Apr 1995, 59 (4) p921-7

Sino-atrial Wenckebach conduction in thyrotoxic periodic paralysis: a case report. Int J Cardiol (IRELAND) Jan 6 1995, 47 (3) p285-9

A possible beneficial effect of selenium administration in antiarrhythmic therapy. J Am Coll Nutr (UNITED STATES) Oct 1994, 13 (5) p496-8

Omega-3 fatty acids and prevention of ventricular fibrillation. Prostaglandins Leukot Essent Fatty Acids (SCOTLAND) Feb-Mar 1995, 52

[Effect of anti-arrhythmia drugs on the beta2 receptor-dependent adenyl cyclase system of lymphocytes in patients with cardiac rhythm disorders]. Kardiologiia (USSR) Jul 1989, 29 (7) p25-9

An expanded concept of "insurance" supplementation—broad-spectrum protection from cardiovascular disease. Med Hypotheses (ENGLAND) Oct 1981, 7 (10) p1287-1302

Italian multicenter study on the safety and efficacy of coenzyme Q10 as adjunctive therapy in heart failure (interim analysis). Clin Investig (GERMANY) 1993, 71 (8 Suppl) pS145-9

Isolated diastolic dysfunction of the myocardium and its response to CoQ10 treatment. Clin Investig (GERMANY) 1993, 71 (8 Suppl) pS140-4

Protective effects of propionyl-L-carnitine during ischemia and reperfusion. Cardiovasc Drugs Ther (UNITED STATES) Feb 1991, 5 Suppl 1 p77-83

Consequences of magnesium deficiency on the enhancement of stress reactions; preventive and therapeutic implications (a review). J Am Coll Nutr (UNITED STATES) Oct 1994

Community-based prevention of stroke: nutritional improvement in Japan. Health Rep (CANADA) 1994, 6 (1)

Effect of dietary magnesium supplementation on intralymphocytic free calcium and magnesium in stroke-prone spontaneously hypertensive rats. Clin Exp Hypertens (UNITED STATES) May 1994

Clinical study of cardiac arrhythmias using a 24-hour continuous electrocardiographic recorder (5th report)—antiarrhythmic action of coenzyme Q10 in diabetics. Tohoku J Exp Med (JAPAN) Dec 1983, 141 Suppl p453-63

Usefulness of coenzyme Q10 in clinical cardiology: a long-term study. Mol Aspects Med (ENGLAND) 1994, 15 Suppl

References

Isolated diastolic dysfunction of the myocardium and its response to CoQ10 treatment. Clin Investig (GERMANY) 1993, 71 (8 Suppl) pS140-4

Effect of coenzyme Q10 on structural alterations in the renal membrane of stroke- prone spontaneously hypertensive rats. Biochem Med Metab Biol (UNITED STATES) Apr 1991

Coenzyme Q10: a new drug for cardiovascular disease. J Clin Pharmacol (UNITED STATES) Jul 1990

[Effects of 2,3-dimethoxy-5-methyl-6-(10'-hydroxydecyl)-1,4-benzoquinone (CV-2619) on adriamycin-induced ECG abnormalities and myocardial energy metabolism in spontaneously hypertensive rats] Nippon Yakurigaku Zasshi (JAPAN) Oct 1982

Bioenergetics in clinical medicine. III. Inhibition of coenzyme Q10-enzymes by clinically used anti-hypertensive drugs. Res Commun Chem Pathol Pharmacol (UNITED STATES) Nov 1975

Bioenergetics in clinical medicine. Studies on coenzyme Q10 and essential hypertension. Res Commun Chem Pathol Pharmacol (UNITED STATES) Jun 1975

[Prevention of cerebrovascular insults] Schweiz Med Wochenschr (SWITZERLAND) Nov 12 1994

[Essential antioxidants in cardiovascular diseases—lessons for Europe] Ther Umsch (SWITZERLAND) Jul 1994

Antioxidant vitamin intake and coronary mortality in a longitudinal population study. Am J Epidemiol (UNITED STATES) Jun 15 1994

Decline in stroke mortality. An epidemiologic perspective. Ann Epidemiol Sep 1993

Can antioxidants prevent ischemic heart disease? J Clin Pharm Ther (ENGLAND) Apr 1993

Antioxidant therapy in the aging process. EXS (SWITZERLAND) 1992, 62

Effect of flosequinan on ischaemia-induced arrhythmias and on ventricular cyclic nucleotide content in the anaesthetized rat. Br J Pharmacol (ENGLAND) Apr 1993, 108 (4) p1111-6

What do the newer inotropic drugs have to offer? CARDIOVASC. DRUGS THER. (USA) , 1992, 6/1 (15-18)

Arrhythmogenic effect of forskolin in the isolated perfused rat heart: Influence of nifedipine reduction of external calcium. CLIN. EXP. PHARMACOL. PHYSIOL. (Australia) , 1989, 16/10 (751-757)

Hormone secretagogues increase cytosolic calcium by increasing cAMP in corticotropin-secreting cells. PROC. NATL ACAD. SCI. U. S. A. (USA) , 1985, 82/23 (8034-8038)

The genesis of arrhythmias during myocardial ischemia. Dissociation between changes in cyclic adenosine monophosphate and electrical instability in the rat. CIRC. RES. (USA) , 1985, 57/5 (668-675) CODEN: CIRUA

Effects of high K on relaxation produced by drugs in the guinea-pig tracheal muscle. RESPIR.

PHYSIOL. (NETHERLANDS) , 1985, 61/1 (43-55)

Forskolin inhibits ouabain-sensitive ATPase in the medulla of rat kidney. IRCS MED. SCI. (ENGLAND) , 1983, 11/11 (957-958)

Arthritis

Treatment of rheumatoid arthritis with blackcurrant seed oil. BR. J. RHEUMATOL. (United Kingdom), 1994, 33/9 (847-852)

Treatment of rheumatoid arthritis with gammalinolenic acid. ANN. INTERN. MED. (USA), 1993, 119/9 (867-873)

Validation of a meta-analysis: The effects of fish oil in rheumatoid arthritis. Journal of Clinical Epidemiology (USA), 1995, 48/11 (1379-1390)

Botanical lipids: Effects on inflammation, immune responses, and rheumatoid arthritis. Seminars in Arthritis and Rheumatism (USA), 1995, 25/2 (87-96)

n-3 Polyunsaturated fatty acids: Update 1995. European Journal of Clinical Investigation (United Kingdom), 1995, 25/9

Marine and botanical lipids as immunomodulatory and therapeutic agents in the treatment of rheumatoid arthritis. Rheumatic Disease Clinics of North America (USA), 1995, 21/3 (759-777)

Attenuation of adjuvant arthritis in rats by treatment with oxygen radical scavengers. IMMUNOL. CELL BIOL. (Australia), 1994, 72/5

Alteration of the cellular fatty acid profile and the production of eicosanoids in human monocytes by gamma-linolenic acid. ARTHRITIS RHEUM. (USA), 1990, 33/10 (1526-1533)

Suppression of acute and chronic inflammation by dietary gamma linolenic acid. J. RHEUMATOL. (Canada), 1989, 16/6 (729-733)

Reactive oxygen species, lipid peroxides and essential fatty acids in patients with rheumatoid arthritis and systemic lupus erythematosus. PROSTAGLANDINS LEUKOTRIENES ESSENT. FATTY ACIDS (United Kingdom), 1991, 43/4

Suppression of acute and chronic inflammation by dietary gamma linolenic acid. J. RHEUMATOL. (Canada), 1989, 16/6 (729-733)

Effects of fish oil supplementation on non-steroidal anti-inflammatory drug requirement in patients with mild rheumatoid arthritis—a double-blind placebo controlled study. Br J Rheumatol (ENGLAND) Nov 1993, 32 (11) p982-9

Association of etretinate and fish oil in psoriasis therapy. Inhibition of hypertriglyceridemia resulting from retinoid therapy after fish oil supplementation. Acta Derm Venereol Suppl (Stockh) (NORWAY) 1994, 186 p151-3

References

Intravenous infusion of n-3 polyunsaturated fatty acids. Proc Soc Exp Biol Med (UNITED STATES) Jun 1992, 200 (2) p171-3

Effects of dietary fish oil lipids on allergic and inflammatory diseases. Allergy Proc (UNITED STATES) Sep-Oct 1991, 12 (5) p299-303

Omega-3 fatty acids in health and disease and in growth and development. Am J Clin Nutr (UNITED STATES) Sep 1991, 54 (3) p438-63

The effect of dietary fish oil supplement upon the content of dihomo-gammalinolenic acid in human plasma phospholipids. Prostaglandins Leukot Essent Fatty Acids (SCOTLAND) May 1990, 40 (1) p9-12

Summary of the NATO advanced research workshop on dietary omega 3 and omega 6 fatty acids: biological effects and nutritional essentiality. J Nutr (UNITED STATES) Apr 1989, 119 (4) p521-8

Health effects and metabolism of dietary eicosapentaenoic acid. Prog Food Nutr Sci (ENGLAND) 1988, 12 (2) p111-50

[Potential value of eicosapentaenoic acid]. Allerg Immunol (Paris) (FRANCE) Oct 1987, 19 (8 Suppl) p12-3

Collagen antibodies in Ross River virus disease (epidemic polyarthritis). Rheumatol Int (GERMANY, WEST) 1987, 7 (6) p267-9

Effects of dietary supplementation with marine fish oil on leukocyte lipid mediator generation and function in rheumatoid arthritis. Arthritis Rheum (UNITED STATES) Sep 1987, 30 (9) p988-97

Low prevalences of coronary heart disease (CHD), psoriasis, asthma and rheumatoid arthritis in Eskimos: are they caused by high dietary intake of eicosapentaenoic acid (EPA), a genetic variation of essential fatty acid (EFA) metabolism or a combination of both? Med Hypotheses (ENGLAND) Apr 1987, 22 (4) p421-8

Inhibition of elastase enzyme release from human polymorphonuclear leukocytes by N-acetyl-galactosamine and N-acetyl-glucosamine. Clin Exp Rheumatol (ITALY) Jan-Feb 1991, 9 (1) p17-21

Severe rheumatoid arthritis: current options in drug therapy. Geriatrics (UNITED STATES) Dec 1990, 45 (12) p43-8

Terminal N-acetylglucosamine in chronic synovitis. Br J Rheumatol (ENGLAND) Feb 1990, 29 (1) p25-31

Membrane N-acetylglucosamine: expression by cells in rheumatoid synovial fluid, and by pre-cultured monocytes. Br J Exp Pathol (ENGLAND) Oct 1989, 70 (5) p567-77

Serum levels of interleukin-2 receptor and activity of rheumatic diseases characterized by immune system activation. Arthritis Rheum (UNITED STATES) Nov 1988, 31 (11) p1358-64

References

[Therapy of gonarthrosis using chondroprotective substances. Prospective comparative study of glucosamine sulphate and glycosaminoglycan polysulphate]. Fortschr Med (GERMANY, EAST) Jun 28 1984, 102 (24) p676-82

Oral glucosamine sulphate in the management of arthrosis: report on a multi-centre open investigation in Portugal. Pharmatherapeutica (ENGLAND) 1982, 3 (3) p157-68

Double-blind clinical evaluation of intra-articular glucosamine in outpatients with gonarthrosis. Clin Ther (UNITED STATES) 1981, 3 (5) p336-43

A double-blind placebo controlled trial of Efamol Marine on skin and joint symptoms of psoriatic arthritis. Br J Rheumatol (ENGLAND) Oct 1994, 33 (10) p954-8

Evening primrose oil in patients with rheumatoid arthritis and side-effects of non- steroidal anti-inflammatory drugs. Br J Rheumatol (ENGLAND) Oct 1991, 30 (5) p370-2

Essential fatty acid and prostaglandin metabolism in Sjogren's syndrome, systemic sclerosis and rheumatoid arthritis. Scand J Rheumatol Suppl (SWEDEN) 1986, 61 p242-5

Beneficial effect of eicosapentaenoic and docosahexaenoic acids in the management of systemic lupus erythematosus and its relationship to the cytokine network. Prostaglandins Leukot Essent Fatty Acids (SCOT) Sep 1994,51 (3) p207-13

Fish-oil fatty acid supplementation in active rheumatoid arthritis. A double-blinded, controlled, crossover study. Ann Intern Med (UNITED STATES) Apr 1987, 106 (4) p497-503

Zonal distribution of chondroitin-4-sulphate/dermatan sulphate and chondroitin-6- sulphate in normal and diseased human synovium. Ann Rheum Dis (ENGLAND) Jan 1994, 53 (1) p35-8

Asthma

Alterations in human leukocyte function induced by ingestion of eicosapentaenoic acid. J Clin Immunol (UNITED STATES) Sep 1986, 6 (5) p402-10

The treatment of asthmatic patients using an alpha-adrenergic receptor blocking agent, co-dergocrine mesylate ('Hydergine'). Pharmatherapeutica (ENGLAND) 1980, 2 (5) p330-6

Plasma vitamin C (ascorbic acid) levels in asthmatic children. Afr J Med Med Sci (ENGLAND) Sep-Dec 1985, 14 (3-4)

Intravenous magnesium sulfate as an adjunct in the treatment of acute asthma. Chest (UNITED STATES) Jun 1995, 107 (6) p1576-81

[Magnesium in lung diseases]. Tidsskr Nor Laegeforen (NORWAY) Mar 10 1995, 115 (7) p827-8

Asthma, inhaled oxidants, and dietary antioxidants. Am J Clin Nutr (UNITED STATES) Mar 1995, 61 (3 Suppl) p625S-630S

References

Relaxant effects of forskolin on guinea pig tracheal smooth muscle. LUNG (GERMANY, WEST), 1987, 165/4 (225-237)

Bronchial asthma: Factors which contribute to 'intractable asthma' and approach to new treatments, from the standpoint of the bronchial pathophysiology. JPN. J. THORAC. DIS. (JAPAN), 1985, 23/9 (971-980)

Bronchodilator and antiallergy activity of forskolin. EUR. J. PHARMACOL. (NETHERLANDS), 1985, 111/1 (1-8)

Activation of cAMP-dependent pathways in human airway smooth muscle cells inhibits TNF-alpha-induced ICAM-1 and VCAM-1 expression and T lymphocyte adhesion. J Immunol (UNITED STATES) Mar 1 1995, 154 (5) p2358-65

Consequences of magnesium deficiency on the enhancement of stress reactions; preventive and therapeutic implications (a review). J Am Coll Nutr (UNITED STATES) Oct 1994, 13 (5) p429-46

Rapid infusion of magnesium sulfate obviates need for intubation in status asthmaticus. Am J Emerg Med (UNITED STATES) Mar 1994, 12 (2)

Magnesium sulfate for the treatment of bronchospasm complicating acute bronchitis in a four-months'-pregnant woman. Ann Emerg Med (UNITED STATES) Aug 1993, 22 (8) p1365-7

Acetylcysteine for life-threatening acute bronchial obstruction. ANN. INTERN. MED. (USA), 1978, 88/5 (656)

Effect of the combination of human thioredoxin and L-cysteine on ischemia- reperfusion injury in isolated rat lungs. European Surgical Research (Switzerland), 1995, 27/6 (363-370)

Effects of N-acetyl-L-cysteine on regional blood flow during endotoxic shock. European Surgical Research (Switzerland), 1995, 27/5 (292-300)

A combination of cefuroxime and N-acetyl-cysteine for the treatment of lower respiratory tract infections in children. INT. J. CLIN. PHARMACOL. THER. TOXICOL. (GERMANY, WEST), 1985, 23/5

Irish general practice study of acetylcysteine (Fabrol) in chronic bronchitis. J. INT. MED. RES. (ENGLAND), 1984, 12/2 (96-101)

Regulation of Ca2+-dependent K+-channel activity in tracheal myocytes by phosphorylation. NATURE (United Kingdom), 1989, 341/6238 (152-154)

Effects of N-acetyl-L-cysteine on regional blood flow during endotoxic shock. European Surgical Research (Switzerland), 1995, 27/5 (292-300)

Irish general practice study of acetylcysteine (Fabrol) in chronic bronchitis. J. INT. MED. RES. (ENGLAND), 1984, 12/2 (96-101)

Atherosclerosis

Vitamin E consumption and the risk of coronary disease in women. NEW ENGL. J. MED. (USA), 1993, 328/20 (1444-1449)

The role of free radicals in disease. Australian and New Zealand Journal of Ophthalmology (Australia), 1995, 23/1

Coenzyme Q10 and coronary artery disease. CLIN. INVEST. SUPPL. (Germany), 1993, 71/8

Dietary antioxidant vitamins and death from coronary heart disease in postmenopausal women. New England Journal of Medicine (USA), 1996, 334/18

Vitamin E and atherosclerosis: Potential role of vitamin E in the prevention of cardiovascular diseases. Nutrition Clinique et Metabolisme (France), 1996, 10/1 (43-44)

Randomized, controlled trial of antioxidant vitamins and cardioprotective diet on hyperlipidemia, oxidative stress, and development of experimental atherosclerosis: The diet and antioxidant trial on atherosclerosis (DATA). Cardiovascular Drugs and Therapy (USA), 1995, 9/6

Serum levels of vitamin E in relation to cardiovascular diseases. Journal of Clinical Pharmacy and Therapeutics (United Kingdom), 1995, 20/6

Oxidative susceptibility of low density lipoprotein from rabbits fed atherogenic diets containing coconut, palm, or soybean oils. Lipids (USA), 1995, 30/12 (1145-1150)

Coantioxidants make alpha-tocopherol an efficient antioxidant for low- density lipoprotein. American Journal of Clinical Nutrition (USA), 1995, 62/6 SUPPL.

Optimal diet for reducing the risk of arteriosclerosis. Canadian Journal of Cardiology (Canada), 1995, 11/SUPPL. G

Effect of vitamin E, vitamin C and beta-carotene on LDL oxidation and atherosclerosis. Canadian Journal of Cardiology (Canada), 1995, 11/SUPPL. G (97G-103G)

Atherosclerosis: Vitamin E protects coronary arteries. Deutsche Apotheker Zeitung (Germany), 1995, 135/41 (42+44)

Effects on health of dietary supplementation with 100 mg d-alpha-tocopheryl acetate, daily for 6 years. Journal of International Medical Research (United Kingdom), 1995, 23/5

Mechanisms of the cardioprotective effect of a diet enriched with omega-3 polyunsaturated fatty acids. Pathophysiology (Netherlands), 1995, 2/3 (131-140)

Prevention of atherosclerosis: The potential role of antioxidants. Postgraduate Medicine (USA), 1995, 98/1

Vitamin E: Metabolism and role in atherosclerosis. ANN. BIOL. CLIN. (France), 1994, 52/7-8

Vitamin C prevents cigarette smoke-induced leukocyte aggregation and adhesion to endothelium in vivo. PROC. NATL. ACAD. SCI. U. S. A. (USA), 1994, 91/16 (7688-7692)

References

Homocysteine and coronary atherosclerosis. J Am Coll Cardiol (UNITED STATES) Mar 1 1996, 27 (3) p517-27

Hyperhomocysteinaemia: a role in the accelerated atherogenesis of chronic renal failure? Neth J Med (NETHERLANDS) May 1995, 46 (5) p244-51

Hyperhomocysteinaemia and endothelial dysfunction in young patients with peripheral arterial occlusive disease. Eur J Clin Invest (ENGLAND) Mar 1995, 25 (3) p176-81

Homocysteine and coronary atherosclerosis. J Am Coll Cardiol (UNITED STATES) Mar 1 1996, 27 (3) p517-27

Vitamin nutrition status and homocysteine: an atherogenic risk factor. Nutr Rev (UNITED STATES) Nov 1994, 52 (11) p383-7

Homocysteine and coronary artery disease. Cleve Clin J Med (UNITED STATES) Nov-Dec 1994, 61 (6) p438-50

Treatment of atherosclerosis and thrombosis with aspirin. Lancet (ENGLAND) Sep 9 1972, 2 (776) p532-4

[Progress in the prevention and treatment of ischemic cerebrovascular diseases with garlic extract] Chung Kuo Chung Hsi I Chieh Ho Tsa Chih (CHINA) Feb 1995, 15 (2) p124-6 (24 Refs.)

Platelets, carotids, and coronaries. Critique on antithrombotic role of antiplatelet agents, exercise, and certain diets. Am J Med (UNITED STATES) Sep 1984, 77 (3) p513-23

Effects of 11-week increases in dietry eicosapentaenoic acid on bleeding time, lipids, and platelet aggregation. Lancet (ENGLAND) Nov 28 1981, 2 (8257) p1190-3

N -3 but not N-6 fatty acids reduce the expression of the combined adhesion and scavenger receptor CD36 in human monocytic cells. Cell Biochem Funct (ENGLAND) Sep 1995, 13 (3) p211-6

Essential fatty acid metabolism in patients with essential hypertension, diabetes mellitus and coronary heart disease. Prostaglandins Leukot Essent Fatty Acids (SCOTLAND) Jun 1995, 52 (6) p387-91

[Changes in fatty acid composition, platelet aggregability and RBC function in elderly subjects with administration of low-dose fish oil concentrate and comparison with younger subjects]. Ronen Igakkai Zasshi (JAPAN) Aug 1994, 31 (8) p596-603

Do fish oils prevent restenosis after coronary angioplasty? Circulation (UNITED STATES) Nov 1994, 90 (5) p2248-57

n-3 fatty acid incorporation into LDL particles renders them more susceptible to oxidation in vitro but not necessarily more atherogenic in vivo. Arterioscler Thromb (UNITED STATES) Jul 1994, 14 (7) p1170-6

Human atherosclerotic plaque contains both oxidized lipids and relatively large amounts of alpha-tocopherol and ascorbate. Arterioscler Thromb Vasc Biol (UNITED STATES) Oct 1995, 15 (10) p1616-24

Attention Deficit Disorder (ADD)

Do nutrient supplements and dietary changes affect learning and emotional reactions of children with learning difficulties? A controlled series of 16 cases. Nutr Health (ENGLAND) 1984, 3 (1-2) p69-77

[Effect of supplementary intake of vitamins for 6 months on physical and mental work capacity of children beginning school education at the age of 6 years]. Vopr Pitan (USSR) Jul-Aug 1988

Nutritional therapy for selected inborn errors of metabolism. J Am Coll Nutr (UNITED STATES) 1989, 8 Suppl

Vitamin supplements and purported learning enhancement in mentally retarded children. J Nutr Sci Vitaminol (Tokyo) (JAPAN) Jun 1989

Vitamin B6 in clinical neurology. Ann N Y Acad Sci (UNITED STATES) 1990, 585 p250-60

[Vitamin B12 deficiency due to abnormal eating habits]. Ned Tijdschr Geneeskd (NETHERLANDS) Feb 26 1994

Use and safety of elevated dosages of vitamin E in infants and children. Int J Vitam Nutr Res Suppl (CANADA) 1989, 30 p69-80

Experience over 17 years with antioxidant treatment in Spielmeyer-Sjogren disease. Am J Med Genet Suppl (UNITED STATES) 1988, 5 p265-74

Vitamin E and the nervous system. Crit Rev Neurobiol (UNITED STATES) 1987, 3 (1)

Clinical uses of vitamin E. Acta Vitaminol Enzymol (ITALY) 1985, 7 Suppl p33-43

Neurologic complications of vitamin E deficiency: case report and review of the literature. Bull Clin Neurosci (UNITED STATES) 1985, 50 p53-60

A progressive neurological syndrome associated with an isolated vitamin E deficiency. Can J Neurol Sci (CANADA) Nov 1984, 11 (4 Suppl) p561-4

[Evaluation of the effectiveness of prophylactic vitamin administration to school children in Moscow]. Vopr Pitan (USSR) May-Jun 1992

The assessment of the vitamin B6 status among Egyptian school children by measuring the urinary cystathionine excretion. Int J Vitam Nutr Res (SWITZERLAND) 1984, 54 (4) p321-7

Dramatic favorable responses of children with learning disabilities or dyslexia and attention deficit disorder to antimotion sickness medications: four case reports. Percept Mot Skills (UNITED STATES) Dec 1991, 73 (3 Pt 1) p723-38

New developments in pediatric psychopharmacology. J Dev Behav Pediatr (UNITED STATES)

References

Sep 1983, 4 (3) p202-9

Dramatic favorable responses of children with learning disabilities or dyslexia and attention deficit disorder to antimotion sickness medications: four case reports. Percept Mot Skills (UNITED STATES) Dec 1991, 73 (3 Pt 1) p723-38

Piracetam in the management of minimal brain dysfunction [letter]. S Afr Med J (SOUTH AFRICA) Aug 7 1976, 50 (34) p1312

Altered dopaminergic function in the prefrontal cortex, nucleus accumbens and caudate-putamen of an animal model of attention-deficit hyperactivity disorder—the spontaneously hypertensive rat. Brain Res (NETHERLANDS) Apr 10 1995, 676 (2) p343-51

Deanol and methylphenidate in minimal brain dysfunction. Clin Pharmacol Ther (UNITED STATES) May 1975, 17 (5) p534-40

Effect of dextroamphetamine and methylphenidate on calcium and magnesium concentration in hyperactive boys. Psychiatry Res (IRELAND) Nov 1994, 54 (2) p199-210

[Deficiency of certain trace elements in children with hyperactivity]. Psychiatr Pol (POLAND) May-Jun 1994, 28 (3) p345-53

[Level of magnesium in blood serum in children from the province of Rzesz'ow]. Wiad Lek (POLAND) Feb 1993, 46 (3-4) p120-2

Gamma-linolenic acid for attention-deficit hyperactivity disorder: placebo-controlled comparison to D-amphetamine. Biol Psychiatry (UNITED STATES) Jan 15 1989, 25 (2) p222-8

Megavitamins and hyperactivity [letter]. Pediatrics (UNITED STATES) Aug 1986, 78 (2) p374-5

Vitamin E and Alzheimer's disease in subjects with Down's syndrome. Journal of Mental Deficiency Research, 1988 Dec Vol 32(6) 479-484

Behavioral disorders, learning disabilities and megavitamin therapy. Adolescence 1987 Fal Vol 22(87) 729-738

Macrocytosis and cognitive decline in Down's syndrome. British Journal of Psychiatry 1986 Dec Vol 149 797-798

Treatment approaches in Down's syndrome: A review. Australia & New Zealand Journal of Developmental Disabilities

A double blind study of vitamin B-sub-6 in Down's syndrome infants: I. Clinical and biochemical results. Journal of Mental Deficiency Research 1985 Sep Vol 29(3) 233-240

A double blind study of vitamin B-sub-6 in Down's syndrome infants: II. Cortical auditory evoked potentials. Journal of Mental Deficiency Research 1985 Sep Vol 29(3) 241-246

Xylose absorption in Down's syndrome. Journal of Mental Deficiency Research 1985 Jun Vol 29(2) 173-177

References

Nutritional aspects of Down's syndrome with special reference to the nervous system. British Journal of Psychiatry 1984 Aug Vol 145 115-120

Children's mental retardation study is attacked: A closer look. International Journal of Biosocial Research 1982 Vol 3(2) 75-86

Effects of nutritional supplementation on IQ and certain other variables associated with Down syndrome. American Journal of Mental Deficiency 1983 Sep Vol 88(2) 214-217

Vitamin A and carotene values of institutionalized mentally retarded subjects with and without Down's syndrome. Journal of Mental Deficiency Research 1977 Mar Vol 21(1) 63-74

Sodium-dependent glutamate binding in senile dementia. Neurobiology of Aging 1987 May-Jun Vol 8(3) 219-223

Alzheimer-like neurotransmitter deficits in adult Down's syndrome brain tissue. Journal of Neurology, Neurosurgery & Psychiatry 1987 Jun Vol 50(6) 775-778

A report on phosphatidylcholine therapy in a Down Syndrome child. Psychological Reports 1986 Feb Vol 58(1) 207-217

Autoimmune Diseases

Androgen and progesterone levels in females with rheumatoid arthritis. REUMATISMO (Italy), 1994, 46/2 (65-69)

Docosahexaenoic and eicosapentaenoic acids inhibit human lymphoproliferative responses in vitro but not the expression of T cell surface activation markers. Scandinavian Journal of Immunology (United Kingdom), 1996, 43/3

Modulation of antioxidant enzymes and programmed cell death by n-3 fatty acids. Lipids (USA), 1996, 31/3 SUPPL. (S91-S96)

Dietary marine lipids suppress continuous expression of interleukin-1beta gene transcription. Lipids (USA), 1996, 31/3 SUPPL. (S23-S31)

Tissue specific regulation of transforming growth factor beta by omega-3 lipid-rich krill oil in autoimmune murine lupus. Nutrition Research (USA), 1996, 16/3 (489-503)

The effects of dietary lipid manipulation on the production of murine T cell-derived cytokines. Cytokine (United Kingdom), 1995, 7/6 (548-553)

Dietary omega-3 lipids delay the onset and progression of autoimmune lupus nephritis by inhibiting transforming growth factor beta mRNA and protein expression. Journal of Autoimmunity (United Kingdom), 1995, 8/3 (381-393)

Fish oil feeding modulates leukotriene production in murine lupus nephritis. PROSTAGLANDINS (USA), 1994, 48/5 (331-348)

Effects of n-3 and n-6 fatty acids on the activities and expression of hepatic antioxidant

References

enzymes in autoimmune-prone NZBxNZW F1 mice. LIPIDS (USA), 1994, 29/8 (561-568)

Increased TGF-beta and decreased oncogene expression by omega-3 fatty acids in the spleen delays onset of autoimmune disease in B/W mice. J. IMMUNOL. (USA), 1994, 152/12 (5979-5987)

Decreased pro-inflammatory cytokines and increased antioxidant enzyme gene expression by omega-3 lipids in murine lupus nephritis. BIOCHEM. BIOPHYS. RES. COMMUN. (USA), 1994, 200/2 (893-898)

Suppression of autoimmune disease by dietary n-3 fatty acids. J. LIPID RES. (USA), 1993, 34/8 (1435-1444)

Role of omega-3 fatty acids in health and disease. NUTR. RES. (USA), 1993, 13/SUPPL. 1 (S19-S45)

Omega-3 polyunsaturated fatty acids: A potential new treatment of immune renal disease. MAYO CLIN. PROC. (USA), 1991, 66/10 (1018-1028)

Practicalities of lipids: ICU patient, autoimmune disease, and vascular disease. J. PARENTER. ENTER. NUTR. (USA), 1990, 14/5 SUPPL.

Dietary marine lipids suppress murine autoimmune disease. J. INTERN. MED. SUPPL. (United Kingdom), 1989, 225/731

Depression of humoral responses and phagocytic functions in vivo and in vitro by fish oil and eicosapentanoic acid. CLIN. IMMUNOL. IMMUNOPATHOL. (USA), 1989, 52/2 (257-270)

The type of dietary fat affects the severity of autoimmune disease in NZB/NZW mice. AM. J. PATHOL. (USA), 1987, 127/1 (106-121)

Effects of dietary supplementation on autoimmunity in the MRL/lpr mouse: A preliminary investigation. ANN. RHEUM. DIS. (UK), 1986, 45/12 (1019-1024)

A fish oil diet rich in eicosapentaenoic acid reduces cyclooxygenase metabolites, and suppresses lupus in MRL-lpr mice. J. IMMUNOL. (USA), 1985, 134/3 (1914-1919)

The protective effect of dietary fish oil on murine lupus. PROSTAGLANDINS (USA), 1985, 30/1 (51-75)

Modulation of antioxidant enzymes and programmed cell death by n-3 fatty acids. Lipids (USA), 1996, 31/3 SUPPL. (S91-S96)

Effect of (n-3) polyunsaturated fatty acids on cytokine production and their biologic function. Nutrition (USA), 1996, 12/1 SUPPL. (S8-S14)

Lipid peroxidase and erythrocyte redox system in systemic vasculitides treated with corticoids. Effect of vitamin E administration. Romanian Journal of Internal Medicine (Romania), 1994, 32/4 (283-289)

Free radical tissue damages in the anterior segment of the eye in experimental autoimmune uveitis. Investigative Ophthalmology and Visual Science (USA), 1996, 37/4

References

Intervention at diagnosis of type I diabetes using either antioxidants or photopheresis. DIA-BETES METAB. REV. (United Kingdom), 1993, 9/4 (329-336)

Free radical theory of aging: Beneficial effect of antioxidants on the life span of male NZB mice: Role of free radical reactions in the deterioration of the immune system with age and in the pathogenesis of systemic lupus erythematosus. AGE (USA), 1980, 3/3 (64-73)

The connective tissue diseases and the overall influence of gender. Int J of Fertility and Menopausal Studies (USA), 1996, 41/2

Blood dehydroepiandrosterone sulphate (DHEAS) levels in pemphigoid/pemphigus and psoriasis. Clinical and Experimental Rheumatology (Italy), 1995, 13/3

Neuroendocrine-immune system interactions and autoimmunity. Annual Review of Immunology (USA), 1995, 13/- (307-338)

Low serum levels of dehydroepiandrosterone may cause deficient IL-2 production by lymphocytes in patients with systemic lupus erythematosus (SLE). Clinical and Experimental Immunology (United Kingdom), 1995, 99/2

Bacterial Infections

Evaluation of the effect of arginine-enriched amino acid solution on tumor growth. J. PARENTER. ENTER. NUTR. (USA), 1985, 9/4 (428-434)

Activation of mouse macrophages by alkylglycerols, inflammation products of cancerous tissues. Cancer Research, 1988 Nov 1, 48(21):6044-9.

Activation of mouse peritoneal macrophages by lysophospholipids and ether derivatives of neutral lipids and phospholipids. Cancer Research, 1987 Apr 15, 47(8):2008-13.

Activation of macrophages by ether analogues of lysophospholipids. Cancer Immunology, Immunotherapy, 1987, 25(3):185-92

Interactions between alkylglycerols and human neutrophil granulocytes. Scandinavian Journal of Clinical and Laboratory Investigation, 1990 Jun, 50(4):363-70

The effect of antioxidants on bleomycin treatment in in vitro and in vivo genotoxicity assays. Mutation Research - Fundamental and Molecular Mechanisms of Mutagenesis (Netherlands), 1995, 329/1 (37-47)

Inhibitory effect of vitamin C on the mutagenicity and covalent DNA binding of the electrophilic and carcinogenic metabolite, 6-sulfooxymethylbenzo(a)pyrene. CARCINOGENESIS (United Kingdom), 1994, 15/5 (917-920)

Few aspects of bacterial colonies in the stomach during the treatment with acidoinhibitors. BOLL. CHIM. FARM. (Italy), 1992, 131/8 (302-303)

The prevention and management of pressure ulcers. MED. CLIN. NORTH AM. (USA), 1989, 73/6 (1511-1524)

References

The inhibition of bacterially mediated N-nitrosation by vitamin C: Relevance to the inhibition of endogenous N-nitrosation in the achlorhydric stomach. CARCINOGENESIS (United Kingdom), 1989, 10/2 (397-399)

Partial purification and some properties of an antibacterial compound from Aloe vera. PHYTOTHER. RES. (United Kingdom), 1988, 2/2 (67-69)

Activation of serum complement leads to inhibition of ascorbic acid transport (42530). PROC. SOC. EXP. BIOL. MED. (USA), 1987, 185/2 (153-157)

Effects of vitamins A, C, and E on aflatoxin Bsub 1-induced mutagenesis in Salmonella typhimurium TA-98 and TA-100. TERATOG. CARCINOG. MUTAG. (USA), 1985, 5/1 (29-40)

Effect of vitamin A supplementation on lectin-induced diarrhoea and bacterial translocation in rats. Nutrition Research (USA), 1996, 16/3 (459-465)

Increased translocation of Escherichia coli and development of arthritis in vitamin A- deficient rats. Infection and Immunity (USA), 1995, 63/8 (3062-3068)

Gastrointestinal infections in children. CURR. OPIN. GASTROENTEROL. (United Kingdom), 1994, 10/1 (88-97)

Intestinal malabsorption presenting with night blindness. BR. J. CLIN. PRACT. (United Kingdom), 1993, 47/5 (275-276)

Etiology of acute lower respiratory tract infection in children from Alabang, Metro Manila. REV. INFECT. DIS. (USA), 1990, 12/SUPPL. 8 (S929-S939)

Effect of vitamin A in enteral formulae for burned guinea-pigs. BURNS (United Kingdom), 1990, 16/4 (265-272)

Vitamin A supplementation improves macrophage function and bacterial clearance during experimental salmonella infection. PROC. SOC. EXP. BIOL. MED. (USA), 1989, 191/1 (47-54)

Inhibition by retinoic acid of multiplication of virulent tubercle bacilli in cultured human macrophages. INFECT. IMMUN. (USA), 1989, 57/3 (840-844)

Corneal ulceration, measles, and childhood blindness in Tanzania. BR. J. OPHTHALMOL. (UK), 1987, 71/5 (331-343)

Impact of vitamin A supplementation on childhood mortality. A randomised controlled community trial. LANCET (UK), 1986, 1/8491 (1169-1173)

Effects of vitamins A, C, and E on aflatoxin Bsub 1-induced mutagenesis in Salmonella typhimurium TA-98 and TA-100. TERATOG. CARCINOG. MUTAG. (USA), 1985, 5/1 (29-40)

Impaired blood clearance of bacteria and phagocytic activity in vitamin A-deficient rats (41999). PROC. SOC. EXP. BIOL. MED. (USA), 1985, 178/2 (204-208)

Chronic salmonella septicemia and malabsorption of vitamin A . AM. J. CLIN. NUTR. (USA), 1979, 32/2 (319-324)

References

Retinol level in patients with psoriasis during treatment with B group vitamins, a bacterial polysaccharide (pyrogenal) and methotrexate (Russian). VESTN.DERM.VENER. (USSR), 1975, 51/1 (55-58)

Essential fatty acids: Biology and their clinical implications. ASIA PAC. J. PHARMACOL. (Singapore), 1991, 6/4 (317-330)

Essential fatty acid deficiency in children. TIJDSCHR. KINDERGENEESKD. (NETHER-LANDS), 1981, 49/1 (10-15)

Nitric oxide-dependent killing of Candida albicans by murine peritoneal cells during an experimental infection . FEMS Immunology and Medical Microbiology (Netherlands), 1995, 11/3 (157-162)

Biosynthesis and interaction of endothelium-derived vasoactive mediators. EICOSANOIDS (Germany), 1991, 4/4 (187-202)

Regulation of macrophage physiology by L-arginine: Role of the oxidative L-arginine deiminase pathway. J. IMMUNOL. (USA), 1989, 143/11 (3641-3646)

Comparative evaluation of aloe vera in the management of burn wounds in guinea pigs. PLAST. RECONSTR. SURG. (USA), 1988, 81/3 (386-389)

Effect of topical zinc oxide on bacterial growth and inflammation in full-thickness skin wounds in normal and diabetic rats. Agren MS; Soderberg TA; Reuterving CO; Hallmans G; Tengrup I, Department of Pathology, University of Linkoping, Sweden. Eur J Surg (SWEDEN) Feb 1991, 157 (2) p97-101.

Antimicrobial activity of some commercial extracts of propolis preparedwith different solvents. Phytotherapy Research (United Kingdom) , 1996, 10/4 (335-336)

Antibacterial action of a formulation containing propolis of Apis mellifera L. REV. FARM. BIO-QUIM. UNIV. SAO PAULO (Brazil) , 1994, 30/1 (19-21)

Electron microscopic and microcalorimetric investigations of the possible mechanism of the antibacterial action of a defined propolis provenance. PLANTA MED. (Germany) , 1994, 60/3 (222-227)

Synergistic effect of ethanolic extract of propolis and antibiotics on the growth of Staphylococcus aureus. ARZNEIM.-FORSCH. DRUG RES. (Germany) , 1993, 43/5 (607-609)

Antibacterial, antifungal, antiamoebic, antiinflammatory and antipyretic studies on propolis bee products. J. ETHNOPHARMACOL. (Ireland) , 1991, 35/1 (77-82)

Antibacterial properties of propolis (bee glue). J. R. SOC. MED. (United Kingdom) , 1990, 83/3 (159-160)

Biological properties and clinical application of propolis. III. Investigation of the sensitivity of staphylococci isolated from pathological cases to ethanol extract of propolis (EEP). ARZNEIM.-FORSCH. (GERMANY, WEST) , 1977, 27/7 (1395)

References

Biological properties and clinical application of propolis. I. Some physico chemical properties of propolis. ARZNEIMITTEL-FORSCH. (GERMANY, WEST) , 1977, 27/4 (889-890)

Balding

United States Patent: [19][11]
Patent Number: 5,352,442
Proctor: [45]
Date of Patent: Oct. 4,1994

Various other U.S. and foreign patents

Further references:

Anderson, Chemical Abstracts, vol. 90, p. 311K (1979).

Ando et al., Chemical Abstracts 93:79872n (1980).

Bazzano et al., Journal of American Academy of Dermatology, vol. 15, pp. 880-883 (1986).

Barry, Pharmacology of the Skin, vol. 1, pp. 121-137 (1987).

Cheng et al., Archives of Dermatological Research, vol. 278, pp. 470-473 (1986).

Cumming. et al., Journal of American Medical Association, vol. 247, pp. 1295-1298 (1982).

Dawber, Dermatologica, vol. 175 suppl. 2, pp. 23-28 (1987).

DeVillez, Archives of Dermatology, vol 121, pp. 197-202, (1985)

Dostert a d., Xenobiotica, vol. 15, No. 10, pp. 799-803 (1985).

Ehman et d., Investigative Radiology, vol. 21, pp. 125-131 (1986).

Feelisch et al., Evr. Journal of Pharmacology, vol. 139, pp. 19-30 (1987).

Feelisch et al., Evr. Journal of Pharmacology, vol. 142, pp. 405-409 (1987).

Fox et al., Annals of the New York Academy of Sciences, vol. 411, pp. 14-19 (1983).

Goffman et al., International Journal of Radiation, Oncology, Biology and Physics, vol. 22, pp. 803-806 (Nov. 4, 1992).

Headington, Current Therapeutic Research, vol. 36, pp. 1098-1105 (1984).

Hearse et al., Circulation Research, vol. 60, pp. 375-383 (1987).

Heschler, Chemical Abstracts, vol. 78, pp. 115-239 (1973). Ignarro et al., Biochemica ct. Biophysica Acta, vol. 631, pp. 221-231 (1980).

J., Soc. Cosmetology Chem., (Italy) vol. 33, pp. 95-96 (Mar./Apr. 1982).

Journal of American Medical Association, vol. 260, No. 20 (1988).

Karlsson et al., Journal of Cyclic Nucleotide and Protein Res., vol. 10, No. 4, pp. 309-315

References

(1985).

Kvedar, Journal of American Academic Dermatology, vol. 12, pp. 215-225 (1985).

Longevity, vol. 2, No. 3, p. 26 (Jan. 1988).

Lucky, Archives of Dermatology, vol. 121, pp.57-62 (1985). Messina, Current Therapeutic Research vol. 34, pp. 319-324 (1983).

Messina, Current Therapeutic Research, vol. 38, pp. 269-282 (1985).

Mitchell et al., IBC USA Conference, South Natick, Mass: (Jun. 27, 1991).

Mittal et al., Proc. of National Academy of Science USA, vol. 74, No. 10 pp. 4360-4364 (1977).

Bladder Conditions

See references under Urinary Tract Infections.

Breast Cancer

Progress on therapy of breast cancer with vitamin Q10 and the regression of metastases. Biochem Biophys Res Commun (UNITED STATES) Jul 6 1995

Apparent partial remission of breast cancer in 'high risk' patients supplemented with nutritional antioxidants, essential fatty acids and coenzyme Q10. Mol Aspects Med (ENGLAND) 1994, 15 Suppl

Effects of isoprenoids (coQ10) on growth of normal human mammary epithelial cells and breast cancer cells in vitro. Anticancer Res (GREECE) Jan-Feb 1994

Partial and complete regression of breast cancer in patients in relation to dosage of coenzyme Q10. Biochem Biophys Res Commun (UNITED STATES) Mar 30 1994

Modulation of the length of the cell cycle time of MCF-7 human breastcancer cells by melatonin. Life Sci (ENGLAND) 1996, 58 (9)

Melatonin blocks the stimulatory effects of prolactin on human breast cancer cell growth in culture. Br J Cancer (ENGLAND) Dec 1995

Melatonin modulation of estrogen-regulated proteins, growth factors, and proto- oncogenes in human breast cancer. J Pineal Res (DENMARK) Mar 1995

Melatonin inhibition of MCF-7 human breast-cancer cells growth: influence of cell proliferation rate. Cancer Lett (IRELAND) Jul 13 1995

Serial transplants of DMBA-induced mammary tumors in Fischer rats as model system for human breast cancer. IV. Parallel changes of biopterin and melatonin indicate interactions between the pineal gland and cellular immunity in malignancy. Oncology (SWITZERLAND)

References

Jul-Aug 1995

Modulation of cancer endocrine therapy by melatonin: a phase II study of tamoxifen plus melatonin in metastatic breast cancer patients progressing under tamoxifen alone. Br J Cancer (ENGLAND) Apr 1995

Modulation of estrogen receptor mRNA expression by melatonin in MCF-7 human breast cancer cells. Mol Endocrinol (UNITED STATES) Dec 1994

Melatonin modulates growth factor activity in MCF-7 human breast cancer cells. J Pineal Res (DENMARK) Aug 1994

Differences between pulsatile or continuous exposure to melatonin on MCF-7 human breast cancer cell proliferation. Cancer Lett (IRELAND) Sep 30 1994

Effects of melatonin on cancer: studies on MCF-7 human breast cancer cells in culture. J Neural Transm Suppl (AUSTRIA) 1986, 21 p433-49

Role of pineal gland in aetiology and treatment of breast cancer. Lancet (ENGLAND) Oct 14 1978

Beta-interferon, retinoids and tamoxifen as maintenance therapy in metastatic breast cancer. A pilot study. Clin Ter (ITALY) Oct 1995

The effects of retinoids on proliferative capacities and macromolecular synthesis in human breast cancer MCF-7 cells. Cancer (UNITED STATES) Nov 15 1980

The anti-proliferative effect of vitamin D3 analogues is not mediated by inhibition of the AP-1 pathway, but may be related to promoter selectivity. Oncogene (ENGLAND) Nov 2 1995

Epidemiology of soy and cancer: perspectives and directions. J Nutr (UNITED STATES) Mar 1995, 125 (3 Suppl)

Effects of tyrosine kinase inhibitors on the proliferation of human breast cancer cell lines and proteins important in the ras signaling pathway. Int J Cancer (UNITED STATES) Jan 17 1996

Selective responsiveness of human breast cancer cells to indole-3-carbinol, a chemopreventive agent. J Natl Cancer Inst (UNITED STATES) Jan 19 1994

Differential stimulatory and inhibitory responses of human MCF-7 breast cancer cells to linoleic acid and conjugated linoleic acid in culture. ANTICANCER RES. (Greece), 1992, 12/6 B

Inhibitory effect of conjugated dienoic derivatives of linoleic acid and beta-carotene on the in vitro growth of human cancer cells. CANCER LETT. (Ireland), 1992, 63/2 (125-133)

Preferential cytotoxicity on tumor cells by caffeic acid phenethyl ester isolated from propolis. EXPERIENTIA (Switzerland) , 1988, 44/3 (230-232)

Effect of caffeic acid esters on carcinogen-induced mutagenicity and human colon adenocarcinoma cell growth. CHEM.-BIOL. INTERACT. (Ireland) , 1992, 84/3 (277-290)

Bursitis

See references under Arthritis.

Cancer Chemotherapy

[Effect of biological membrane stabilizing drugs (coenzyme Q10, dextran sulfate and reduced glutathione) on adriamycin (doxorubicin)-induced toxicity and microsomal lipid peroxidation in mice] Gan To Kagaku Ryoho. 1996 Jan. 23(1). P 93-8

Coenzyme Q10, plasma membrane oxidase and growth control. Mol Aspects Med. 1994. 15 SupplP s1-11

Protective effects of various drugs on adriamycin (doxorubicin)-induced toxicity and microsomal lipid peroxidation in mice and rats. Biol Pharm Bull. 1993 Nov. 16(11). P 1114-7

Tissue concentration of doxorubicin (adriamycin) in mouse pretreated with alpha- tocopherol or coenzyme Q10. Acta Med Okayama. 1991 Jun. 45(3). P 195-9

[Electrocardiogram analysis of adriamycin cardiotoxicity in 160 cases] Chung Hua Chung Liu Tsa Chih. 1991 Jan. 13(1). P 71-3

Adriamycin-Fe3+-induced mitochondrial protein damage with lipid peroxidation. Biol Pharm Bull. 1995 Apr. 18(4). P 514-7

Effect of antioxidants on adriamycin-induced microsomal lipid peroxidation. Biol Trace Elem Res. 1995 Jan-Mar. 47(1-3). P 111-6

Alpha tocopherol improves focal glomerulosclerosis in rats with adriamycin-induced progressive renal failure. Nephron. 1994. 68(3). P 347-52

Adriamycin-induced oxidative stress in rat central nervous system. Biochem Mol Biol Int. 1993 Apr. 29(5). P 807-20

[Cardioprotection in chemo- and radiotherapy for malignant diseases—an echocardiographic pilot study] Schweiz Rundsch Med Prax. 1995 Oct 24. 84(43). P 1220-3

Randomised comparison of fluorouracil, epidoxorubicin and methotrexate (FEMTX) plus supportive care with supportive care alone in patients with non-resectable gastric cancer. Br J Cancer. 1995 Mar. 71(3). P 587-91

Enhancement of the antineoplastic effect of anticarcinogens on benzo[a]pyrene- treated Wistar rats, in relation to their number and biological activity. Cancer Lett. 1994 Jul 29. 82(2). P 153-65

Critical reappraisal of vitamins and trace minerals in nutritional support of cancer patients. Support Care Cancer. 1993 Nov. 1(6). P 295-7

The effects of chemotherapy including cisplatin on vitamin D metabolism. Endocr J. 1993 Dec. 40(6). P 737-42

References

Vitamin A, a useful biochemical modulator capable of preventing intestinal damage during methotrexate treatment. Pharmacol Toxicol. 1993 Aug. 73(2). P 69-74

Chemotherapy-induced alopecia: new developments South Med J. 1993 May. 86(5). P 489-96

Vitamin E enhances the chemotherapeutic effects of adriamycin on humanprostatic carcinoma cells in vitro. J. UROL. (BALTIMORE) (USA), 1986, 136/2 (529-531)

Hematological aspects of vitamin E, continued. Adriamycin cardiotoxicity amelioration by alpha-tocopherol. AM. J. PEDIATR. HEMATOL. ONCOL. (USA), 1979, 1/2 (151-153)

Treatment of cancer-related thrombocytopenia by low-dose subcutaneous Interleukin- 2 plus the pineal hormone melatonin: A biological phase II study. Journal of Biological Regulators and Homeostatic Agents (Italy), 1995, 9/2 (52-54)

Type 2 Th cells as target of the circadian melatonin signal: Relevance in local immunity. Regional Immunology (USA), 1995, 6/5-6 (350-354)

Hematopoietic rescue via T-cell-dependent, endogenous granulocyte- macrophage colony-stimulating factor induced by the pineal neurohormone melatonin in tumor-bearing mice. CANCER RES. (USA), 1994, 54/9 (2429-2432)

Randomized study with the pineal hormone melatonin versus supportive care alone in advanced nonsmall cell lung cancer resistant to a first-line chemotherapy containing cis-platin. ONCOLOGY (SWITZERLAND) (Switzerland), 1992, 49/5 (336-339)

Preliminary studies on melatonin in the treatment of myelodysplastic syndromes following cancer chemotherapy. J. PINEAL RES. (Denmark), 1990, 8/4 (347-354)

Melatonin increase as predictor for tumor objective response to chemotherapy in advanced cancer patients. TUMORI (Italy), 1988, 74/3 (339-345)

Cancer Radiation Therapy

Taurine deficiency after intensive chemotherapy and/or radiation. Am J Clin Nutr; 55(3):708-11 1992

Effect of glutaurine and its derivatives and their combinations with radiation protective substances upon irradiated mice. Acta Radiol Oncol Radiat Phys Biol; 20(5):319-324 1981

[Effect of mixed gamma-neutron irradiation on taurine penetration through cellular membranes of rat peripheral blood leukocytes] Res. Inst. Biology and Biophysics, V. V. Kuibyshev Tomsk State Univ., Tomsk, USSR

[Sources of taurine hyperexcretion in irradiated rats] Radiobiologiia; 20(3):455-459 1980

[Taurine and sh-group content in the platelets of irradiated rats] Radiobiologiia; 18(2):271-274

References

Biological Effects of Alkylglycerolsl. Prog Biochem Pharmacol; 22:48-57 1988, (37 Refs)

Effect of alkoxyglycerols on the frequency of injuries following radiation therapy for carcinoma of the uterine cervix. Acta Obstet Gynecol Scand; 56(4):441-448 1977

In vivo radioprotective activity of Panax ginseng and diethyldithiocarbamate. In Vivo; 7(5):467-70 1993

Inhibition of mutagenesis and transformation by root extracts of panax ginseng in vitro. Planta Med; 57(2):125-8 1991

Restoration of radiation injury by ginseng. Ii. Some properties of the radioprotective substances. J Radiat Res (Tokyo); 22(3):336-343

Restoration of radiation injury by ginseng. I. Responses of x-irradiated mice to ginseng extract. J Radiat Res (Tokyo); 22(3):323-335

[Substances stimulating recovery from radiation injury]. Radioisotopes; 27(11):666-675 1978

Acemannan Immunostimulant in combination with surgery and radiation therapy on spontaneous canine and feline fibrosarcomas. J Am Anim Hosp Assoc; 31(5):439-47 1995

Acemannan-containing wound dressing gel reduces radiation-induced skin reactions in C3H mice. Int J Radiat Oncol Biol Phys; 32(4):1047-52 1995

Cancer Surgery

Interleukin 2 treatment in colorectal cancer: current results and future prospects. Eur J Surg Oncol; 20(6):622-9 1994

Perioperative immunomodulation in cancer surgery. Am J Surg; 167(1):174-9 1994

Immune defects in patients with head and neck cancer. Anticancer Res; 13(6B):2507-19 1993

Effects of alprazolam on cellular immune response to surgical stress in mice. Cancer Lett; 73(2-3):155-60 1993

Morphine attenuates surgery-induced enhancement of metastatic colonization in rats. Pain; 54(1):21-8 1993

Narcotic-induced suppression of natural killer cell activity in ventilated and nonventilated rats. Clin Immunol Immunopathol; 64(2):173-6 1992

The impact of surgery on natural killer cell cytotoxicity and tumor metastasis in rats. Diss Abstr Int [B]; 53(4):1776 1992

Altered lymphocyte subsets and natural killer cells of patients with obstructive jaundice in perioperative period. J Tongji Med Univ; 11(3):145-9 1991

Hierarchical immunosuppression of regional lymph nodes in patients with head and neck

References

squamous cell carcinoma. Otolaryngol Head Neck Surg; 105(4):517-27 1991

Effects of alprazolam on t-cell immunosuppressive response to surgical stress in mice. Cancer Lett; 58(3):183-7 1991

Blood transfusion and survival after laryngectomy for laryngeal carcinoma. J Laryngol Otol; 105(4):293-4 1991

[The effect of surgical intervention on the state of the immune system in brain tumors]. Klin Khir; (12):4-6 1990

[Dynamics of various indicators of immunity in relation to the type of anesthesia during surgical treatment of patients with lung cancer after irradiation]. Vestn Khir Im I I Grek; 145(8):99-102 1990

Mechanism of surgical stress impairment of murine natural killer cell cytotoxicity. Diss Abstr Int [B]; 51(6):2809 1990

Highly immunogenic regressor tumor cells can prevent development of postsurgical tumor immunity. Cell Immunol; 119(1):101-13 1989

General concepts in cancer treatment. Surgical Oncology: A European Handbook, p. 121-305, 1989

Effects of low dose perioperative interferon on the surgically induced suppression of antitumour immune responses. Br J Surg; 75(10):976-81 1988

Lymphocyte subsets, natural killer cytotoxicity, and perioperative blood transfusion for elective colorectal cancer surgery. Cancer Detect Prev Suppl; 1:571-6 1987

Effect of surgical stress on murine natural killer cell cytotoxicity. J Immunol; 138(1):171-8 1987

Immune suppression: therapeutic alterations. Principles of Cancer Biotherapy, p. 93-162, 1987

Suppression of natural killer cell activity by surgical stress in cancer patients and the underlying mechanisms. Acta Med Okayama; 40(2):113-9 1986

Surgical stress-mediated suppression of murine natural killer cell cytotoxicity. Cancer Res; 44(9):3888-91 1984

Surgery, trauma and immune suppression. Evolving the mechanism. Ann Surg; 197(4):434-8 1983

Surgical essentials in the care of the elderly cancer patient. Aging; 24:57-61 1983

[Postoperative treatment of malignant brain tumors with acnu and psk-particularly immunological follow-up research]. Gan To Kagaku Ryoho; 9(6):1081-90 1982

Principles of pathology in surgery. Principles of Pathology in Surgery, 453 pp., 1980

Small cell carcinoma of the lung. Ann Thorac Surg; 30(6):602-610 1980

References

Cancer and immunocompetence. Acta Chir Scand Suppl; (498):146-150 1980

Alteration of lymphocyte function due to anesthesia: in vivo and in vitro suppression of mitogen-induced blastogenesis by sodium pentobarbital. Surgery; 87(5):573-580 1980

A mechanism of suppression of antitumor immunity (lai reactivity) by surgery. Cancer Immunol Immunother; 7(4):263-269 1980

[The state of immune responsiveness in various course of stomach cancer]. Vopr Onkol; 23(4):72-76 1977

Effects of operation on immune response in cancer patients: sequential evaluation of in vitro lymphocyte function. Surgery; 79(1):46-51 1976

[Surgery, hormone therapy, and irradiation in a patient with metastasizing mammary carcinoma]. Fortschr Med; 92(14):615-616 1974

Renal impairment associated with the pre-operative administration of recombinant interleukin-2. Clin Sci (Colch); 87(5):513-8 1994

Cancer Treatment Protocol

T-cell adjuvants. Int J Immunopharmacol; 16(9):703-10 1994

Therapy of secondary t-cell immunodeficiencies with biological substances and drugs. Med Oncol Tumor Pharmacother; 6(1):11-7 1989

Immunological effects of isoprinosine as a pulse immunotherapy in melanoma and arc patients. Cancer Detect Prev Suppl; 1:457-62 1987

Isoprinosine as an immunopotentiator in an animal model of human osteosarcoma. Int J Immunopharmacol; 3(4):383-389 1981

Immune effects of preoperative immunotherapy with high-dose subcutaneous interleukin-2 versus neuroimmunotherapy with low-dose interleukin-2 plus the neurohormone melatonin in gastrointestinal tract tumor patients. J Biol Regul Homeost Agents; 9(1):31-3 1995

The immunoneuroendocrine role of melatonin. J Pineal Res; 14(1):1-10 1993

Endocrine and immune effects of melatonin therapy in metastatic cancer patients. Eur J Cancer Clin Oncol; 25(5):789-95 1989

Potential of tyrosine kinase receptors as therapeutic targets in cancer. Cancer Therapy in the Twenty-First Century, Vol 1, p.49-81, 1994.

In vitro inhibition of proliferation of MDA-MB-435 human breast cancer cells by combinations of tocotrienols and flavonoids (Meeting abstract). FASEB J; 9(4):A868 1995

Effects of tyrosine kinase inhibitors on the proliferation of human breast cancer cell lines and proteins important in the ras signaling pathway. Int J Cancer; 65(2):186-91 1996

References

Reversal of multidrug resistance in vivo by dietary administration of the phytochemical indole-3-carbinol. Cancer Res; 56(3):574-81 1996

Differential sensitivity of human prostatic cancer cell lines to the effects of protein kinase and phosphatase inhibitors. Cancer Lett; 98(1):103-10 1995

Growth regulation of the human papillary thyroid cancer cell line by protein tyrosine kinase and cAMP-dependent protein kinase. Endocr J; 41(4):399-407 1994

The effects of different combinations of flavonoids on the proliferation of MDA-MB-435 human breast cancer cells (Meeting abstract). Proc Annu Meet Am Assoc Cancer Res; 36:A3538 1995

Preferential requirement for protein tyrosine phosphatase activity in the 12-O- tetrade-canoylphorbol-13-acetate-induced differentiation of human colon cancer cells. Biochem Pharmacol; 50(8):1217-22 1995

Bioactive organosulfur phytochemicals in Brassica oleracea vegetables—a review. Food Chem Toxicol; 33(6):537-43 1995

[Growth and invasion of differentiated thyroid gland carcinoma: importance of signal trans-duction]. Langenbecks Arch Chir; 380(2):96-101 1995

Nerve growth factor stimulates clonal growth of human lung cancer cell lines and a human glioblastoma cell line expressing high-affinity nerve growth factor binding sites involving tyro-sine kinase signaling. Cancer Res; 55(10):2212-9 1995

Evaluation of the biochemical targets of genistein in tumor cells. J Nutr; 125(3 Suppl):784S-789S 1995

In vitro hormonal effects of soybean isoflavones. J Nutr; 125(3 Suppl):751S-756S 1995

Resistance of melanoma cell lines to interferons correlates with reduction of IFN- induced tyrosine phosphorylation. Induction of the anti-viral state by IFN is prevented by tyrosine kinase inhibitors. J Immunol; 154(5):2248-56 1995

Biotherapy of B-cell precursor leukemia by targeting genistein to CD19-associated tyrosine kinases. Science; 267(5199):886-91 1995

Genistein inhibits the growth of prostate cancer cells. What is the mechanism? Proc Annu Meet Am Assoc Cancer Res; 36:A2310 1995

Growth-inhibitory effects of the natural phyto-oestrogen genistein in MCF-7 human breast cancer cells. Eur J Cancer; 30A(11):1675-82 1994

Natural flavonoids and lignans are potent cytostatic agents against human leukemic HL-60 cells. Life Sci; 55(13):1061-9 1994

The natural tyrosine kinase inhibitor genistein produces cell cycle arrest and apoptosis in Jurkat T-leukemia cells. Leuk Res; 18(6):431-9 1994

Selective responsiveness of human breast cancer cells to indole-3-carbinol, a chemopreventive agent. J Natl Cancer Inst; 86(2):126-31 1994

Genistein is an effective stimulator of sex hormone-binding globulin production in hepato-carcinoma human liver cancer cells and suppresses proliferation of these cells in culture. Steroids; 58(7):301-4 1993

Lycopene is a more potent inhibitor of human cancer cell proliferation than either alpha-carotene or beta-carotene. Nutr Cancer; 24(3):257-66 1995

Inhibitory effect of 220-oxa-1,25-dihydroxyvitamin D3 on the proliferation of pancreatic cancer cell lines. Gastroenterology; 110(5):1605-13 1996

Antiproliferative responses to two human colon cancer cell lines to vitamin D3 are differently modified by 9-cis-retinoic acid. Cancer Res; 56(3):623-32 1996

Vitamin D: a modulator of cell proliferation and differentiation. J Steroid Biochem Mol Biol; 37(6):873-6 1990

Preferential cytotoxicity on tumor cells by caffeic acid phenethyl ester isolated from propolis. EXPERIENTIA (Switzerland) , 1988, 44/3 (230-232)

Effect of caffeic acid esters on carcinogen-induced mutagenicity and human colon adeno-carcinoma cell growth. CHEM.-BIOL. INTERACT. (Ireland) , 1992, 84/3 (277-290)

Candida (Fungal, Yeast) Infections

[Fecal microflora in healthy young people]. Zh Mikrobiol Epidemiol Immunobiol (USSR) Feb 1983, (2) p36-40

Biotherapeutic agents. A neglected modality for the treatment and prevention of selected intestinal and vaginal infections. JAMA (UNITED STATES) Mar 20 1996, 275 (11) p870-6

Influence of lactobacilli on the adhesion of Staphylococcus aureus and Candida albicans to fibers and epithelial cells. J Ind Microbiol (ENGLAND) Sep 1995, 15 (3) p248-53

Effect of Lactobacillus acidophilus on antibiotic-associated gastrointestinal morbidity: a prospective randomized trial. J Otolaryngol (CANADA) Aug 1995, 24 (4) p230-3

Inhibition of Candida albicans by Lactobacillus acidophilus: evidence for the involvement of a peroxidase system. Microbios (ENGLAND) 1994, 80 (323) p125-33

Ingestion of yogurt containing Lactobacillus acidophilus as prophylaxis for candidal vaginitis [see comments]. Ann Intern Med (UNITED STATES) Mar 1 1992, 116 (5) p353-7

Evidence for the involvement of thiocyanate in the inhibition of Candida albicans by Lactobacillus acidophilus. Microbios (ENGLAND) 1990, 62 (250) p37-46

Viricidal effects of Lactobacillus and yeast fermentation. Appl Environ Microbiol (UNITED STATES) Aug 1983, 46 (2) p452-8

Inhibition of Candida albicans by Lactobacillus acidophilus. J Dairy Sci (UNITED STATES)

References

May 1980, 63 (5) p830-2

Thrush bowel infection: existence, incidence, prevention and treatment, particularly by a Lactobacillus acidophilus preparation. Curr Med Drugs (ENGLAND) Dec 1967, 8 (4) p3-11

[Candida infection of the female genitalia. Complaints and clinical findings] Candidainfektion des weiblichen dGenitales. Beschwerden und Befund. Med Klin (GERMANY, WEST) Jan 31 1969, 64 (5) p203-6

Dietary supplement of neosugar alters the fecal flora and decreases activities of some reductive enzymes in human subjects. Am J Clin Nutr (UNITED STATES) May 1996, 63 (5) p709-16

In vitro fructooligosaccharide utilization and inhibition of Salmonella spp. by selected bacteria. Poult Sci (UNITED STATES) Sep 1995, 74 (9) p1418-25

Dietary fructooligosaccharide, xylooligosaccharide and gum arabic have variable effects on cecal and colonic microbiota and epithelial cell proliferation in mice and rats. J Nutr (UNITED STATES) Oct 1995, 125 (10) p2604-9

A comparison of susceptibility to five antifungal agents of yeast cultures from burn patients. Burns (ENGLAND) May 1995, 21 (3) p167-70

[A trial of the use of diflucan (fluconazole) in patients with vaginal candidiasis]. Antibiot Khimioter. 1993 Dec. 38(12). P 39-41

[Fluconazole—a new antifungal agent]. Tidsskr Nor Laegeforen. 1992 Jun 10. 112(15). P 1961-3

[Endogenous candida endophthalmitis: a new therapy]. Klin Monatsbl Augenheilkd. 1991 Dec. 199(6). P 446-9

Perspective Evaluation of Candida Antigen Detection Test For Invasive Candidiasis and Immunocompromised Adult Patients With Cancer. The American Journal of Medicine, December 1989;87(621-627)

Pathogenesis of Candidiasis: Immunosuppression By Cell Wall Mannan Catabolites, Archives of Surgery, November 1989; 124:1290-1294

Ingestion of Yogurt Containing Lactobacillus Acidophilus as Prophylaxis for Candidal Vaginitis. Annals of Internal Medicine, March 1, 1992;116(5):353-357

Garlic: A Review of Its Relationship to Malignant Disease. Preventive Medicine, May 1990;19(3):346-361

Anticandidal and Anticarcinogenic Potentials For Garlic. International Clinical Nutrition Review, October 1990;10(4):423-429.

Vaginal Flora and Urinary Tract Infections. Current Opinion in Infectious Disease, 1991;4:37-41

Regulation of The Immune Response to Candida Albicans by Monocyte and Progesterone.

American Journal of Obstetrics and Gynecology, 1991;164:1351-4

Hydrogen Peroxide-Producing Organisms Toxic To Vaginal Bacteria. Infectious Disease News, August 8, 1991;5

The Vaginal Ecosystem. Mardh, Per-Anders, M.D., American Journal of Obstetrics and Gynecology, October 1991;165(4): Part II:1163-1168.

Ingestion of Yogurt Containing Lactobacillus Acidophilus as Prophylaxis for Candidal Vaginitis. Annals of Internal Medicine, March 1, 1992;116(5);353-357

Catabolic Wasting

Feeding conjugated linoleic acid to animals partially overcomes catabolic responses due to endotoxin injection. Biochem Biophys Res Commun (UNITED STATES) Feb 15 1994, 198

Inhibition of lipolysis and muscle protein degradation by EPA in cancer cachexia. Nutrition (USA), 1996, 12/1 SUPPL. (S31-S33)

The effect of polyunsaturated fatty acids on the progress of cachexia in patients with pancreatic cancer. Nutrition (USA), 1996, 12/1 SUPPL. (S27-S30)

Comparison of the effectiveness of eicosapentaenoic acid administered as either the free acid or ethyl ester as an anticachectic and antitumour agent. PROSTAGLANDINS LEUKOTRIENES ESSENT. FATTY ACIDS (United Kingdom), 1994, 51/2 (141-145)

Kinetics of the inhibition of tumour growth in mice by eicosapentaenoic acid-reversal by linoleic acid. BIOCHEM. PHARMACOL. (United Kingdom), 1993, 45/11 (2189-2194)

Anticachectic and antitumor effect of eicosapentaenoic acid and its effect on protein turnover. CANCER RES. (USA), 1991, 51/22 (6089-6093)

Muscle wasting and dedifferentiation induced by oxidative stress in a murine model of cachexia is prevented by inhibitors of nitric oxide synthesis and antioxidants. EMBO Journal (United Kingdom), 1996, 15/8 (1753-1765)

Modulation of immune function and weight loss by L-arginine in obstructive jaundice in the rat. BR. J. SURG. (United Kingdom), 1994, 81/8 (1199-1201)

Effects of L-carnitine on serum triglyceride and cytokine levels in rat models of cachexia and septic shock. British Journal of Cancer (United Kingdom), 1995, 72/5

L-carnitine deficiency in AIDS patients. AIDS (United Kingdom), 1992, 6/2 (203-205)

The enzymatic activities of branched-chain amino acid catabolism in tumour-bearing rats. CANCER LETT. (Ireland), 1992, 61/3 (239-242)

Branched chain amino acids as the protein component of parenteral nutrition in cancer cachexia. BR. J. SURG. (United Kingdom), 1989, 76/2 (149-153)

Zinc in different tissues: Relation to age and local concentrations in cachexia, liver cirrhosis and long-term intensive care. INFUSIONSTHER. KLIN. ERNAHR. (SWITZERLAND), 1979, 6/4 (225-229)

The role of serum protein in congestive heart failure. Nutritional support in organ failure: proceedings of the International Symposium, 1990, -/- (45- 52)

Clinical rise of a combination containing phosphocreatinine as adjuvant to physiokinesiotherapy. RIABILITAZIONE (ITALY), 1976, 9/2 (51-62)

Myopathy and HIV infection. Current Opinion in Rheumatology (USA), 1995, 7/6 (497-502)

Effects of L-carnitine on serum triglyceride and cytokine levels in rat models of cachexia and septic shock. British Journal of Cancer (United Kingdom), 1995, 72/5

Cataract

Stereospecific effects of R-lipoic acid on buthionine sulfoximine-induced cataract formation in newborn rats. Biochem Biophys Res Commun (UNITED STATES) Apr 16 1996, 221 (2) p422-9

Alpha-Lipoic acid as a biological antioxidant. Free Radic Biol Med (UNITED STATES) Aug 1995, 19 (2) p 227-50

Alpha-lipoic acid supplementation prevents symptoms of vitamin E deficiency. Biochem Biophys Res Commun (UNITED STATES) Oct 14 1994

A review of the evidence supporting melatonin's role as an antioxidant. J Pineal Res (DENMARK) Jan 1995, 18 (1) p1-11

Glutathione deficiency decreases tissue ascorbate levels in newborn rats: ascorbate spares glutathione and protects against oxidative damage. Proc Natl Acad Sci U S A (UNITED STATES) Jun 1 1991, 88 (11) p4656-60

51Cr release and oxidative stress in the lens. Lens Eye Toxic Res (UNITED STATES) 1989, 6 (1-2) p183-202

Free radical tissue damage: protective role of antioxidant nutrients. FASEB J (UNITED STATES) Dec 1987, 1 (6) p441-5

Oxidative damage and defense. Am J Clin Nutr (US) Jun 1996, 63 (6) p985S-990S

[Antioxidative vitamins and cataracts in the elderly]. Z Ernahrungswiss (GERMANY) Sep 1995, 34 (3) p167-76

Alpha-lipoic acid prevents buthionine sulfoximine-induced cataract formation in newborn rats. Free Radic Biol Med (UNITED STATES) Apr 1995, 18 (4) p823-9

Prevention of cataracts by nutritional and metabolic antioxidants. Crit Rev Food Sci Nutr (UNITED STATES) 1995, 35 (1-2) p111-29

Free radicals, exercise, and antioxidant supplementation. Int J Sport Nutr (UNITED STATES)

References

Sep 1994, 4 (3) p205-20, Comment in Int J Sport Nutr 1994 Sep;4(3):203-4

The use of vitamin supplements and the risk of cataract among US male physicians. Am J Public Health (UNITED STATES) May 1994, 84 (5) p788-92

Modelling cortical cataractogenesis VII: Effects of vitamin E treatment on galactose- induced cataracts. Exp Eye Res (ENGLAND) Feb 1985, 40 (2) p213-22

Modeling cortical cataractogenesis. V. Steroid cataracts induced by solumedrol partially prevented by vitamin E in vitro. Exp Eye Res (ENGLAND) Jul 1983, 37 (1) p65-76

Antioxidant vitamins in cataract prevention. Z Ernahrungswiss (GERMANY, WEST) Mar 1989, 28 (1) p56-75

Biochemical and morphological changes in the lenses of selenium and/or vitamin E deficient rats. Biomed Environ Sci (UNITED STATES) Jun 1994, 7 (2) p109-15

Biochemical changes and cataract formation in lenses from rats receiving multiple, low doses of sodium selenite. Exp Eye Res (ENGLAND) Nov 1992, 55 (5) p671-8

Defense system of the lens against oxidative damage: effect of oxidative challenge on cataract formation in glutathione peroxidase deficient-acatalasemic mice. Exp Eye Res (ENGLAND) Oct 1980, 31 (4) p425-33 (no abstract)

Intraocular irrigating solutions and lens clarity. AMER.J.OPHTHAL. (USA), 1976, 82/4 (594-597)

Intraocular irrigating solutions. Their effect on the corneal endothelium. ARCH.OPHTHAL. (USA), 1975, 93/8 (648-657)

Cerebral Vascular Disease

The effect of hypertension on cerebral atherosclerosis in the cynomolgus monkey. STROKE (USA), 1993, 24/8 (1218-1227)

The case for intravenous magnesium treatment of arterial disease in general practice: Review of 34 years of experience. J. NUTR. MED. (United Kingdom), 1994, 4/2 (169-177)

Neuropsychiatric complications of cardiac surgery. J. CARDIOTHORAC. VASC. ANESTH. (USA), 1994, 8/1 SUPPL. 1 (13-18)

Effects of the dipyridamol-dihydroergotoxine (Hydergine) methane sulphonate associations on pOsub 2 and its incidence in brain tissue. GEN. PHARMACOL. (ENGLAND), 1983, 14/6 (579-583)

The protective effects of dietary fish oil on focal cerebral infarction. PROSTAGLANDINS MED. (USA), 1979, 3/5 (257-268)

What causes infarction in ischemic brain? NEUROLOGY (USA), 1983, 33/2 (222-233)

Effects of antihypertensive drugs on blood velocity: implications for prevention of cerebral vascular disease. CANAD.J.NEUROL.SCI. (CANADA), 1977, 4/2 (93-97)

Oxygen radicals in cerebral vascular injury. CIRC. R RES. (USA), 1985, 57/4 (508-516)

Postischemic tissue injury by iron-mediated free radical lipid peroxidation. USA ANN. EMERG. MED. (USA), 1985, 14/8 (804-809)

Role of iron ions in the genesis of reperfusion injury following successful cardiopulmonary resuscitation: Preliminary data and a biochemical hypothesis. ANN. EMERG. MED. (USA), 1985, 14/8 (777-783)

Cortical pOsub 2 distribution during oligemic hypotension and its pharmacological modifications (Hydergine). SWITZERLAND ARZNEIM.-FORSCH. (GERMANY, WEST), 1978, 28/5 (768-770)

The use of piracetam (Nootropil) in post-anesthetic recovery of elderly patients. (A preliminary study). GREECE ACTA ANAESTHESIOL. HELL. (GREECE), 1981, 15/1-2 (76-80)

Free radical reaction products and antioxidant capacity in arterial plasma during coronary artery bypass grafting. J. THORAC. CARDIOVASC. SURG. (USA), 1994, 108/1 (140-147)

Biochemical studies of cerebral ischemia in the rat - Changes in cerebral free amino acids, catecholamines and uric acid. JAPAN BRAIN NERVE (JAPAN), 1986, 38/3 (253-258)

Free radicals scavenging action and anti-enzyme activities of procyanidines from Vitis vinifera. A mechanism for their capillary protective action. Arzneimittelforschung (GERMANY) May 1994, 44 (5) p592-601

Prevention of postischemic cardiac injury by the orally active iron chelator 1,2- dimethyl-3-hydroxy-4-pyridone (L1) and the antioxidant (+)-cyanidanol-3. CIRCULATION (USA), 1989, 80/1 (158-164)

Iron-load increases the susceptibility of rat hearts to oxygen reperfusion damage. Protection by the antioxidant (+)-cyanidanol-3 and deferoxamine. CIRCULATION (USA), 1988, 78/2 (442-449)

Cholesterol Reduction

Clinical trials with gugulipid. A new hypolipidaemic agent. J Assoc Physicians India (INDIA) May 1989, 37 (5) p323-8

Hypolipidemic and antioxidant effects of Commiphora mukul as an adjunct to dietary therapy in patients with hypercholesterolemia. Cardiovasc Drugs Ther (UNITED STATES) Aug 1994, 8 (4) p659-64

Beneficial effects of Allium sativum (garlic), Allium cepa and Commiphora mukul on experimental hyperlipidemia and atherosclerosis—a comparative evaluation. J Postgrad Med (INDIA) Jul 1991, 37 (3) p132-5

Curcumin, a major component of food spice turmeric (Curcuma longa) inhibits aggregation

References

and alters eicosanoid metabolism in human blood platelets. Prostaglandins Leukotrienes and Essential Fatty Acids (United Kingdom), 1995, 52/4 (223- 227)

Influence of capsaicin, eugenol, curcumin and ferulic acid on sucrose-induced hypertriglyceridemia in rats. NUTR. REP. INT. (USA), 1988, 38/3 (571-581)

Inhibitory effect of curcumin, an anti-inflammatory agent, on vascular smooth muscle cell proliferation. EUR. J. PHARMACOL. (Netherlands), 1992, 221/2-3 (381-384)

Polyphenols as cancer chemopreventive agents. J Cell Biochem Suppl (UNITED STATES) 1995, 22 p169-80

Anti-tumour and antioxidant activity of natural curcuminoids. Cancer Lett (IRELAND) Jul 20 1995, 94 (1) p79-83

Phospholipid epitopes for mouse antibodies against bromelain-treated mouse erythrocytes. Immunology (ENGLAND) Sep 1987, 62 (1) p11-6

The effect of spices on cholesterol 7 alpha-hydroxylase activity and on serum and hepatic cholesterol levels in the rat. Int J Vitam Nutr Res (SWITZERLAND) 1991, 61 (4) p364-9

Effect of gugulipid on bioavailability of diltiazem and propranolol. J Assoc Physicians India (INDIA) Jun 1994, 42 (6) p454-5

Clinical trials with gugulipid. A new hypolipidaemic agent. J Assoc Physicians India (INDIA) May 1989, 37 (5) p323-8

Biological effects of isoflavones in young women: Importance of the chemical composition of soyabean products. British Journal of Nutrition (United Kingdom), 1995, 74/4 (587-601)

Overview of proposed mechanisms for the hypocholesterolemic effect of soy. Journal of Nutrition (USA), 1995, 125/3 SUPPL. (606S-611S)

Biological effects of a diet of soy protein rich in isoflavones on the menstrual cycle of pre-menopausal women. AM. J. CLIN. NUTR. (USA), 1994, 60/3 (333-340)

A review of the clinical effects of phytoestrogens. Obstetrics and Gynecology (USA), 1996, 87/5 II SUPPL. (897-904)

Nutritional interest of flavonoids. Medecine et Nutrition (France), 1996, 32/1 (17-27)

Inhibition of protein tyrosine kinase alters the effect of serum basic protein I on triacylglycerols and cholesterol differently in normal and hyperapoB fibroblasts. Arteriosclerosis, Thrombosis, and Vascular Biology (USA), 1995, 15/8 (1195-1203)

Influence of dietary curcumin and cholesterol on the progression of experimentally induced diabetes in albino rat. Molecular and Cellular Biochemistry (USA), 1995, 152/1 (13-21)

Effect of retinol deficiency and curcumin or turmeric feeding on brain $Na+-K+$ adenosine triphosphatase activity. MOL. CELL. BIOCHEM. (USA), 1994, 137/2 (101-107)

Bioactive substances in food: Identification and potential uses. CAN. J. PHYSIOL. PHARMA-

COL. (Canada), 1994, 72/4 (423-434)

Mechanism of antiinflammatory actions of curcumine and boswellic acids. J. ETHNOPHAR-MACOL. (Ireland), 1993, 38/2-3 (113-119)

Influence of dietary spices on adrenal steroidogenesis in rats. NUTR. RES. (USA), 1993, 13/4 (435-444)

Differential effects of dietary lipids and curcumin on kidney microsomal fatty acids and Na+, K+ - ATPase activity in rat. NUTR. RES. (USA), 1992, 12/7 (893-904)

Chronic Fatigue Syndrome

Isolated diastolic dysfunction of the myocardium and its response to CoQ10 treatment. Clin Investig (GERMANY) 1993, 71 (8 Suppl) pS140-4

Analysis of dietary intake and selected nutrient concentrations in patients with chronic fatigue syndrome. J Am Diet Assoc (UNITED STATES) Apr 1996, 96 (4) p383-6

[Chronic fatigue syndrome]. Nippon Naika Gakkai Zasshi (JAPAN) Sep 10 1993, 82 (9) p1571-6

Electron-microscopic investigation of muscle mitochondria in chronic fatigue syndrome. Neuropsychobiology (SWITZERLAND) 1995, 32 (4) p175-81

Serum levels of carnitine in chronic fatigue syndrome: clinical correlates. Neuropsychobiology (SWITZERLAND) 1995, 32 (3) p132-8

Acylcarnitine deficiency in chronic fatigue syndrome. Clin Infect Dis (UNITED STATES) Jan 1994, 18 Suppl 1 pS62-7

Cirrhosis

See references under Liver (Cirrhosis)

Common Cold

Vitamin C and the common cold: a retrospective analysis of Chalmers' review. J Am Coll Nutr (UNITED STATES) Apr 1995

Interrelation of vitamin C, infection, haemostatic factors, and cardiovascular disease. BMJ (ENGLAND) Jun 17 1995, 310 (6994) p1559-63

Does vitamin C alleviate the symptoms of the common cold?—a review of current evidence. Scand J Infect Dis (SWEDEN) 1994, 26 (1) p1-6

Recommended dietary allowance: support from recent research. J Nutr Sci Vitaminol (Tokyo) (JAPAN) 1992, Spec No p173-6

References

Vitamin C and the common cold. Br J Nutr (ENGLAND) Jan 1992, 67 (1) p3-16

Vitamin C and the common cold: using identical twins as controls. Med J Aust (AUSTRALIA) Oct 17 1981, 2 (8) p411-2

The effects of ascorbic acid and flavonoids on the occurrence of symptoms normally associated with the common cold. Am J Clin Nutr (UNITED STATES) Aug 1979, 32 (8) p1686-90

Winter illness and vitamin C: the effect of relatively low doses. Can Med Assoc J (CANADA) Apr 5 1975, 112 (7) p823-6

Acetylcysteine: a drug with an interesting past and a fascinating future. Respiration (SWITZERLAND) 1986, 50 Suppl 1 p26-30

[Effect of Astragalus membranaceus on Ca2+ influx and coxsackie virus B3 RNA replication in cultured neonatal rat heart cells]. Chung Kuo Chung Hsi I Chieh Ho Tsa Chih (CHINA) Aug 1995

The inhibitory effect of astragalus membranaceus on coxsackie B-3 virus RNA replication. Chin Med Sci J (CHINA) Sep 1995, 10 (3) p146-50

[The effect of astragalus polysaccharides (APS) on cell mediated immunity (CMI) in burned mice]. Chung Hua Cheng Hsing Shao Shang Wai Ko Tsa Chih (CHINA) Mar 1994

Immunomodulating Chinese herbal medicines. Mem Inst Oswaldo Cruz (BRAZIL) 1991, 86 Suppl 2 p159-64

[The effect of vitamin A and Astragalus on the splenic T lymphocyte-CFU of burned mice]. Chung Hua Cheng Hsing Shao Shang Wai Ko Tsa Chih (CHINA) Jun 1989

Nutritional antioxidants and the modulation of inflammation: theory and practice. New Horiz (UNITED STATES) May 1994

Evaluation of zinc complexes on the replication of rhinovirus 2 in vitro. Res Commun Chem Pathol Pharmacol (UNITED STATES) Dec 1989

Zinc gluconate and the common cold: a controlled clinical study. J Int Med Res (ENGLAND) Jun 1992, 20 (3) p234-46

Prophylaxis and treatment of rhinovirus colds with zinc gluconate lozenges. J Antimicrob Chemother (ENGLAND) Dec 1987

Reduction in duration of common colds by zinc gluconate lozenges in a double-blind study. Antimicrob Agents Chemother (UNITED STATES) Jan 1984, 25 (1) p20-4

Antivirals for the chemoprophylaxis and treatment of influenza. Semin Respir Infect (UNITED STATES) Mar 1992

Utilization of pulse oximetry for the study of the inhibitory effects of antiviral agents on influenza virus in mice. Antimicrob Agents Chemother (UNITED STATES) Feb 1992

Further studies with short duration ribavirin aerosol for the treatment of influenza virus infec-

References

tion in mice and respiratory syncytial virus infection in cotton rats. Antiviral Res (NETHER-LANDS) Jan 1992

High dose-short duration ribavirin aerosol treatment—a review. Bull Int Union Tuberc Lung Dis (FRANCE) Jun-Sep 1991

Viral pneumonia. Infect Dis Clin North Am (UNITED STATES) Sep 1991

Aerosol and intraperitoneal administration of ribavirin and ribavirin triacetate: pharmacokinetics and protection of mice against intracerebral infection with influenza A/WSN virus. Antimicrob Agents Chemother (UNITED STATES) Jul 1991

Antiviral drug therapy. Am Fam Physician (UNITED STATES) Jan 1991

Molecular mechanisms of action of ribavirin. Rev Infect Dis (UNITED STATES) Nov-Dec 1990

New acquisitions in the chemotherapy of viral infections. Verh K Acad Geneeskd Belg (BELGIUM) 1990

Comparison of oral and aerosol ribavirin regimens in the high risk elderly. J Clin Pharmacol (UNITED STATES) Dec 1989

Comparative activities of several nucleoside analogs against influenza A, B, and C viruses in vitro. Antimicrob Agents Chemother (UNITED STATES) Jun 1988

Antiviral drugs for common respiratory diseases. What's here, what's to come. Postgrad Med (UNITED STATES) Feb 1 1988, 83 (2) p136-9, 142-3, 146-8

Oral ribavirin treatment of influenza A and B. Antimicrob Agents Chemother (UNITED STATES) Aug 1987

Clinical review of ribavirin. Infect Control (UNITED STATES) May 1987, 8 (5) p215-8

Clinical use of antiviral drugs. Drug Intell Clin Pharm (UNITED STATES) May 1987

Protection of mice from lethal influenza virus infection with high dose-short duration ribavirin aerosol. Antimicrob Agents Chemother (UNITED STATES) Dec 1986, 30 (6) p942-4

Ribavirin: a clinical overview. Eur J Epidemiol (ITALY) Mar 1986

Effect of ribavirin triphosphate on primer generation and elongation during influenza virus transcription in vitro. Antiviral Res (NETHERLANDS) Feb 1985, 5 (1) p39-48

Ribavirin. Drug Intell Clin Pharm (UNITED STATES) Feb 1984

[Immunomodulating activity of ethanol-water extracts of the roots of Echinacea gloriosa L., Echinacea angustifolia DC. and Rudbeckia speciosa Wenderoth tested on the immune system in C57BL6 inbred mice]. Cesk Farm (CZECH REPUBLIC) Aug 1993

Application of purified polysaccharides from cell cultures of the plant Echinacea purpurea to mice mediates protection against systemic infections with Listeria monocytogenes and Candida albicans. Int J Immunopharmacol (ENGLAND) 1991, 13 (1)

Macrophage activation by the polysaccharide arabinogalactan isolated from plant cell cul-

References

tures of Echinacea purpurea. J Natl Cancer Inst (UNITED STATES) May 3 1989

Macrophage activation and induction of macrophage cytotoxicity by purified polysaccharide fractions from the plant Echinacea purpurea. Infect Immun (UNITED STATES) Dec 1984

Combined antiviral and antimediator treatment of rhinovirus colds. J Infect Dis (UNITED STATES) Oct 1992, 166 (4)

[Common cold: diagnostic steps? Antibiotics?]. Ther Umsch (SWITZERLAND) Apr 1992, 49 (4)

Alpha 2-interferon for the common cold. Ann Pharmacother (UNITED STATES) Mar 1992, 26 (3) (no abstract)

Managing viral upper respiratory infections. Aust Fam Physician (AUSTRALIA) May 1991, 20 (5)

Immunological barriers in the nose and paranasal sinuses. Acta Otolaryngol (Stockh) (SWEDEN) May-Jun 1987, 103

Interferon for the treatment of infections. Annu Rev Med (UNITED STATES) 1987, 38 p51-9

Effect of Astragalus membranaceus on electrophysiological activities of acute experimental coxsackie B-3 viral myocarditis in mice.CHIN. MED. SCI. J. (China) , 1993, 8/4 (203-206)

Efficacy and safety of the standardized ginseng extract G 115 for potentiating vaccination against common cold and/or influenza syndrome. Drugs under Experimental and Clinical Research (Switzerland) , 1996, 22/2 65-72)

An emerging green pharmacy: Modern plant medicines and health. Gruber J.W.; DerMarderosian A. Laboratory Medicine (USA) , 1996, 27/3 (170-176)

Immunity in myocardiac hypertrophy rat and effect of total saponins of panax ginseng in vivo and in vitro. Chinese Pharmacological Bulletin (China) , 1996, 12/1 (84-86)

Treatment of experimental coxsackie B-3 viral myocarditis with astragalus membranaceus in mice. CHIN. MED. J. (CHINA) (China) , 1990, 103/1 (14-18)

Effect of Astragalus membranaceus injecta on coxsackie b-2 virus infected rat beating heart cell culture.CHIN. MED. J. (PEKING) (CHINA) , 1987, 100/7 (595-602)

Sambucol Inhibited Several Strains of Influenza Virus And Reduced Symptoms During an Outbreak of Influenza B Panama.Weizmann Institute of Science 2-15-94

The Effect of Sambucol on HIV Infection in Vitro. Congress of Microbiology 2-6-95

Congestive Heart Failure/Cardiomyopathy

Pharmacology and inotropic potential of FORSKOLIN in the human heart. J Clin Invest (UNITED STATES) Jul 1984, 74 (1) p212-23

[Effects of FORSKOLIN on canine congestive heart failure]. Nippon Yakurigaku Zasshi (JAPAN) Nov 1986, 88 (5) p389-94

Italian multicenter study on the safety and efficacy of COENZYME Q10 as adjunctive therapy in heart failure. CoQ10 Drug Surveillance Investigators. Mol Aspects Med (ENGLAND) 1994, 15 Suppl ps287-94

[Coenzyme Q10 (ubiquinone) in the treatment of heart failure. Are any positive effects documented?]. Tidsskr Nor Laegeforen (NORWAY) Mar 20 1994, 114 (8) p939-42

Italian multicenter study on the safety and efficacy of COENZYME Q10 as adjunctive therapy in heart failure (interim analysis). The CoQ10 Drug Surveillance Investigators. Clin Investig (GERMANY) 1993, 71 (8 Suppl) pS145-9

Isolated diastolic dysfunction of the myocardium and its response to CoQ10 treatment. Clin Investig (GERMANY) 1993, 71 (8 Suppl) pS140-4

Effect of coenzyme Q10 therapy in patients with congestive heart failure: a long-term multicenter randomized study. Clin Investig (GERMANY) 1993, 71 (8 Suppl) pS134-6

Role of metabolic therapy in cardiovascular disease. Clin Investig (GERMANY) 1993, 71 (8 Suppl) pS124-8

Usefulness of TAURINE in chronic congestive heart failure and its prospective application. Jpn Circ J (JAPAN) Jan 1992, 56 (1) p95-9

Coenzyme Q10: a new drug for cardiovascular disease. J Clin Pharmacol (UNITED STATES) Jul 1990, 30 (7) p596-608

Coenzyme Q10: a new drug for myocardial ischemia? Med Clin North Am (UNITED STATES) Jan 1988, 72 (1) p243-58

Cardiac performance and coenzyme Q10 in thyroid disorders. Endocrinol Jpn (JAPAN) Dec 1984, 31 (6) p755-61

A clinical study of the effect of COENZYME Q on congestive heart failure. Jpn Heart J (JAPAN) Jan 1976, 17 (1) p32-42

[MAGNESIUM in cardiology]. Schweiz Rundsch Med Prax (SWITZERLAND) May 2 1995, 84 (18) p526-32

MAGNESIUM therapy in acute myocardial infarction when patients are not candidates for thrombolytic therapy. J Cardiol (UNITED STATES) Feb 15 1995, 75 (5) p321-3

[Oral MAGNESIUM supplementation to patients receivingdiuretics — normalization of MAGNESIUM, POTASSIUM and sodium, and POTASSIUM pumps in the skeletal muscles]. Ugeskr

References

Laeger (DENMARK) Jul 4 1994, 156 (27) p4007-10, 4013

Effects of intravenous MAGNESIUM sulfate on arrhythmias in patients with congestive heart failure. Am Heart J (UNITED STATES) Jun 1993, 125 (6) p1645-50

MAGNESIUM-POTASSIUM interactions in cardiac arrhythmia. Examples of ionic medicine. Magnes Trace Elem (SWITZERLAND) 92 1991, 10 (2-4) p193-204

Clinical clues to MAGNESIUM deficiency. Isr J Med Sci (ISRAEL) Dec 1987, 23 (12) p1238-41

Platelet TAURINE in patients with arterial hypertension, myocardial failure or infarction. Acta Med Scand Suppl (SWEDEN) 1980, 642 p79-84

Physiological and experimental regulation of TAURINE content in the heart. Fed Proc (UNITED STATES) Jul 1980, 39 (9) p2685-90

A relation between myocardial TAURINE contest and pulmonary wedge pressure in dogs with heart failure. Physiol Chem Phys (UNITED STATES) 1977, 9 (3) p259-63

Adrenergic stimulation of TAURINE transport by the heart. Science (UNITED STATES) Oct 28 1977, 198 (4315) p409-11

Effects of L-CARNITINE administration on left ventricular remodeling after acute anterior myocardial infarction. J Am Coll Cardiol (UNITED STATES) Aug 1995, 26 (2) p380-7

The myocardial distribution and plasma concentration of CARNITINE in patients with mitral valve disease. Surg Today (JAPAN) 1994, 24 (4) p313-7

Myocardial CARNITINE metabolism in congestive heart failure induced by incessant tachycardia. Basic Res Cardiol (GERMANY) Jul-Aug 1993, 88 (4) p362-70

[The clinical and hemodynamic effects of propionyl-L-CARNITINE in the treatment of congestive heart failure]. Clin Ter (ITALY) Nov 1992, 141 (11) p379-84

L-CARNITINE treatment for congestive heart failure—experimental and clinical study. Jpn Circ J (JAPAN) Jan 1992, 56 (1) p86-94

The therapeutic potential of CARNITINE in cardiovascular disorders. Clin Ther (UNITED STATES) Jan-Feb 1991, 13 (1) p2-21; discussion 1

[Dilated cardiomyopathy due to primary CARNITINE deficiency] Cardiomiopatia dilatativa da deficit primitivo di carnitina. Squarcia. Pediatr Med Chir (ITALY) Mar-Apr 1986, 8 (2) p157-61

Characterization of inwardly rectifying K+ channel in human cardiac myocytes. Alterations in channel behavior in myocytes isolated from patients with idiopathic dilated cardiomyopathy. Circulation (UNITED STATES) Jul 15 1995, 92 (2) p164-74

Impaired forearm vasodilation to hyperosmolal stimuli in patients with congestive heart failure secondary to idiopathic dilated cardiomyopathy or to ischemic cardiomyopathy. Am J Cardiol (UNITED STATES) Nov 15 1992, 70 (15) p1315-9

Usefulness of coenzyme Q10 in clinical cardiology: a long-term study. Mol Aspects Med (ENGLAND) 1994, 15 Suppl

Co-enzyme Q10: a new drug for cardiovascular disease. J Clin Pharmacol (UNITED STATES) Jul 1990

Bioenergetics in clinical medicine. Studies on coenzyme Q10 and essential hypertension. Res Commun Chem Pathol Pharmacol (UNITED STATES) Jun 1975

Can antioxidants prevent ischemic heart disease? J Clin Pharm Ther (ENGLAND) Apr 1993

Antioxidant therapy in the aging process. EXS (SWITZERLAND) 1992, 62

Constipation

Comparison of the effects of magnesium hydroxide and a bulk laxative on lipids, carbohydrates, vitamins A and E, and minerals in geriatric hospital patients in the treatment of constipation. J Int Med Res (ENGLAND) Sep-Oct 1989, 17 (5) p442-54

[Magnesium: current concepts of its physiopathology, clinical aspects and therapy]. Acta Vitaminol Enzymol (ITALY) 1982, 4 (1-2) p87-97

[Treatment of constipation with vitamin B5 or dexpanthenol] Med Chir Dig (FRANCE) 1979, 8 (7) p671-4

Endogenous nitric oxide modulates morphine-induced constipation. Biochem Biophys Res Commun (UNITED STATES) Dec 16 1991, 181 (2) p889-93

Effectiveness of bran supplement on the bowel management of elderly rehabilitation patients. J Gerontol Nurs (UNITED STATES) Oct 1995, 21 (10) p21-30

Mechanisms of constipation in older persons and effects of fiber compared with placebo. J Am Geriatr Soc (UNITED STATES) Jun 1995, 43 (6)

Deafness

See references under Hearing Loss.

Depression

Natural product formulations available in europe for psychotropic indications. Psychopharmacology Bulletin (USA), 1995, 31/4 (745-751)

Antidepressive effectiveness of a highly dosed hypericum extract. Munchener Medizinische Wochenschrift (Germany) , 1996, 138/3 (35-39)

St. John's Wort in the treatment of depression. Johanniskraut zur antidepressiven therapie. Fortschritte der Medizin (Germany), 1995, 113/25 (32-33)

References

Hypericum perforatum. Fitoterapia (Italy), 1995, 66/1 (43-68)

Psychomotoric performance improvement: Antidepressant therapy with St John's wort. THERAPIEWOCHE (Germany), 1995, 45/2 (106+108+110+112)

Hypericum in the treatment of seasonal affective disorders. J. GERIATR. PSYCHIATRY NEUROL. (Canada), 1994, 7/SUPPL. 1 (S29-S33)

Effectiveness and tolerance of the hypericum extract LI 160 compared to maprotiline: A multicenter double-blind study. J. GERIATR. PSYCHIATRY NEUROL. (Canada), 1994, 7/SUPPL. 1 (S24-S28)

Effectiveness and tolerance of the hypericum extract LI 160 in comparison with imipramine: Randomized double-blind study with 135 outpatients. J. GERIATR. PSYCHIATRY NEUROL. (Canada), 1994, 7/SUPPL. 1 (S19-S23)

Multicenter double-blind study examining the antidepressant effectiveness of the hypericum extract LI 160. J. GERIATR. PSYCHIATRY NEUROL. (Canada), 1994, 7/SUPPL. 1 (S15-S18)

Hypericum treatment of mild depressions with somatic symptoms. J. GERIATR. PSYCHIATRY NEUROL. (Canada), 1994, 7/SUPPL. 1 (S12-S14)

St. Johns' wort: A prescription from nature against depressions. Johanniskraut: ein rezept der natur gegen depressionen. THERAPIEWOCHE (Germany), 1994, 44/14 (808+811-815)

Psychopharmacological therapy after acquired brain damage. MUNCH. MED. WOCHENSCHR. (Germany), 1994, 136/4 (51-55)

Extract of St. John's wort in the treatment of depression - Attention and reaction remain unimpaired. FORTSCHR. MED. (Germany), 1993, 111/19 (37-40)

Investigations of the antidepressive effects of St. Johns Wort. PZ WISS. (Germany), 1993, 138/2 (50-54)

Experimental animal studies of the psychotropic activity of a Hypericum extract. ARZNEIM.-FORSCH./DRUG RES. (GERMANY, WEST), 1987, 37/1 (10-13)

Plasma tryptophan and five other amino acids in depressed and normal subjects. Archives of General Psychiatry 38(6):642-646, 1981

Trace amine deficit in depressive illness: the phenylalanine connexion. Acta Psychiatrica Scandinavica 61(Suppl. 280):29-39, 1980

Phenylalanine levels in endogenous psychoses. Psychiatrie, Neurologie und Medizinische Psychologie 32(10):631-633, 1980

Evaluation of the relative potency of individual competing amino acids to tryptophan transport in endogenously depressed patients. Psychiatry Research 3(2):141-150, 1980

Amino acids in mental illness. Biological psychiatry today. Vol. B Amsterdam, Elsevier/North Holland, 1979, p1581-4

References

Lithium prevention of amphetamine-induced 'manic' excitement and of reserpine- induced 'depression' in mice: possible role of 2-phenylethylamine. Psychopharmacology (Berlin) 59(3):259-262, 1978

Depression, pregnancy and phenylalanine. Neuropisiquiatria (Buenos Aires) 8(1):60-64, 1977

Theoretical and therapeutic potential of indoleamine precursors in affective disorders. Neuropsychobiology (Basel) 3(4):199-233, 1977

Phenylethylamine and glucose in true depression. Journal of Orthomolecular Psychiatry (Regina) 5(3):199-202, 1976

Therapeutic action of D-phenylalanine in Parkinson's disease. Arzneimittel-Forschung (Aulendorf) 26(4):577-579, 1976

Effects of D-phenylalanine on clinical picture and phenethylaminuria in depression. Biological Psychiatry 10(2):235-239, 1975

Phenylalanine for endogenous depression. Journal of Orthomolecular Psychiatry (Regina) 3(2):80-81, 1974

Rapidity of onset of the antidepressant effect of parenteral S-adenosyl-L-methionine. Psychiatry Research (Ireland), 1995, 56/3

The clinical potential of ademetionine (S-adenosylmethionine) in neurological disorders. DRUGS (New Zealand), 1994, 48/2 (137-152)

Primary fibromyalgia is responsive to S-adenosyl-L-methionine. CURR. THER. RES. CLIN. EXP. (USA), 1994, 55/7

S-adenosyl-L-methionine in Sjogren's syndrome and fibromyalgia. CURR. THER. RES. CLIN. EXP. (USA), 1994, 55/6

Effects of S-adenosyl-L-methionine on cognitive and vigilance functions in the elderly. CURR. THER. RES. CLIN. EXP. (USA), 1994, 55/6

Results of treatment with s-adenosyl-l-methionine in patients with major depression and internal illnesses. CURR. THER. RES. CLIN. EXP. (USA), 1994, 55/6

S-adenosyl-l-methionine (SAM) as antidepressant: Meta-analysis of clinical studies. ACTA NEUROL. SCAND. SUPPL. (Denmark), 1994, 89/154

S-adenosyl-L-methionine in the treatment of major depression complicating chronic alcoholism. CURR. THER. RES. CLIN. EXP. (USA), 1994, 55/1

Clinical evaluation of S-adenosyl-L-methionine versus transcutaneous electrical nerve stimulation in primary fibromyalgia. CURR. THER. RES. CLIN. EXP. (USA), 1993, 53/2

Double blind, placebo-controlled study of S-adenosyl-L-methionine in depressed postmenopausal women. PSYCHOTHER. PSYCHOSOM. (Switzerland), 1993, 59/1

S-Adenosyl-methionine (SAM) as antidepressant. NEW TRENDS CLIN. NEUROPHARMA-

References

COL. (Italy), 1992, 6/1-4

Efficacy of S-adenosyl-L-methionine in speeding the onset of action of imipramine. PSYCHI-ATRY RES. (Ireland), 1992, 44/3

Oral S-adenosyl-L-methionine in depression. CURR. THER. RES. CLIN. EXP. (USA), 1992, 52/3

Neuroendocrine effects of S-adenosyl-(L)-methionine, a novel putative antidepressant. J. PSYCHIATR. RES. (United Kingdom), 1990, 24/2

The antidepressant potential of oral S-adenosyl-l-methionine. ACTA PSYCHIATR. SCAND. (Denmark), 1990, 81/5

S-Adenosyl-L-methionine. A review of its pharmacological properties and therapeutic potential in liver dysfunction and affective disorders in relation to its physiological role in cell metabolism. DRUGS (New Zealand), 1989, 38/3

Antidepressants: A Comparative review of the clinical pharmacology and therapeutic use of the 'newer' versus the 'older' drugs. DRUGS (New Zealand), 1989, 37/5 (713-738)

Neuropharmacology of S-adenosyl-L-methionine. AM. J. MED. (USA), 1987, 83/5 A (95-103)

Vitamins in psychiatry. Do they have a role?. DRUGS (AUSTRALIA), 1985, 30/1

S-adenosyl-L-methionine (SAM) in clinical practice: Preliminary report on 75

minor depressives. CURR. THER. RES., CLIN. EXP. (USA), 1985, 37/4

S-Adenosyl-L-Methionine (SAM) treatment in psychogeriatry: a controlled clinical trial in depressed patients. G.GERONTOL. (ITALY), 1977, 25/3

A methyl donor, adenosylmethionine, in depression. FOLIA NEUROPSYCHIAT.(LECCE) (ITALY), 1973, 16/4

Therapeutic effects and mechanism of action of S adenosyl l methionine in depressive syndromes. MINERVA MED. (ITALY), 1973, 64/29 (1515-1529)

S-Adenosyl-methionine (SAM) as antidepressant. NEW TRENDS CLIN. NEUROPHARMA-COL. (Italy), 1992, 6/1-4

Antidepressants: A Comparative review of the clinical pharmacology and therapeutic use of the 'newer' versus the 'older' drugs. DRUGS (New Zealand), 1989, 37/5 (713-738)

Monitoring S-adenosyl-methionine blood levels and antidepressant effect. ACTA NEUROL. (ITALY), 1980, 35/6 (488-495)

Long-term high dose treatment of depression with St John's wort extract. TW Neurologie Psychiatrie (Germany), 1995, 9/4 (220-221)

Effective phytotherapy for depressive patients. Effiziente phytotherapie fur depressive. Munchener Medizinische Wochenschrift (Germany), 1996, 138/7 (58)

St John's wort - An effective alternative with almost no side-effects for the treatment of depression. Depressionen: johanniskraut - die effektive und nebenwirkungsarme alternative. Zeitschrift fur Allgemeinmedizin (Germany), 1996, 72/1 (63)

Hypericum perforatum (Saint Johns wort) in the treatment of depression. THERAPIEWOCHE (Germany), 1993, 43/17 (962)

Good results with Hypericum perforatum in the treatment of depressions. FORTSCHR. MED. (Germany), 1993, 111/8 (57-58)

The efficacy of hypericum extract is double-blind verified. PRAX. MAG. MED. (Germany), 1993, -/4 (46)

Medicinal plants improve the results of brain performance test. FORTSCHR. MED. (Germany), 1993, 111/6 (50)

The efficacy of Hypericum extract in the treatment of depression. MÜNCH. MED. WOCHEN-SCHR. (Germany), 1993, 135/8 (65)

Phytotherapeutic antidepressive agent with few side-effects. FORTSCHR. MED. (Germany), 1993, 111/3 (54+56)

Depression - To brighten up the mind with Saint-John's-Wort. TW NEUROL. PSYCHIATR. (Germany), 1992, 6/12 (793-794)

Saint Johns wort in the treatment of depressions. THERAPIEWOCHE (Germany), 1992, 42/51-52 (3074-3075)

Saint Johns wort (Hypericum perforatum extract) in the treatment of depressions. FORTSCHR. MED. (Germany), 1992, 110/31 (68-69)

Herbal medicine in depressions? PHARM. ZTG. (Germany), 1992, 137/41 (78-79)

Identification of selective MAO-type-A inhibitors in Hypericum perforatum. PHARMACOPSY-CHIATRY (Germany, Federal Republic of), 1989, 22/5 (194)

Diabetes Type I (Juvenile Diabetes)

Oral alpha lipoic acid preparation proves good bioavailability in diabetic polyneuropathy. Therapiewoche (Germany), 1995, 45/23 (1367-1370)

Lipoic acid improves nerve blood flow, reduces oxidative stress, and improves distal nerve conduction in experimental diabetic neuropathy. Diabetes Care (USA), 1995, 18/8 (1160-1167)

Thioctic (lipoic) acid: A therapeutic metal-chelating antioxidant? Biochemical Pharmacology (United Kingdom), 1995, 50/1 (123-126)

Diabetic polyneuropathy. Most effective measure: Keep blood sugar close to normal from the start. Munchener Medizinische Wochenschrift (Germany), 1995, 137/6

Primary preventive and secondary interventionary effects of acetyl-L-carnitine on diabetic neuropathy in the bio-breeding Worcester rat. Journal of Clinical Investigation (USA), 1996, 97/8 (1900-1907)

Effects of acetyl- and proprionyl-L-carnitine on peripheral nerve function and vascular supply in experimental diabetes. Metabolism: Clinical and Experimental (USA), 1995, 44/9

Acetyl-L-carnitine corrects the altered peripheral nerve function of experimental diabetes. Metabolism: Clinical and Experimental (USA), 1995, 44/5

Diabetic neuropathy in the rat: 1. Alcar augments the reduced levels and axoplasmic transport of substance P. J. NEUROSCI. RES. (USA), 1995, 40/3 (414-419)

Hypothesis: the role of vitamin C in diabetic angiopathy. PERSPECT.BIOL.MED. (USA), 1974, 17/2 (210-217)

Treatment of symptomatic diabetic peripheral neuropathy with the anti-oxidant alpha- lipoic acid. A 3-week multicentre randomized controlled trial (ALADIN Study). Diabetologia (Germany), 1995, 38/12 (1425-1433)

Alternative therapeutic principles in the prevention of microvascular and Neuropathic complications. Diabetes Research and Clinical Practice (Ireland), 1995, 28/SUPPL.

Effects of aminoguanidine on rat pancreatic islets in culture and on the pancreatic islet blood flow of anaesthetized rats. Biochemical Pharmacology (USA), 1996, 51/12 (1711-1717)

Aminoguanidine prevents the decreased myocardial compliance produced by streptozotocin-induced diabetes mellitus in rats. Circulation (USA), 1996, 93/10 (1905-1912)

Slowing of peripheral motor nerve conduction was ameliorated by aminoguanidine in streptozocin-induced diabetic rats. European Journal of Endocrinology (Norway), 1996, 134/4 (467-473)

Thiamine pyrophosphate and pyridoxamine inhibit the formation of antigenic advanced glycation end-products: Comparison with aminoguanidine. Biochemical and Biophysical Research Communications (USA), 1996, 220/1

Advanced glycosylation end products in diabetic renal and vascular disease. American Journal of Kidney Diseases (USA), 1995, 26/6 (875-888)

Aminoguanidine treatment inhibits the development of experimental diabetic retinopathy. PROC. NATL ACAD. SCI. U. S. A. (USA), 1991, 88/24 (11555-11558)

Aminoguanidine effects on nerve blood flow, vascular permeability, electrophysiology, and oxygen free radicals. PROC. NATL. ACAD. SCI. U. S. A. (USA), 1991, 88/14 (6107-6111)

Diabetes Type II (Adult Onset Diabetes)

Homologous physiological effects of phenformin and chromium picolinate. Med Hypotheses (ENGLAND) Oct 1993, 41 (4) p316-24

[The effect of chromium picolinate on the liver levels of trace elements] Efecto del picolinato de cromo en los niveles hepaticos de algunos elementos traza. Nutr Hosp (SPAIN) Nov-Dec 1995, 10 (6) p373-6

Anabolic effects of insulin on bone suggest a role for chromium picolinate in preservation of bone density. Med Hypotheses (ENGLAND) Sep 1995, 45 (3) p241-6

Longevity effect of chromium picolinate—'rejuvenation' of hypothalamic function? Med Hypotheses(ENGLAND) Oct 1994, 43 (4) p253-65

Thiamine pyrophosphate and pyridoxamine inhibit the formation of antigenic advanced glycation end-products: comparison with aminoguanidine. Biochem Biophys Res Commun (UNITED STATES) Mar 7 1996, 220 (1) p113-9

Loss of glucose-induced insulin secretion and GLUT2 expression in transplanted beta- cells. Diabetes (UNITED STATES) Jan 1995, 44 (1) p75-9

Case report: amelioration of insulin resistance in diabetes with dehydroepiandrosterone. Am J Med Sci (UNITED STATES) Nov 1993, 306 (5) p320-4

Therapeutic effects of dehydroepiandrosterone metabolites in diabetes mutant mice (C57BL/KsJ-db/db). Endocrinology (UNITED STATES) Jul 1984, 115 (1) p239-43

The endocrine pancreas in pyridoxine deficient rats. Med (JAPAN) Jul 1981, 134 (3) p331-6

Vitamin B6 metabolism and diabetes. Biochem Med Metab Biol (UNITED STATES) Jun 1994, 52 (1) p10-7

A deficiency of vitamin B6 is a plausible molecular basis of the retinopathy of patients with diabetes mellitus. Biochem Biophys Res Commun (UNITED STATES) Aug 30 1991, 179 (1) p615-9

Erythrocyte O2 transport and metabolism and effects of vitamin B6 therapy in type II diabetes mellitus. Diabetes (UNITED STATES) Jul 1989, 38 (7) p881-6

Diabetes and adrenal disease. Baillieres Clin Endocrinol Metab (ENGLAND) Oct 1992, 6 (4) p829-47

[Preventive treatment of diabetic microangiopathy: blocking the pathogenic mechanisms] Diabete Metab (FRANCE) 1994, 20 (2 Pt 2) p219-28

Alternative therapeutic principles in the prevention of microvascular and neuropathic complications. Diabetes Res Clin Pract (IRELAND) Aug 1995, 28 Suppl pS201-7

Enhancement of glucose disposal in patients with type 2 diabetes by alpha-lipoic acid. Arzneimittelforschung (GERMANY) Aug 1995, 45 (8) p872-4

References

Inhibition with N-acetylcysteine of enhanced production of tumor necrosis factor in strepto-zotocin-induced diabetic rats. Clin Immunol Immunopathol (UNITED STATES) Jun 1994, 71 (3) p333-7

Effects of acetyl- and proprionyl-L-carnitine on peripheral nerve function and vascular supply in experimental diabetes. Metabolism (UNITED STATES) Sep 1995, 44 (9) p1209-14

Acetyl-L-carnitine for symptomatic diabetic neuropathy [letter] Diabetologia (GERMANY) Jan 1995, 38 (1) p123

Peptide alterations in autonomic diabetic neuropathy prevented by acetyl-L-carnitine. Int J Clin Pharmacol Res (SWITZERLAND) 1992, 12 (5-6) p225-30

Prevention of cardiovascular and renal pathology of aging by the advanced glycation inhibitor aminoguanidine. Proc Natl Acad Sci U S A (UNITED STATES) Apr 30 1996, 93 (9) p3902-7

Prevention of long-term complications of non-insulin-dependent diabetes mellitus. Clin Invest Med (CANADA) Aug 1995, 18 (4) p332-9

Secondary intervention with aminoguanidine retards the progression of diabetic retinopathy in the rat model. Diabetologia (GERMANY) Jun 1995, 38 (6) p656-60

Prevention of glomerular basement membrane thickening by aminoguanidine in experimen-tal diabetes mellitus. Metabolism (UNITED STATES) Oct 1991, 40 (10) p1016-9

Can metformin reduce insulin resistance in polycystic ovary syndrome? Fertil Steril (UNITED STATES) May 1996, 65 (5) p946-9

Effects of diet and metformin administration on sex hormone-binding globulin, androgens, and insulin in hirsute and obese women. J Clin Endocrinol Metab (UNITED STATES) Jul 1995, 80 (7) p2057-62

[The value of metformin in therapy of type 2 diabetes: effect on insulin resistance, diabetic control and cardiovascular risk factors] Wien Klin Wochenschr (AUSTRIA) 1994, 106 (24) p793-802

Oral vanadyl sulfate improves insulin sensitivity in NIDDM but not in obese nondiabetic sub-jects. Diabetes (UNITED STATES) May 1996, 45 (5) p659-66

Oral vanadyl sulfate improves hepatic and peripheral insulin sensitivity in patients with non-insulin-dependent diabetes mellitus. J Clin Invest (UNITED STATES) Jun 1995, 95 (6) p2501-9

Toxicity studies on one-year treatment of non-diabetic and streptozotocin-diabetic rats with vanadyl sulphate. Pharmacol Toxicol (DENMARK) Nov 1994, 75 (5) p265-73

Antidiabetic action of vanadyl in rats independent of in vivo insulin-receptor kinase activity. Diabetes (UNITED STATES) Apr 1991, 40 (4) p492-8

Digestive Disorders

Digestive processes in the human colon. Nutrition (USA) , 1995, 11/1 (37-45)

The ileum and carbohydrate-mediated feedback regulation of postprandial pancreaticobiliary secretion in normal humans.PANCREAS (USA) , 1991, 6/5 (495-505)

Factors influencing carbohydrate digestion: Acute and long-term consequences.DIABETES NUTR. METAB. CLIN. EXP. (Italy) , 1990, 3/3 (251-258): Two distinct adaptive responses in the synthesis of exocrine pancreatic enzymes to inverse changes in protein and carbohydrate in the diet. AM. J. PHYSIOL. (USA) , 1984, 10/6 (G611-G616)

Carbohydrate absorption.MED.CLIN.N.AMER. (USA) , 1974, 58/6 (1387-1395)

Dietary carbohydrates. Their indications and contraindications in clinical medicine.PRACTI-TIONER (ENGLAND) , 1974, 212/1270 (448-453)

An analysis on fat digestion in the upper small intestine after intragastric infusion of a test meal in patients with exocrine pancreatic insufficiency.Japanese Journal of Gastroenterology (Japan) , 1995, 92/8 (1169-1177)

Pancreatic triglyceride lipase and colipase: Insights into dietary fat digestion.GASTROEN-TEROLOGY (USA) , 1994, 107/5 (1524-1536)

Role of nonpancreatic lipolytic activity in exocrine pancreatic insufficiency.GASTROEN-TEROLOGY (USA) , 1987, 92/1 (125-129)

Rat lingual lipase: Effect of proteases, bile, and pH on enzyme stability Roberts I.M. AM. J. PHYSIOL. (USA) , 1985, 12/4 (G496-G500)

Fat digestion by lingual lipase: Mechanism of lipolysis in the stomach and upper small intestine. PEDIATR. RES. (USA) , 1984, 18/5 (402-409)

Fat digestion in the stomach: Stability of lingual lipase in the gastric environment.PEDIATR. RES. (USA) , 1984, 18/3 (248-254)

Colipase and lipase secretion in childhood-onset pancreatic insufficiency. Delineation of patients with steatorrhea secondary to relative colipase deficiency.GASTROENTEROLOGY (USA) , 1984, 86/1 (1-7)

New results about the role of lipase, colipase and bile acids in the fat digestion.DTSCH. Z. VERDAU.-STOFFWECHSELKR. (GERMANY, EAST) , 1980, 40/6 (246-252)

Lipases, bile salts and fat digestion: New insights. ITAL. J. GASTROENTEROL. (ITALY) , 1980, 12/2 (140-145)

Congenital pancreatic lipase deficiency. J. PEDIATR. (USA) , 1980, 96/3I (412-416)

Controlled, double-blind multicenter trial of alyophilized total pancreas preparation against placebo in functional digestive disorders. FRANCE MED. CHIR. DIG. (FRANCE) , 1987, 16/2 (137-141)

Down Syndrome

Vitamin E and Alzheimer's disease in subjects with Down syndrome. Journal of Mental Deficiency Research 1988 Dec Vol 32(6) 479-484

Behavioral disorders, learning disabilities and megavitamin therapy. Adolescence 1987 Fal Vol 22(87) 729-738

Macrocytosis and cognitive decline in Down syndrome. British Journal of Psychiatry 1986 Dec Vol 149 797-798

Treatment approaches in Down syndrome: A review. Australia & New Zealand Journal of Developmental Disabilities

A double blind study of vitamin B-sub-6 in Down syndrome infants: I. Clinical and biochemical results. Journal of Mental Deficiency Research 1985 Sep Vol 29(3) 233-240

A double blind study of vitamin B-sub-6 in Down syndrome infants: II. Cortical auditory evoked potentials. Journal of Mental Deficiency Research 1985 Sep Vol 29(3) 241-246

Xylose absorption in Down syndrome. Journal of Mental Deficiency Research 1985 Jun Vol 29(2) 173-177

Nutritional aspects of Down syndrome with special reference to the nervous system. British Journal of Psychiatry 1984 Aug Vol 145 115-120

Children's mental retardation study is attacked: A closer look. International Journal of Biosocial Research 1982 Vol 3(2) 75-86

Effects of nutritional supplementation on IQ and certain other variables associated with Down syndrome. American Journal of Mental Deficiency 1983 Sep Vol 88(2) 214-217

Vitamin A and carotene values of institutionalized mentally retarded subjects with and without Down syndrome. Journal of Mental Deficiency Research 1977 Mar Vol 21(1) 63-74

Sodium-dependent glutamate binding in senile dementia. Neurobiology of Aging 1987 May-Jun Vol 8(3) 219-223

Alzheimer-like neurotransmitter deficits in adult Down syndrome brain tissue. Journal of Neurology, Neurosurgery & Psychiatry 1987 Jun Vol 50(6) 775-778

A report on phosphatidylcholine therapy in a Down Syndrome child. Psychological Reports 1986 Feb Vol 58(1) 207-217

Emphysema And Chronic Obstructive Pulmonary Disease

Muscle and serum magnesium in pulmonary intensive care unit patients. Crit Care Med (UNITED STATES) Aug 1988, 16 (8) p751-60

Fluid and electrolyte considerations in diuretic therapy for hypertensive patients with chronic obstructive pulmonary disease. Arch Intern Med (UNITED STATES) Jan 1986, 146 (1) p129-33

Safety and effectiveness of ticarcillin plus clavulanate potassium in treatment of lower respiratory tract infections. Am J Med (UNITED STATES) Nov 29 1985, 79 (5B) p78-80

Frequently nebulized beta-agonists for asthma: effects on serum electrolytes. Ann Emerg Med (UNITED STATES) Nov 1992, 21 (11) p1337-42

Effect of nebulized albuterol on serum potassium and cardiac rhythm in patients with asthma or chronic obstructive pulmonary disease. Pharmacotherapy (UNITED STATES) Nov-Dec 1994, 14 (6) p729-33

The intrabronchial microbial flora in chronic bronchitis patients: a target for N-acetylcysteine therapy? Eur Respir J (DENMARK) Jan 1994, 7 (1) p94-101

[The influence of n-acetylcysteine on chemiluminescence of granulocytes in peripheral blood of patients with chronic bronchitis] Pneumonol Alergol Pol (POLAND) 1993, 61 (11-12)

Effects of coenzyme Q10 administration on pulmonary function and exercise performance in patients with chronic lung diseases. Clin Investig (GERMANY) 1993, 71 (8 Suppl) pS162-6

Protection by N-acetylcysteine of the histopathological and cytogenetical damage produced by exposure of rats to cigarette smoke. Cancer Lett (NETHERLANDS) Jun 15 1992, 64 (2) p123-31

Investigation of the protective effects of the antioxidants ascorbate, cysteine, and dapsone on the phagocyte-mediated oxidative inactivation of human alpha-1-protease inhibitor in vitro. Am Rev Respir Dis (UNITED STATES) Nov 1985, 132 (5) p1049-54

The role of dornase alfa (PULMOZYME) in the treatment of cystic fibrosis. Annals of Pharmacotherapy (USA), 1996, 30/6 (656-661)

Inhalation therapy with recombinant human deoxyribonuclease I Gonda I (PULMOZYME). Advanced Drug Delivery Reviews (Netherlands), 1996, 19/1 (37-46)

Aerosolized dornase alpha (rhDNase-PULMOZYME)) in cystic fibrosis. Journal of Clinical Pharmacy and Therapeutics (United Kingdom), 1995, 20/6

New pharmacologic approaches: rhDNase. Revue de Pneumologie Clinique (France), 1995, 51/3 (193-200)

Taurine and serine supplementation modulates the metabolic response to tumor necrosis factor alpha in rats fed a low protein diet. J. NUTR. (USA), 1992, 122/7 (1369-1375)

L-Carnitine and its role in medicine: A current consideration of its pharmacokinetics, its role in fatty acid metabolism and its use in ischaemic cardiac disease and primary and secondary L-carnitine deficiencies. Epitheorese Klinikes Farmakologias kai Farmakokinetikes (Greece), 1996, 14/1 (11-64)

Esophageal Reflux (Heartburn)

Prevention of esophageal cancer: the nutrition intervention trials in Linxian, China. Linxian Nutrition Intervention Trials Study Group. Cancer Res. 1994 Apr 1. 54(7 Suppl). P 2029s-2031s

Effects of vitamin/mineral supplementation on the proliferation of esophageal squamous epithelium in Linxian, China. Cancer Epidemiol Biomarkers Prev. 1994 Apr-May. 3(3). P 277-9

[Preliminary report on the results of nutrition prevention trials of cancer and other common diseases among residents in Linxian, China] Chung Hua Chung Liu Tsa Chih. 1993 May. 15(3). P 165-81

Chemoprevention of oral leukoplakia and chronic esophagitis in an area of high incidence of oral and esophageal cancer. Ann Epidemiol. 1993 May. 3(3). P 225-34

[Clinical aspects, diagnosis and treatment of esophageal spasm] Grud Serdechnososudistaia Khir. 1991 Jun. (6). P 57-60

Association of esophageal cytological abnormalities with vitamin and lipotrope deficiencies in populations at risk for esophageal cancer. ANTICANCER RES. (Greece), 1988, 8/4 (711-716)

The effect of gamma-linolenic acid on clinical status, red cell fatty acid composition and membrane microviscosity in infants with atopic dermatitis. SO:Drugs Exp Clin Res. 1994. 20(2). P 77-84

Fatty acid compositions of plasma lipids in atopic dermatitis/asthma patients. SO:Arerugi. 1994 Jan. 43(1). P 37-43

Possible immunologic involvement of antioxidants in cancer prevention. Am J Clin Nutr. 1995 Dec. 62(6 Suppl). P 1477S-1482S

Estrogen Replacement Therapy

A review of the clinical effects of phytoestrogens. Obstetrics and Gynecology (USA), 1996, 87/5 II SUPPL. (897-904)

Molecular effects of genistein on estrogen receptor mediated pathways. Carcinogenesis (United Kingdom), 1996, 17/2 (271-275)

Rationale for the use of genistein-containing soy matrices in chemoprevention trials for breast

References

and prostate cancer. Journal of Cellular Biochemistry (USA), 1995, 58/SUPPL. 22

Dietary flour supplementation decreases post-menopausal hot flushes: Effect of soy and wheat. Maturitas (Ireland), 1995, 21/3 (189-195)

Soy and experimental cancer: Animal studies. Journal of Nutrition (USA), 1995, 125/3 SUPPL.

Aromatase in bone cell: Association with osteoporosis in postmenopausal women. Journal of Steroid Biochemistry and Molecular Biology (United Kingdom), 1995, 53/1-6 (165-174)

Estrogen replacement therapy and fatal ovarian cancer. Am J Epidemiol (UNITED STATES) May 1 1995

Inhibition of breast cancer cell growth by combined treatment with vitamin D3 analogues and tamoxifen. Cancer Res (UNITED STATES) Nov 1 1994, 54 (21) p5711-7

Melatonin modulation of estrogen-regulated proteins, growth factors, and proto-oncogenes in human breast cancer. J Pineal Res (DENMARK) Mar 1995

Melatonin inhibition of MCF-7 human breast-cancer cells growth: influence of cell proliferation rate. Cancer Lett (IRELAND) Jul 13 1995

Modulation of cancer endocrine therapy by melatonin: a phase II study of tamoxifen plus melatonin in metastatic breast cancer patients progressing under tamoxifen alone. Br J Cancer (ENGLAND) Apr 1995

Modulation of estrogen receptor mRNA expression by melatonin in MCF-7 human breast cancer cells. Mol Endocrinol (UNITED STATES) Dec 1994

Melatonin modulates growth factor activity in MCF-7 human breast cancer cells. J Pineal Res (DENMARK) Aug 1994

Role of pineal gland in aetiology and treatment of breast cancer. Lancet (ENGLAND) Oct 14 1978

3beta-hydroxysteroid dehydrogenase/isomerase and aromatase activity in primary cultures of developing zebra finch telencephalon: Dehydroepiandrosterone as substrate for synthesis of androstenedione and estrogens. General and Comparative Endocrinology (USA), 1996, 102/3 (342- 350)

Aromatase in bone cell: Association with osteoporosis in postmenopausal women. Journal of Steroid Biochemistry and Molecular Biology (United Kingdom), 1995, 53/1-6 (165-174)

Abnormal production of androgens in women with breast cancer. ANTICANCER RES. (Greece), 1994, 14/5 B (2113-2117)

Endogenous sex hormones: Impact on lipids, lipoproteins, and insulin. AM. J. MED. (USA), 1995, 98/1 A (40S-47S)

Dehydroepiandrosterone antiestrogenic action through androgen receptor in MCF-7 human breast cancer cell line. ANTICANCER RES. (Greece), 1993, 13/6 A (2267-2272)

Effect of flax seed ingestion on the menstrual cycle. J. CLIN. ENDOCRINOL. METAB. (USA), 1993, 77/5 (1215-1219)

Transdermal estrogen replacement therapy in normal perimenopausal women: Effects on pituitary- ovarian function. Gynecological Endocrinology (United Kingdom), 1996, 10/1 (49-53)

Hormone replacement therapy, hormone levels, and lipoprotein cholesterol concentrations in elderly women. American Journal of Obstetrics and Gynecology (USA), 1996, 174/3

Estrogen and nerve growth factor-related systems in brain. Effects on basal forebrain cholinergic neurons and implications for learning and memory processes and aging. ANN. NEW YORK ACAD. SCI. (USA), 1994, 743/- (165-199)

Postmenopausal estrogen replacement: A long-term cohort study. AM. J. MED. (USA), 1994, 97/1 (66-77)

Impact of the menopause on the epidemiology and risk factors of coronary artery heart disease in women. EXP. GERONTOL. (USA), 1994, 29/3-4 (357-375)

Hormone therapy and endometrium cancer. REPROD. HUM. HORM. (France), 1994, 7/4 (137-139)

Progestin replacement in the menopause: Effects on the endometrium and serum lipids. CURR. OPIN. OBSTET. GYNECOL. (USA), 1994, 6/3 (284-292)

Effects of hormone replacement therapy on lipoprotein(a) and lipids in postmenopausal women. ARTERIOSCLER. THROMB. (USA), 1994, 14/2 (275-281)

Fibrinogen and Cardiovascular Disease

Effects of various fatty acids alone or combined with vitamin E on cell growth and fibrinogen concentration in the medium of HepG2 cells. Thromb Res (UNITED STATES) Oct 1 1995, 80 (1) p75-83

[The role of platelets in the protective effect of a combination of vitamins A, E, C and P in thrombinemia] Gematol Transfuziol (RUSSIA) Sep-Oct 1995, 40 (5) p9-11

[Improvement of hemorheology with ginkgo biloba extract. Decreasing a cardiovascular risk factor] Fortschr Med (GERMANY) May 10 1992, 110 (13) p247-50

On the pharmacology of bromelain: an update with special regard to animal studies on dose-dependent effects. Planta Med (GERMANY, WEST) Jun 1990, 56 (3) p249-53

Effects of various fatty acids alone or combined with vitamin E on cell growth and fibrinogen concentration in the medium of HepG2 cells. Thromb Res (UNITED STATES) Oct 1 1995, 80 (1) p75-83

Protein/platelet interaction with an artificial surface: effect of vitamins and platelet inhibitors. Thromb Res (UNITED STATES) Jan 1 1986, 41 (1) p9-22

[Preventive effects of green tea extract on lipid abnormalities in serum, liver and aorta of mice fed a atherogenic diet] Nippon Yakurigaku Zasshi (JAPAN) Jun 1991, 97 (6) p329-37

Relationship between plasma essential fatty acids and smoking, serum lipids, blood pressure and haemostatic and rheological factors. Prostaglandins Leukot Essent Fatty Acids (SCOTLAND) Aug 1994, 51 (2) p101-8

Omega-3 fatty acids in health and disease and in growth and development Am J Clin Nutr (UNITED STATES) Sep 1991, 54 (3) p438-63

Fibromyalgia

Oral S-adenosylmethionine in primary fibromyalgia—Double-blind clinical evaluation. Scand J Rheumatol (SWEDEN) 1991, 20 (4) p294-302,

Cerebrospinal fluid S-adenosylmethionine in depression and dementia: effects of treatment with parenteral and oral S-adenosylmethionine. J Neurol Neurosurg Psychiatry (ENGLAND) Dec 1990, 53 (12) p1096-8

The antidepressant potential of oral S-adenosyl-l-methionine. Acta Psychiatr Scand (DENMARK) May 1990, 81 (5) p432-6,

Oral S-adenosylmethionine in depression: a randomized, double-blind, placebo- controlled trial. Am J Psychiatry (UNITED STATES) May 1990, 147 (5) p591-5,

Disability and impairment in fibromyalgia syndrome: Possible pathogenesis and etiology. Critical Reviews in Physical and Rehabilitation Medicine (USA) , 1995, 7/3 (189-232)

Primary fibromyalgia is responsive to S-adenosyl-L-methionine. CURR. THER. RES. CLIN. EXP. (USA) , 1994, 55/7 (797-806)

S-adenosyl-L-methionine in Sjogren's syndrome and fibromyalgia. CURR. THER. RES. CLIN. EXP. (USA) , 1994, 55/6 (699-706)

Clinical evaluation of S-adenosyl-L-methionine versus transcutaneous electrical nerve stimulation in primary fibromyalgia. CURR. THER. RES. CLIN. EXP. (USA) , 1993, 53/2 (222-229)

Oral S-adenosylmethionine in primary fibromyalgia. Double-blind clinical evaluation. SCAND. J. RHEUMATOL. (Sweden) , 1991, 20/4 (294-302)

Evaluation of S-adenosylmethionine in primary fibromyalgia. A double-blind crossover study. AM. J. MED. (USA) , 1987, 83/5 A (107-110)

S-adenosylmethionine blood levels in major depression: Changes with drug treatment. ACTA NEUROL. SCAND. SUPPL. (Denmark) , 1994, 89/154 (15-18)

Psychological distress during puerperium: A novel therapeutic approach using S-adenosyl-methionine. CURR. THER. RES. CLIN. EXP. (USA) , 1993, 53/6 (707-716)

References

Double blind, placebo-controlled study of S-adenosyl-L-methionine in depressed post-menopausal women. PSYCHOTHER. PSYCHOSOM. (Switzerland) , 1993, 59/1 (34-40)

S-adenosylmethionine treatment of depression: A controlled clinical trial. AM. J. PSYCHIA-TRY (USA) , 1988, 145/9 (1110-1114)

Treatment of depression in rheumatoid arthritic patients. A comparison of S-adenosylme-thionine (Samyr) and placebo in a double-blind study. CLIN. TRIALS J. (UK) , 1987, 24/4 (305-310)

Monitoring S-adenosyl-methionine blood levels and antidepressant effect. ACTA NEUROL. (ITALY) , 1980, 35/6 (488-495)

Evaluation of S-adenosylmethionine (SAM) effectiveness on depression. CURR. THER. RES., CLIN. EXP. (USA) , 1980, 27/6II (908-918)

Flu-Influenza Virus

Efficacy and safety of aerosolized ribavirin in young children hospitalized with influenza: a dou-ble-blind, multicenter, placebo-controlled trial. J Pediatr (UNITED STATES) Jul 1994

Antivirals for the chemoprophylaxis and treatment of influenza. Semin Respir Infect (UNITED STATES) Mar 1992

Utilization of pulse oximetry for the study of the inhibitory effects of antiviral agents on influen-za virus in mice. Antimicrob Agents Chemother (UNITED STATES) Feb 1992

Further studies with short duration ribavirin aerosol for the treatment of influenza virus infec-tion in mice and respiratory syncytial virus infection in cotton rats. Antiviral Res (NETHER-LANDS) Jan 1992

High dose-short duration ribavirin aerosol treatment—a review. Bull Int Union Tuberc Lung Dis (FRANCE) Jun-Sep 1991

Molecular mechanisms of action of ribavirin. Rev Infect Dis (UNITED STATES) Nov-Dec 1990

Ribavirin aerosol treatment of influenza. Infect Dis Clin North Am (UNITED STATES) Jun 1987

Comparative activities of several nucleoside analogs against influenza A,B, and C viruses in vitro. Antimicrob Agents Chemother (UNITED STATES) Jun 1988

Ribavirin aerosol in the elderly. Chest (UNITED STATES) Jun 1988

Favorable outcome after treatment with amantadine and ribavirin in a pregnancy complicat-ed by influenza pneumonia. A case report. Department of Obstetrics and Gynecology, Baylor College of Medicine, Houston, TX 77030

Oral ribavirin treatment of influenza A and B. Antimicrob Agents Chemother (UNITED STATES) Aug 1987

References

Ribavirin: a clinical overview. Eur J Epidemiol (ITALY) Mar 1986

Ribavirin small-particle aerosol treatment of infections caused by influenza virus strains A/Victoria/7/83 (H1N1) and B/Texas/1/84. Antimicrob Agents Chemother (UNITED STATES) Mar 1985

Effect of ribavirin triphosphate on primer generation and elongation during influenza virus transcription in vitro. Antiviral Res (NETHERLANDS) Feb 1985, 5 (1) p39-48

Ribavirin aerosol treatment of influenza B virus infection. Trans Assoc Am Physicians (UNITED STATES) 1983, 96

Treatment of influenza A (H1N1) virus infection with ribavirin aerosol. Antimicrob Agents Chemother (UNITED STATES) Aug 1984

Immune modulating properties of root extracts of different Echinacea species. Zeitschrift fur Phytotherapie (Germany) , 1995, 16/3 (157-162+165-166)

Echinacea. PHARM. J. (United Kingdom) , 1994, 253/6806 (342-343)

Host-resistance increasing activity of root extracts from Echinacea species. PLANTA MED. (Germany) , 1993, 59/7 SUPPL. (A672-A673)

Echinacea combinations; efficacy and acceptability in 'flu' and nasopharyngeal inflammations. DTSCH. APOTH.-ZTG (GERMANY, WEST) , 1987, 127/16 (853-854)

Papilloma virus infections of the skin. Universitats-Hautklinik, D-7800 Freinburg i. Breisgau GERMANY, WEST

Direct characterization of caffeoyl esters with antihyaluronidase activity in crude extracts from Echinacea angustifolia roots by fast atom bombardment tandem mass spectrometry. FARMACO (Italy) , 1993, 48/10 (1447-1461)

Anti-inflammatory activity of Echinacea angustifolia fractions separated on the basis of molecular weight. PHARMACOL. RES. COMMUN. (United Kingdom) , 1988, 20/SUPPL. 5 (87-90)

In vitro activity of Mercurius cyanatus against relevant pathogenic bacteria isolates. Arzneimittel-Forschung/Drug Research (Germany) , 1995, 45/9 (1018-1020)

Immune modulating properties of root extracts of different Echinacea species. Zeitschrift fur Phytotherapie (Germany) , 1995, 16/3 (157-162+165-166)

Mechanisms of propolis water extract antiherpetic activity. II. Activity of propolis water extract lectines. REV. ROUM. VIROL. (Romania) , 1993, 44/1-2 (49-54)

Comparison of the anti-herpes simplex virus activities of propolis and 3- methyl-but-2- enyl caffeate. J. NAT. PROD. LLOYDIA (USA) , 1994, 57/5 (644-647)

Synergistic effect of flavones and flavonols against herpes simplex virus type 1 in cell culture. Comparison with the antiviral activity of propolis. J. NAT. PROD. LLOYDIA (USA), 1992, 55/12 (1732-1740)

Recent advances in the chemotherapy of herpes virus infections. REV. ROUM. MED. (RUMANIA) , 1981, 32/1 (57-77)

Anti-influenza virus effect of some propolis constituents and their analogues (esters of substituted cinnamic acids). J. NAT. PROD. LLOYDIA (USA) , 1992, 55/3 (294-297)

The effect of an aqueous propolis extract, of rutin and of a rutin-quercetin mixture on experimental influenza virus infection in mice. REV. ROUM. MED. (RUMANIA) , 1981, 32/3 (213-215)

Gingivitis

Vitamin C, oral scurvy and periodontal disease. S Afr Med J (SOUTH AFRICA) May 26 1984, 65 (21)

[Anticalculus dentifrices. A new era in preventive dentistry?] Ned Tijdschr Tandheelkd (NETHERLANDS) Dec 1989, 96 (12)

Effect of tea polyphenols on glucan synthesis by glucosyltransferase from Streptococcus mutans. Chem Pharm Bull (Tokyo) (JAPAN) Mar 1990, 38 (3)

Green Tea to Prevent Dental Cares. Chung Hua Kou Chiang Hsueh Tsa Chih (CHINA) Jul 1993, 28 (4) p197-9 54

[Management of gingival inflammation with active ingredients in toothpaste] Dtsch Zahnarztl Z (GERMANY, WEST) Jun 1975, 30 (6) p382-4

Evidence for enhanced treatment of periodontal disease by therapy with coenzyme Q. Int J Vitam Nutr Res (SWITZERLAND) Apr 1973, 43 (4) p537-48

Zinc in etiology of periodontal disease. Med Hypotheses (ENGLAND) Mar Stomatological Clinic, Medical 1993, 40 (3) p182-5

Diabetes and periodontal diseases. Possible role of vitamin c deficiency: an hypothesis. J Periodontol (UNITED STATES) May 1981, 52 (5) p251-4

Relationship of mineral status and intake to periodontal disease. Am J Clin Nutr (UNITED STATES) Jul 1976, 29 (7)

Comparative In Vitro Activity of Sanguinarine Against Oral. ANTIMICROBIAL AGENTS AND CHEMOTHEROPY, Apr. 1985, p. 663-65 Vol. 27, No. 4

MICs of sanguinarine were determined for 52 oral reference strains and 129 fresh isolates from human dental plaque. Sanguinarine was found to completely inhibit the growth of 98% of the isolates at a concentration of 16 ,ug/ml.

Zinc And Sanguinaria. J Periodontol 60(2):91-5, 1989)

Supplementation or local application may reduce gingival exudate from inflammed and infected gums - which suggests improved tissue health. (Folate mouthwash appears to to be more effective than oral folate.) J Clin Periodonlol 14(6):315-9, 1987)

Effects on established gingivitis in periodontal patients. J Clin Periodontol 11:619-28, 1984).

Effects of extended systemic and topical folate supplementation on gingivitis of pregnancy. J Clin periodontal 9(3):27580, 1982).

Effects of topical and systemic folic acid supplementation on gingivitis in pregnancy. J Clin Periodontol 7(5):402-14, 1980).

The effect of topical application of folic acid on gingival health. J Oral Med 33(1):20-22,1978).

The effect of folic acid on gingival health. J periodontol 47(11):667-8, 1976).

Glaucoma

Neurotransmitters and intraocular pressure. FUNDAM. CLIN. PHARMACOL. (France), 1988, 2/4 (305-325)

HP 663: A novel compound for the treatment of glaucoma. DRUG DEV. RES. (USA), 1988, 12/3-4 (197-209)

Intraocular pressure effects of multiple doses of drugs applied to glaucomatous monkey eyes. ARCH. OPHTHALMOL. (USA), 1987, 105/2 (249-252)

Laser-induced glaucoma in rabbits. EXP. EYE RES. (UK), 1986, 43/6 (885-894)

Regulation of aqueous flow by the adenylate cyclase receptor complex in the ciliary epithelium. AM. J. OPHTHALMOL. (USA), 1985, 100/1 (194-198)

Forskolin suppresses sympathetic neuron function and causes ocular hypotension. CURR. EYE RES. (ENGLAND), 1985, 4/2 (87-96)

Forskolin lowers intraocular pressure by reducing aqueous inflow. INVEST. OPHTHALMOL. VISUAL SCI. (USA), 1984, 25/3 (268-276)

Indomethacin and epinephrine effects on outflow facility and cyclic adenosine monophosphate formation in monkeys. Investigative Ophthalmology and Visual Science (USA), 1996, 37/7 (1348-1359)

Hair Loss

See references under Balding

Hearing Loss

[Hydergine in pathology of the inner ear] An Otorrinolaringol Ibero Am (SPAIN) 1990, 17 (1) p85-98

[Ginkgo extract EGb 761 (tenobin)/HAES versus naftidrofuryl A randomized study of therapy of sudden deafness] Laryngorhinootologie (GERMANY) Mar 1994, 73 (3) p149-52,

[Therapeutic trial in acute cochlear deafness. A comparative study of Ginkgo biloba extract and nicergoline] Presse Med (FRANCE) Sep 25 1986, 15 (31) p1559-61,

[The influence on sound damages by an extract of ginkgo biloba] Arch Otorhinolaryngol (UNITED STATES) Jul 8 1975, 209 (3) p203-15

Results of combined low-power laser therapy and extracts of Ginkgo biloba in cases of sensorineural hearing loss and tinnitus. Adv Otorhinolaryngol (SWITZERLAND) 1995, 49 p101-4

Trial of an extract of Ginkgo biloba (EGB) for tinnitus and hearing loss [letter]. Clin Otolaryngol (ENGLAND) Dec 1988, 13 (6) p501-2,

Hemochromatosis

Biological markers of oxidative stress induced by ethanol and iron overload in rat. Int J Occup Med Environ Health (POLAND) 1994, 7 (4) p355-63

Antioxidant status and lipid peroxidation in hereditary haemochromatosis. Free Radic Biol Med (UNITED STATES) Mar 1994, 16 (3)

Iron storage, lipid peroxidation and glutathione turnover in chronic anti-HCV positive hepatitis. J Hepatol (DENMARK) Apr 1995, 22 (4) p449-56

Induction of oxidative single- and double-strand breaks in DNA by ferric citrate. Free Radic Biol Med (UNITED STATES) Aug 1993

A unique rodent model for both the cardiotoxic and hepatotoxic effects of prolonged iron overload. Lab Invest (UNITED STATES) Aug 1993, 69 (2) p217-22

Biochemical and biophysical investigations of the ferrocene-iron-loaded rat. An animal model of primary haemochromatosis. Eur J Biochem (GERMANY) Dec 5 1991, 202 (2) p405-10

Antioxidant and iron-chelating activities of the flavonoids catechin, quercetin and diosmetin on iron-loaded rat hepatocyte cultures. BIOCHEM. PHARMACOL. (United Kingdom), 1993

Iron absorption and phenolic compounds: Importance of different phenolic structures. EUROP. J. CLIN. NUTR. (United Kingdom), 1989

Inhibition of the tobacco-specific nitrosamine-induced lung tumorigenesis by compounds derived from cruciferous vegetables and green tea. ANN. NEW YORK ACAD. SCI. (USA), 1993, 686

References

The effects of caffeic acid and its related catechols on hydroxyl radical formation by 3-hydroxyanthranilic acid, ferric chloride, and hydrogen peroxide. ARCH. BIOCHEM. BIOPHYS. (USA), 1990, 276/1

A novel antioxidant flavonoid (IdB 1031) affecting molecular mechanisms of cellular activation. FREE RADIC. BIOL. MED. (USA), 1994, 16/5 (547-553)

Prevention of postischemic cardiac injury by the orally active iron chelator 1,2- dimethyl-3-hydroxy-4-pyridone (L1) and the antioxidant (+)-cyanidanol-3. CIRCULATION (USA), 1989, 80/1 (158-164)

Hepatotoxicity of menadione predominates in oxygen-rich zones of the liver lobule. J. PHARMACOL. EXP. THER. (USA), 1989, 248/3 (1317-1322)

Iron-load increases the susceptibility of rat hearts to oxygen reperfusion damage. Protection by the antioxidant (+)-cyanidanol-3 and deferoxamine. CIRCULATION (USA), 1988, 78/2 (442-449)

Hepatocyte injury resulting from the inhibition of mitochondrial respiration at low oxygen concentrations involves reductive stress and oxygen activation. Chemico-Biological Interactions (Ireland), 1995, 98/1 (27-44)

Modulating hypoxia-induced hepatocyte injury by affecting intracellular redox state. Biochimica et Biophysica Acta - Molecular Cell Research (Netherlands), 1995, 1269/2 (153-161)

Protection of rat myocardial phospholipid against peroxidative injury through superoxide-(xanthine oxidase)-dependent, iron-promoted fenton chemistry by the male contraceptive gossypol. BIOCHEM. PHARMACOL. (United Kingdom), 1988, 37/17 (3335-3342)

Protective effect of tea polyphenol on rat myocardial injury induced by isoproterenol. Chinese Traditional and Herbal Drugs (China)(Apr) 1995

Effect of the interaction of tannins with coexisting substances. Part 2. reduction of heavy metal ions and solubilization of precipitates. Journal of the Pharmaceutical Society of Japan (Japan), V102, (8), 1982

Free radicals scavenging action and anti-enzyme activities of procyanidines from Vitis vinifera. A mechanism for their capillary protective action. Arzneimittelforschung (GERMANY) May 1994, 44 (5) p592-601

The inhibitory action of chlorogenic acid on the intestinal iron absorption in rats. Acta Physiol Pharmacol Ther Latinoam (ARGENTINA) 1992, 42 (3)

Inhibition of tobacco-specific nitrosamine-induced lung tumorigenesis by compounds derived from cruciferous vegetables and green tea. Ann N Y Acad Sci (UNITED STATES) May 28 1993, 686

Ascorbic acid prevents the dose-dependent inhibitory effects of polyphenols and phytates on nonheme-iron absorption. Am J Clin Nutr (UNITED STATES) Feb 1991, 53 (2)

Phytic acid. A natural antioxidant. J Biol Chem (UNITED STATES) Aug 25 1987, 262 (24)

[Effect of polyphenols of coffee pulp on iron absorption]. Arch Latinoam Nutr (VENEZUELA) Jun 1985, 35 (2)

Factors affecting the absorption of iron from cereals. Br J Nutr (ENGLAND) Jan 1984, 51 (1) p37-46

The effect of red and white wines on nonheme-iron absorption in humans. Am J Clin Nutr (UNITED STATES) Apr 1995

Prevention of iron deficiency. Baillieres Clin Haematol (ENGLAND) Dec 1994, 7 (4)

Iron absorption and phenolic compounds: importance of different phenolic structures. Eur J Clin Nutr (ENGLAND) Aug 1989, 43 (8) p547-57

Hepatitis B

[Markers of chronic hepatitis B in children after completion of therapywith isoprinosine] Pol Tyg Lek (POLAND) Mar 15-29 1993, 48 (11-13) p263-4

[Course of chronic virus hepatitis B in children and attempts at modifying its treatment] Pol Tyg Lek (POLAND) Mar 15-29 1993, 48 (11-13) p258-60

Isoprinosine in the treatment of chronic active hepatitis type B. Scand J Infect Dis (SWEDEN) 1990, 22 (6) p645-8

[Evaluation of the treatment of chronic active hepatitis (HBsAg+) with isoprinosine. II. Immunological studies] Pol Tyg Lek (POLAND) Apr 16-30 1990, 45 (16-18) p347-51

In vitro studies on the effect of certain natural products against hepatitis B virus. Indian J Med Res (INDIA) Apr 1990, 92 p133-8

Effects of glycyrrhizin on hepatitis B surface antigen: a biochemical and morphological study. J Hepatol (DENMARK) Oct 1994, 21 (4) p601-9

Glycyrrhizin withdrawal followed by human lymphoblastoid interferon in the treatment of chronic hepatitis B. Gastroenterol Jpn (JAPAN) Dec 1991, 26 (6) p742-6

Combination therapy of glycyrrhizin withdrawal and human fibroblast Interferon for chronic hepatitis B. Clin Ther (UNITED STATES) 1989, 11 (1) p161-9

Alpha-interferon combined with immunomodulation in the treatment of chronic hepatitis B. J Gastroenterol Hepatol (AUSTRALIA) 1991, 6 Suppl 1 p13-4

Improvement of liver fibrosis in chronic hepatitis C patients treated with natural interferon alpha. J Hepatol (DENMARK) Feb 1995, 22 (2) p135-42

Diagnosis and treatment of the major hepatotropic viruses. Am J Med Sci (UNITED STATES) Oct 1993, 306 (4) p248-61

References

Treatment of chronic viral hepatitis.J Antimicrob Chemother (ENGLAND) Jul 1993, 32 Suppl A p107-20

[Mechanisms of the effect of interferon (IFN) therapy in patients with type B and C chronic hepatitis] Hokkaido Igaku Zasshi (JAPAN) May 1993, 68 (3) p297-309

A pilot study of ribavirin therapy for recurrent hepatitis C virus infection after liver transplantation. Transplantation (UNITED STATES) May 27 1996, 61 (10) p1483-8

Ribavirin as therapy for chronic hepatitis C. A randomized, double- blind, placebo-controlled trial. Ann Intern Med (UNITED STATES) Dec 15 1995, 123 (12) p897-903

Treatment with ribavirin+alpha interferon in HCV chronic active hepatitis non-responders to interferon alone: preliminary results. J Chemother (ITALY) Feb 1995, 7 (1) p58-61

Combined treatment with interferon alpha-2b and ribavirin for chronic hepatitis C in patients with a previous non-response or non-sustained response to interferon alone. J Med Virol (UNITED STATES) May 1995, 46 (1) p43-7

Increase in hepatic iron stores following prolonged therapy with ribavirin in patients with chronic hepatitis C. J Hepatol (DENMARK) Dec 1994, 21 (6) p1109-12

Therapy for chronic hepatitis C. Gastroenterol Clin North Am (UNITED STATES) Sep 1994, 23 (3) p603- 13

Treatment of chronic viral hepatitis. Baillieres Clin Gastroenterol (ENGLAND) Jun 1994, 8 (2) p233-53

Elevated serum iron predicts poor response to interferon treatment in patients with chronic HCV infection. Dig Dis Sci (UNITED STATES) Nov 1995, 40 (11) p2431-3

Distribution of iron in the liver predicts the response of chronic hepatitis C infection to interferon therapy [published erratum appears in Am J Clin Pathol 1995 Aug;104(2):232] Am J Clin Pathol (UNITED STATES) Apr 1995, 103 (4) p419-24

Increased serum iron and iron saturation without liver iron accumulation distinguish chronic hepatitis C from other chronic liver diseases. Dig Dis Sci (UNITED STATES) Dec 1994, 39 (12) p2656-9

Response related factors in recombinant interferon alfa-2b treatment of chronic hepatitis C. Gut (ENGLAND) 1993, 34 (2 Suppl) pS139-40

Measurements of iron status in patients with chronic hepatitis [see comments] Gastroenterology (UNITED STATES) Jun 1992, 102 (6) p2108-13

[Effect of green tea on iron absorption in elderly patients with iron deficiency anemia] Nippon Ronen Igakkai Zasshi (JAPAN) Sep 1990, 27 (5) p555-8

[Current knowledge in the treatment of chronic hepatitis C] Acquisitions recentes dans le traitement de l'hepatite C chronique. Rev Med Liege (BELGIUM) Dec 1995, 50 (12) p501-4

Hepatitis C

Ribavirin as therapy for chronic hepatitis C. A randomized, double- blind, placebo-controlled trial. Ann Intern Med (UNITED STATES) Dec 15 1995, 123 (12) p897-903

Treatment with ribavirin+alpha interferon in HCV chronic active hepatitis non-responders to interferon alone: preliminary results. J Chemother (ITALY) Feb 1995, 7 (1) p58-61

Combined treatment with interferon alpha-2b and ribavirin for chronic hepatitis C in patients with a previous non-response or non-sustained response to interferon alone. J Med Virol (UNITED STATES) May 1995, 46 (1) p43-7

[Evaluation of the treatment of chronic active hepatitis (HBsAg+) with isoprinosine. II. Immunological studies] Pol Tyg Lek (POLAND) Apr 16-30 1990, 45 (16-18) p347-51

In vitro studies on the effect of certain natural products against hepatitis B virus. Indian J Med Res (INDIA) Apr 1990, 92 p133-8

Effects of glycyrrhizin on hepatitis B surface antigen: a biochemical and morphological study. (DENMARK) Oct 1994, 21 (4) p601-9

Glycyrrhizin withdrawal followed by human lymphoblastoid interferon in the treatment of chronic hepatitis B. Gastroenterol Jpn (JAPAN) Dec 1991, 26 (6) p742-6

Combination therapy of glycyrrhizin withdrawal and human fibroblast interferon for chronic hepatitis B. Clin Ther (UNITED STATES) 1989, 11 (1) p161-9

Alpha-interferon combined with immunomodulation in the treatment of chronic hepatitis B. J Gastroenterol Hepatol (AUSTRALIA) 1991, 6 Suppl 1 p13-4

Improvement of liver fibrosis in chronic hepatitis C patients treated with natural interferon alpha. J Hepatol (DENMARK) Feb 1995, 22 (2) p135-42

Diagnosis and treatment of the major hepatotropic viruses. Am J Med Sci (UNITED STATES) Oct 1993, 306 (4) p248-61

Treatment of chronic viral hepatitis. J Antimicrob Chemother (ENGLAND) Jul 1993, 32 Suppl A p107-20

[Mechanisms of the effect of interferon (IFN) therapy in patients with type B and C chronic hepatitis] Hokkaido Igaku Zasshi (JAPAN) May 1993, 68 (3) p297-309

A pilot study of ribavirin therapy for recurrent hepatitis C virus infection after liver transplantation. Transplantation (UNITED STATES) May 27 1996, 61 (10) p1483-8

Therapy for chronic hepatitis C. Gastroenterol Clin North Am (UNITED STATES) Sep 1994, 23 (3) p603-13

Treatment of chronic viral hepatitis. Baillieres Clin Gastroenterol (ENGLAND) Jun 1994, 8 (2) p233-53

Elevated serum iron predicts poor response to interferon treatment in patients with chronic

References

HCV infection. Dig Dis Sci (UNITED STATES) Nov 1995, 40 (11) p2431- 3

Distribution of iron in the liver predicts the response of chronic hepatitis C infection to interferon therapy [published erratum appears in Am J Clin Pathol 1995 Aug;104(2):232] Am J Clin Pathol (UNITED STATES) Apr 1995, 103 (4) p419-24

Increased serum iron and iron saturation without liver iron accumulation distinguish chronic hepatitis C from other chronic liver diseases. Dig Dis Sci (UNITED STATES) Dec 1994, 39 (12) p2656- 9

Response related factors in recombinant interferon alfa-2b treatment of chronic hepatitis C. Gut (ENGLAND) 1993, 34 (2 Suppl) pS139-40

Measurements of iron status in patients with chronic hepatitis. Gastroenterology (UNITED STATES) Jun 1992, 102 (6) p2108-13

[Markers of chronic hepatitis B in children after completion of therapy with isoprinosine] Pol Tyg Lek (POLAND) Mar 15-29 1993, 48 (11-13) p263-4

[Course of chronic virus hepatitis B in children and attempts at modifying its treatment] Pol Tyg Lek (POLAND) Mar 15-29 1993, 48 (11-13) p258-60

Isoprinosine in the treatment of chronic active hepatitis type B. Scand J Infect Dis (SWEDEN) 1990, 22 (6) p645-8

Antioxidant and iron-chelating activities of the flavonoids catechin, quercetin and diosmetin on iron-loaded rat hepatocyte cultures. BIOCHEM. PHARMACOL. (United Kingdom), 1993

Iron absorption and phenolic compounds: Importance of different phenolic structures. EUROP. J. CLIN. NUTR. (United Kingdom), 1989

Inhibition of the tobacco-specific nitrosamine-induced lung tumorigenesis by compounds derived from cruciferous vegetables and green tea. ANN. NEW YORK ACAD. SCI. (USA), 1993, 686

The effects of caffeic acid and its related catechols on hydroxyl radical formation by 3-hydroxyanthranilic acid, ferric chloride, and hydrogen peroxide. ARCH. BIOCHEM. BIOPHYS. (USA), 1990, 276/1

A novel antioxidant flavonoid (IdB 1031) affecting molecular mechanisms of cellular activation. FREE RADIC. BIOL. MED. (USA), 1994, 16/5 (547-553)

Prevention of postischemic cardiac injury by the orally active iron chelator 1,2-dimethyl-3-hydroxy-4-pyridone (L1) and the antioxidant (+)-cyanidanol-3. CIRCULATION (USA), 1989, 80/1 (158-164)

Hepatotoxicity of menadione predominates in oxygen-rich zones of the liver lobule. J. PHARMACOL. EXP. THER. (USA), 1989, 248/3 (1317-1322)

HIV Infection (AIDS)
(Opportunistic Infections)

Selenium and HIV in Pediatrics. J. NUTR. IMMUNOL. (USA), 1994, 3/1 (41-49)

N-Acetylcysteine enhances T cell functions and T cell growth in culture. INT. IMMUNOL. (United Kingdom), 1993, 5/1 (97-101

Cysteine and glutathione deficiency in HIV-infected patients. The basis for treatment with N-acetyl-cysteine. AIDS-FORSCHUNG (Germany), 1992, 7/4 (197-199)

N-acetylcysteine (NAC) enhances interleukin-2 but suppresses interleukin-4 secretion from normal and HIV+ CD4+ T-cells. Cell Mol Biol (Noisy-le-grand) (FRANCE) 1995, 41 Suppl 1 pS35-40

N-acetylcysteine enhances antibody-dependent cellular cytotoxicity in neutrophils and mononuclear cells from healthy adults and human immunodeficiency virus-infected patients. J Infect Dis (UNITED STATES) Dec 1995, 172 (6) p1492-502

Glutathione precursor and antioxidant activities of N-acetylcysteine and oxothiazolidine carboxylate compared in in vitro studies of HIV replication. AIDS Res Hum Retroviruses (UNITED STATES) Aug 1994, 10 (8) p961-7

Role for oxygen radicals in self-sustained HIV-1 replication in monocyte-derived macrophages: enhanced HIV-1 replication by N-acetyl-L-cysteine. J Leukoc Biol (UNITED STATES) Dec 1994, 56 (6) p702- 7

Effects of glutathione precursors on human immunodeficiency virus replication. Chem Biol Interact (IRELAND) Jun 1994, 91 (2-3) p217-24

Effect of glutathione depletion and oral N-acetyl-cysteine treatment on CD4+ and CD8+ cells. FASEB J (UNITED STATES) Apr 1 1994, 8 (6) p448-51

N-acetylcysteine enhances T cell functions and T cell growth in culture. Int Immunol (ENGLAND) Jan 1993, 5 (1) p97-101

Comparative study of the anti-HIV activities of ascorbate and thiol- containing reducing agents in chronically HIV-infected cells. Am J Clin Nutr (UNITED STATES) Dec 1991, 54 (6 Suppl) p1231S-1235S

Role for oxygen radicals in self-sustained HIV-1 replication in monocyte-derived macrophages: Enhanced HIV-1 replication by N-acetyl-L-cysteine. J. LEUKOCYTE BIOL. (USA), 1994, 56/6 (702-707)

Effects of glutathione precursors on human immunodeficiency virus replication. CHEM.-BIOL. INTERACT. (Ireland), 1994, 91/2-3 (217- 224)

Antioxidant status and lipid peroxidation in patients infected with HIV. CHEM.-BIOL. INTERACT. (Ireland), 1994, 91/2-3 (165- 180)

N-acetylcysteine inhibits latent HIV expression in chronically infected cells. AIDS RES. HUM.

References

RETROVIRUSES (USA), 1991, 7/6 (563- 567)

Selenium mediated inhibition of transcription factor NF-kappaB and HIV-1 LTR promoter activity. Archives of Toxicology (Germany), 1996, 70/5 (277- 283)

Release of nitric oxide from astroglial cells: A key mechanism in neuroimmune disorders. Advances in Neuroimmunology (United Kingdom), 1995, 5/4 (421-430)

Carnitine depletion in peripheral blood mononuclear cells from patients with AIDS: Effect of oral L-carnitine. AIDS (United Kingdom), 1994, 8/5 (655-660)

High dose L-carnitine improves immunologic and metabolic parameters in AIDS patients. IMMUNOPHARMACOL. IMMUNOTOXICOL. (USA), 1993, 15/1 (1-12)

Stress, Immunity and Ageing. A role for acetyl-L-carnitine: proceedings of the workshop. ICS844. Universita degli Studi dell'Aquila degli Abruzzi, L'Aquila Italy

Vitamin B-12 abnormalities in HIV-infected patients. EUR. J. HAEMATOL. (Denmark), 1991, 47/1 (60-64)

HIV-infected patients with vitamin B-12 deficiency and autoantibodies to intrinsic factor: Disease pathogenesis and therapy. AIDS PATIENT CARE (USA), 1991, 5/3 (125-128)

One-year follow-up on the safety and efficacy of isoprinosine for human immunodeficiency virus infection. J. INTERN. MED. (United Kingdom), 1992, 231/6 (607- 615)

Immunotherapy of human immunodeficiency virus infection. TRENDS PHARMACOL. SCI. (United Kingdom), 1991, 12/3 (107-111)

The efficacy of inosine pranobex in preventing the acquired immunodeficiency syndrome in patients with human immunodeficiency virus infection. NEW ENGL. J. MED. (USA), 1990, 322/25 (1757-1763)

The activities of coenzyme Q10 and vitamin B6 for immune responses. BIOCHEM. BIOPHYS. RES. COMMUN. (USA), 1993, 193/1 (88-92)

Coenzyme Q10 increases T4/T8 ratios of lymphocytes in ordinary subjects and relevance to patients having the AIDS related complex. BIOCHEM. BIOPHYS. RES. COMMUN. (USA), 1991, 176/2 (786-791)

Biochemical deficiencies of coenzyme Q10 in HIV-infection and exploratory treatment. BIOCHEM. BIOPHYS. RES. COMMUN. (USA), 1988, 153/2 (888-896)

Coenzyme Q10 increases T4/T8 ratios of lymphocytes in ordinary subjects and relevance to patients having the AIDS related complex. BIOCHEM. BIOPHYS. RES. COMMUN. (USA), 1991, 176/2 (786-791)

Relationship between sex steroid hormone levels and CD4 lymphocytes in HIV infected men. Experimental and Clinical Endocrinology and Diabetes (Germany),1996,104

Inhibition of 3'azido-3'deoxythymidine-resistant HIV-1 infection by dehydroepiandrosterone in vitro. BIOCHEM. BIOPHYS. RES. COMMUN. (USA), 1994, 201/3 (1424-1432)

Inhibition of HIV-1 latency reactivation by dehydroepiandrosterone (DHEA) and an analog of DHEA. AIDS RES. HUM. RETROVIRUSES (USA), 1993, 9/8 (747- 754)

Evidence for changes in adrenal and testicular steroids during HIV infection. J. ACQUIRED IMMUNE DEFIC. SYNDR. (USA), 1992, 5/8 (841-846)

Dehydroepiandrosterone as predictor for progression to AIDS in asymptomatic human immunodeficiency virus-infected men. J. INFECT. DIS. (USA), 1992, 165/3 (413-418)

Decreased serum dehydroepiandrosterone is associated with an increased progression of human immunodeficiency virus infection in men with CD4 cell counts of 200-499. J. INFECT. DIS. (USA), 1991, 164/5 (864-868)

Hypertension (High Blood Pressure)

Treatment of essential hypertension with coenzyme Q10. Mol Aspects Med (ENGLAND) 1994, 15 Suppl

Coenzyme Q10 in essential hypertension. Mol Aspects Med (ENGLAND) 1994, 15 Suppl

Usefulness of coenzyme Q10 in clinical cardiology: a long-term study. Mol Aspects Med (ENGLAND) 1994, 15 Suppl

Influence of coenzyme Q-10 on the hypotensive effects of enalapril and nitrendipine in spontaneously hypertensive rats. Pol J Pharmacol (POLAND) Sep-Oct 1994, 46 (5) p457- 61

Isolated diastolic dysfunction of the myocardium and its response to CoQ10 treatment. Clin Investig (GERMANY) 1993, 71 (8 Suppl)

Effect of coenzyme Q10 on structural alterations in the renal membrane of stroke-prone spontaneously hypertensive rats. Biochem Med Metab Biol (UNITED STATES) Apr 1991

Coenzyme Q10: a new drug for cardiovascular disease. J Clin Pharmacol (UNITED STATES) Jul 1990

Coenzyme Q10: a new drug for myocardial ischemia? Med Clin North Am (UNITED STATES) Jan 1988

Bioenergetics in clinical medicine. XVI. Reduction of hypertension in patients by therapy with coenzyme Q10. Res Commun Chem Pathol Pharmacol (UNITED STATES) Jan 1981

Bioenergetics in clinical medicine. VIII. Adminstration of coenzyme Q10 to patients with essential hypertension. Res Commun Chem Pathol Pharmacol (UNITED STATES) Aug 1976

Bioenergetics in clinical medicine. III. Inhibition of coenzyme Q10- enzymes by clinically used anti-hypertensive drugs. Res Commun Chem Pathol Pharmacol (UNITED STATES) Nov 1975

Bioenergetics in clinical medicine. Studies on coenzyme Q10 and essential hypertension. Res Commun Chem Pathol Pharmacol (UNITED STATES) Jun 1975

[Garlic (Allium sativum)—a potent medicinal plant] Fortschr Med (GERMANY) Jul 20 1995

References

A meta-analysis of the effect of garlic on blood pressure. J Hypertens (ENGLAND) Apr 1994

Patient preferences for novel therapy: an N-of-1 trial of garlic in the treatment for hypertension. J Gen Intern Med (UNITED STATES) Nov 1993

Can garlic lower blood pressure? A pilot study. Pharmacotherapy (UNITED STATES) Jul-Aug 1993

Hypertension and hyperlipidaemia: garlic helps in mild cases. Br J Clin Pract Symp Suppl (ENGLAND) Aug 1990

Defective renal adenylate cyclase response to prostaglandin E2 in spontaneously hypertensive rats. J Hypertens (ENGLAND) Apr 1985, 3 (2)

Renal response to L-arginine in salt-sensitive patients with essential hypertension. Hypertension (UNITED STATES) Mar 1996

L-arginine restores dilator responses of the basilar artery to acetylcholine during chronic hypertension. Hypertension (UNITED STATES) Apr 1996

Vitamin C deficiency and low linolenate intake associated with elevated blood pressure: the Kuopio Ischaemic Heart Disease Risk Factor Study. J Hypertens Suppl (ENGLAND) Dec 1987

Regulation of blood pressure by nitroxidergic nerve. J Diabetes Complications (UNITED STATES) Oct-Dec 1995

[Endothelial function and arterial hypertension] Ann Ital Med Int (ITALY) Oct 1995, 10 Suppl

Contrasting effect of antihypertensive treatment on the renal response to L-arginine. Hypertension (UNITED STATES) Dec 1995

Prospective study of nutritional factors, blood pressure, and hypertension among US women. Hypertension (UNITED STATES) May 1996

[Overview—suppression effect of essential trace elements on arteriosclerotic development and it's mechanism] Nippon Rinsho (JAPAN) Jan 1996

[Interrelationship between dietary intake of minerals and prevalence of hypertension] Vopr Pitan (RUSSIA) 1995, (6)

Potassium depletion and salt-sensitive hypertension in Dahl rats: effect on calcium, magnesium, and phosphate excretions. Clin Exp Hypertens (UNITED STATES) Aug 1995

Consequences of magnesium deficiency on the enhancement of stress reactions; preventive and therapeutic implications (a review). J Am Coll Nutr (UNITED STATES) Oct 1994

Relationship of magnesium intake and other dietary factors to blood pressure: the Honolulu heart study. Am J Clin Nutr (UNITED STATES) Feb 1987

[Role of electrolytes in the development and maintenance of hypertension] Nippon Naibunpi Gakkai Zasshi (JAPAN) May 20 1994

Effect of dietary magnesium supplementation on intralymphocytic free calcium and magnesium in stroke-prone spontaneously hypertensive rats. Clin Exp Hypertens (UNITED STATES) May 1994

Vasorelaxant properties of n-3 polyunsaturated fatty acids in aortas from spontaneously hypertensive and normotensive rats. J Cardiovasc Risk (ENGLAND) Jun 1994

Effects of a combination of evening primrose oil (gamma linolenic acid) and fish oil (eicosapentaenoic + docahexaenoic acid) versus magnesium, and versus placebo in preventing pre-eclampsia. Women Health (UNITED STATES) 1992, 19 (2-3)

Antithrombotic activity of garlic: its inhibition of the synthesis of thromboxane-B2 during infusion of arachidonic acid and collagen in rabbits. Prostaglandins Leukot Essent Fatty Acids (SCOTLAND) Oct 1990

Bulgarian traditional medicine: a source of ideas for phytopharmacological investigations. J Ethnopharmacol (SWITZERLAND) Feb 1986

Garlic as a natural agent for the treatment of hypertension: a preliminary report. Cytobios (ENGLAND) 1982, 34 (135-36)

The decline in stroke mortality. An epidemiologic perspective. Ann Epidemiol (UNITED STATES) Sep 1993

Antioxidant therapy in the aging process. EXS (SWITZERLAND) 1992, 62

Antioxidants show an anti-hypertensive effect in diabetic and hypertensive subjects. Clin Sci (Colch) (ENGLAND) Dec 1991

[Relation between vitamin C consumption and risk of ischemic heart disease] Vopr Pitan (USSR) Nov-Dec 1983

Blood pressure and nutrient intake in the United States. Science (UNITED STATES) Jun 29 1984

Hypoglycemia

Preventing Hypoglycemia. Anti-Aging News, January 1982 Vo.2, No. 1 pg 6-7

Glutathione protects against hypoxic/hypoglycemic decreases in 2- deoxyglucose uptake and presynaptic spikes in hippocampal slices. Eur J Pharmacol (NETHERLANDS) Jan 24 1995, 273 (1-2) p191-5

Glutathione protects against hypoxic/hypoglycemic decreases in 2- deoxyglucose uptake and presynaptic spikes in hippocampal slices. Eur J Pharmacol (NETHERLANDS) Jan 24 1995, 273 (1-2) p191-5

Immune Enhancement

Vitamins and immunity: II. Influence of L-carnitine on the immune system. Acta Vitaminol Enzymol (ITALY) 1982, 4 (1-2)

Suppression of tumor growth and enhancement of immune status with high levels of dietary vitamin B6 in BALB/c mice. J Natl Cancer Inst (UNITED STATES) May 1987

The activities of coenzyme Q10 and vitamin B6 for immune responses. Biochem Biophys Res Commun (UNITED STATES) May 28 1993, 193 (1)

Research on coenzyme Q10 in clinical medicine and in immunomodulation. Drugs Exp Clin Res (SWITZERLAND) 1985, 11 (8) p539- 45

Immunoenhancing effect of flavonoid compounds on lymphocyte proliferation and immunoglobulin synthesis. Int J Immunopharmacol (ENGLAND) 1984, 6 (3) p205-15

Immunological senescence in mice and its reversal by coenzyme Q10. Mech Ageing Dev (SWITZERLAND) Mar 1978, 7 (3)

Immune effects of preoperative immunotherapy with high-dose subcutaneous interleukin-2 versus neuroimmunotherapy with low-dose interleukin-2 plus the neurohormone melatonin in gastrointestinal tract tumor patients. J Biol Regul Homeost Agents (ITALY) Jan-Mar 1995, 9 (1) p31-3

Pineal-opioid system interactions in the control of immunoinflammatory responses. Ann N Y Acad Sci (UNITED STATES) Nov 25 1994

Evidence for a direct action of melatonin on the immune system. Biol Signals (SWITZER-LAND) Mar-Apr 1994

The immuno-reconstituting effect of melatonin or pineal grafting and its relation to zinc pool in aging mice. Neuroimmunol (NETHERLANDS) Sep 1994

The immunoneuroendocrine role of melatonin. J Pineal Res (DENMARK) Jan 1993, 14 (1) p1-10

The pineal neurohormone melatonin stimulates activated CD4+, Thy-1+ cells to release opi-oid agonist(s) with immunoenhancing and anti-stress properties. J Neuroimmunol (NETHER-LANDS) Jul 1990, 28 (2)

Endocrine and immune effects of melatonin therapy in metastatic cancer patients. Eur J Cancer Clin Oncol (ENGLAND) May 1989

Dehydroepiandrosterone (DHEA) treatment reverses the impaired immune response of old mice to influenza vaccination and protects from influenza infection. Vaccine (ENGLAND) 1995, 13 (15) p1445-8

Dehydroepiandrosterone modulation of lipopolysaccharide-stimulated monocyte cytotoxicity. J Immunol (UNITED STATES) Jan 1 1996, 156 (1)

References

Administration of dehydroepiandrosterone reverses the immune suppression induced by high dose antigen in mice. Immunol Invest (UNITED STATES) May 1995

Pregnenolone and dehydroepiandrosterone as precursors of native 7-hydroxylated metabolites which increase the immune response in mice. J Steroid Biochem Mol Biol (ENGLAND) Jul 1994

The relationship of serum DHEA-S and cortisol levels to measures of immune function in human immunodeficiency virus-related illness. Am J Med Sci (UNITED STATES) Feb 1993

Dehydroepiandrosterone enhances IL2 production and cytotoxic effector function of human T cells. Clin Immunol Immunopathol (UNITED STATES) Nov 1991

Protection from glucocorticoid induced thymic involution by dehydroepiandrosterone. Life Sci (ENGLAND) 1990, 46 (22)

Immune development in young-adult C.RF-hyt mice is affected by congenital and maternal hypothyroidism. Proc Soc Exp Biol Med (UNITED STATES) Oct 1993

Binding and functional effects of thyroid stimulating hormone on human immune cells. J Clin Immunol (UNITED STATES) Jul 1990

Immunorestoration in children with recurrent respiratory infections treated with isoprinosine. Int J Immunopharmacol (ENGLAND) 1987, 9 (8)

Isoprinosine abolishes the blocking factor-mediated inhibition of lymphocyte responses to Epstein-Barr virus antigens and phytohemagglutinin. Int J Immunopharmacol (ENGLAND) 1986, 8 (1)

Isoprinosine as an immunopotentiator in an animal model of human osteosarcoma. Int J Immunopharmacol (ENGLAND) 1981, 3 (4)

The effect of Biostim (RU-41740) on the expression of cytokine mRNAs in murine peritoneal macrophages in vitro. Toxicol Lett (NETHERLANDS) Oct 1990

Isoprinosine (INOSINE PRANOBEX BAN, INPX) in the treatment of Aids and other acquired immunodeficiencies of importance. Cancer Detect Prev Suppl; 1:597-609 1987

Immunological effests of Isoprinosine as a pulse immunotherapy in melanoma and ARC patients in melanoma and ARC patients. Cancer Detect Prev Suppl; 1:457-62 1987

A modified determination of coenzyme Q10 in human blood and CoQ10 blood levels in diverse patients with allergies. Biofactors (ENGLAND) Dec 1988, 1 (4)

Carnitine in human immunodeficiency virus type 1 infection/acquired immune deficiency syndrome. J Child Neurol (UNITED STATES) Nov 1995, 10 Suppl

Oxidative damage and mitochondrial decay in aging. Proc Natl Acad Sci U S A (UNITED STATES) Nov 8 1994

Carnitine depletion in peripheral blood mononuclear cells from patients with AIDS: effect of oral L-carnitine. AIDS (UNITED STATES) May 1994, 8 (5) p655-60

Immunological parameters in aging: studies on natural immunomodulatory and immuno-protective substances. Int J Clin Pharmacol Res (SWITZERLAND) 1990, 10 (1- 2)

Insomnia

Melatonin replacement therapy of elderly insomniacs. Sleep (USA), 1995, 18/7 (598-603)

Improvement of sleep equality in elderly people by controlled-release melatonin. Lancet (United Kingdom), 1995, 346/8974 (541-544)

Sleep-inducing effects of low doses of melatonin ingested in the evening. Clinical Pharmacology and Therapeutics (USA), 1995, 57/5 (552-558)

Light, melatonin and the sleep-wake cycle. J. PSYCHIATRY NEUROSCI. (Canada), 1994, 19/5 (345-353)

Melatonin rhythms in night shift workers. SLEEP (USA), 1992, 15/5 (434-441)

Effect of melatonin replacement on serum hormone rhythms in a patient lacking endogenous melatonin. BRAIN RES. BULL. (USA), 1991, 27/2 (181-185)

Melatonin administration in insomnia. NEUROPSYCHOPHARMACOLOGY (USA), 1990, 3/1 (19-23)

Melatonin replacement therapy of elderly insomniacs. Sleep (UNITED STATES) Sep 1995, 18 (7) p598-603

Melatonin replacement corrects sleep disturbances in a child with pineal tumor. Neurology (USA), 1996, 46/1 (261-263)

Use of melatonin in circadian rhythm disorders and following phase shifts. Acta Neurobiologiae Experimentalis (Poland), 1996, 56/1 (359-362)

Treatment of delayed sleep phase syndrome. General Hospital Psychiatry (USA), 1995, 17/5 (335-345)

Nutritional factors in the etiology of the premenstrual tension syndromes. J Reprod Med (UNITED STATES) Jul 1983, 28 (7) p446-64

Effects of intravenously administered vitamin B12 on sleep in the rat. Physiol Behav (UNITED STATES) Jun 1995, 57 (6) p1019-24

Treatment of persistent sleep-wake schedule disorders in adolescents with methylcobalamin (vitamin B12). Sleep (UNITED STATES) Oct 1991, 14 (5) p414-8

Treatment of persistent sleep-wake schedule disorders in adolescents with methylcobalamin (vitamin B12). Sleep (UNITED STATES) Oct 1991, 14 (5) p414-8,

Vitamin B12 treatment for sleep-wake rhythm disorders. Sleep (UNITED STATES) Feb 1990, 13 (1) p15-23

[Folate and the nervous system (author's transl)] Folates et systeme nerveux. Sem Hop (FRANCE) Sep 18-25 1979, 55 (31-32) p1383-7

The effects of nicotinamide upon sleep in humans. Biol Psychiatry (UNITED STATES) Feb 1977, 12 (1) p139-43

Jet Lag

A double-blind trial of MELATONIN as a treatment for jet lag in international cabin crew. Biol Psychiatry (UNITED STATES) Apr 1 1993

MELATONIN and jet lag: confirmatory result using a simplified protocol. Biol Psychiatry (UNITED STATES) Oct 15 1992, 32 (8) p705-11

Role of biological clock in human pathology] Presse Med (FRANCE) Jun 17 1995, 24 (22) p1041-6

Melatonin marks circadian phase position and resets the endogenous circadian pacemaker in humans. Ciba Found Symp (NETHERLANDS) 1995, 183 p303-17; discussion 317-21

The role of pineal gland in circadian rhythms regulation. Bratisl Lek Listy (SLOVAKIA) Jul 1994, 95 (7) p295- 303

Light, melatonin and the sleep-wake cycle. J Psychiatry Neurosci (CANADA) Nov 1994, 19 (5) p345-53

Circadian rhythms, jet lag, and chronobiotics: an overview. Chronobiol Int (UNITED STATES) Aug 1994, 11 (4) p253-65

[Chronobiological sleep disorders and their treatment possibilities] Ther Umsch (SWITZER-LAND) Oct 1993, 50 (10) p704-8

Chronopharmacological actions of the pineal gland. Drug Metabol Drug Interact (ENGLAND) 1990, 8 (3-4) p189-201

Some effects of MELATONIN and the control of its secretion in humans. Ciba Found Symp (NETHERLANDS) 1985, 117 p266-83

Kidney Disease

Kidney stone clinic: Ten years of experience. Nederlands Tijschrift voor de Klinische Chemie (Netherlands), 1996, 21/1

Magnesium in the physiopathology and treatment of renal calcium stones. PRESSE MED. (FRANCE), 1987, 16/1 (25-27)

Urinary factors of kidney stone formation in patients with Crohn's disease. KLIN. WOCHEN-SCHR. (Germany, Federal Republic of), 1988, 66/3 (87-91)

Renal stone formation in patients with inflammatory bowel disease. SCANNING MICROSC. (USA), 1993, 7/1 (371-380)

Calcium and calcium magnesium carbonate specimens submitted as urinary tract stones. J. UROL. (USA), 1993, 149/2 (244-249)

Etiology and treatment of urolithiasis. AM. J. KIDNEY DIS. (USA), 1991, 18/6 (624-637)

Pathogenesis of nephrolithiasis post-partial ileal bypass surgery: Case-control study. KIDNEY INT. (USA), 1991, 39/6 (1249-1254)

The effect of glucose intake on urine saturation with calcium oxalate, calcium phosphate, uric acid and sodium urate. INT. UROL. NEPHROL. (Netherlands), 1988, 20/6

Magnesium metabolism in health and disease. DIS. MON. (USA), 1988, 34/4 (166-218)

Prophylaxis of recurring urinary stones: hard or soft mineral water. MINERVA MED. (Italy), 1987, 78/24 (1823-1829)

Urothelial injury to the rabbit bladder from various alkaline and acidic solutions used to dissolve kidney stones. J. UROL. (BALTIMORE) (USA), 1986, 136/1 (181-183)

Kidney stones, magnesium and spa treatment. PRESSE THERM. CLIM. (FRANCE), 1983, 120/1 (33-35)

Learning Disorders

Refer to references under Attention Deficit Disorder (ADD), or Age Associated Mental Impairment (Brain Aging).

Leukemia-Lymphoma
(And Hodgkin's Disease)

Retinoids in cancer treatment. J Clin Pharmacol. 1992 Oct. 32(10). P 868-88

Induction of differentiation and enhancement of vincristine sensitivity of human erythroleukemia HEL cells by vesnarinone, a positive inotropic agent. Exp Hematol. 1996 Jan. 24(1). P 37-42

1,25-dihydroxyvitamin D3 primes acute promyelocytic cells for TPA- induced monocytic differentiation through both PKC and tyrosine phosphorylation cascades. Exp Cell Res. 1996 Jan 10. 222(1). P 61-9

Probing the pathobiology of response to all-trans retinoic acid in cute promyelocytic leukemia: premature chromosome condensation/fluorescence in situ hybridization analysis. Blood. 1996 Jan 1. 87(1). P 218-26

Acute renal failure associated with the retinoic acid syndrome in acute promyelocytic leukemia. Am J Kidney Dis. 1996 Jan. 27(1). P 134-7

References

[Synthesis of retinoids with a modified polar ·group and their antitumor activity. Report I] Bioorg Khim. 1995 Dec. 21(12). P 941-9

Induction of differentiation in murine erythroleukemia cells by 1 alpha,25-dihydroxy vitamin D3. Cancer Lett. 1995 Apr 14. 90(2). P 225-30

Synergistic differentiation of U937 cells by all-trans retinoic acid and 1 alpha, 25-dihydroxyvitamin D3 is associated with the expression of retinoid X receptor alpha. Biochem Biophys Res Commun. 1994 Aug 30. 203(1). P 272-80

1,25(OH)2-16ene-vitamin D3 is a potent antileukemic agent with low potential to cause hypercalcemia. Leuk Res (1994 Jun) 18(6):453-63

Genistein enhances the ICAM-mediated adhesion by inducing the expression of ICAM-1 and its counter-receptors. Biochem Biophys Res Commun (1994 Aug 30) 203(1):443-9

Induction of differentiation and dna breakage in human hl-60 and k- 562 leukemia cells by genistein. Proc Annu Meet Am Assoc Cancer Res (1990) 31:A2605

Tretinoin. A review of its pharmacodynamic and pharmacokinetic properties and use in the management of acute promyelocytic leukaemia. Drugs. 1995 Nov. 50(5). P 897-923

[Treatment of acute promyelocytic leukemia with trans-retinoic acid. Experience of the Santa Maria Hospital, Medical School of Lisbon] Acta Med Port. 1994 Dec. 7(12). P 717-24

Vitamin A preserves the cytotoxic activity of adriamycin while counteracting its peroxidative effects in human leukemic cells in vitro. Biochem Mol Biol Int. 1994 Sep. 34(2). P 329-35

In vitro all-trans retinoic acid (ATRA) sensitivity and cellular retinoic acid binding protein (CRABP) levels in relapse leukemic cells after remission induction by ATRA in acute promyelocytic leukemia. Leukemia. 1994 Jun. 8(6). P 914-7

Mechanisms of protection of hematopoietic stem cells from irradiation. Leuk Lymphoma. 1994 Mar. 13(1-2). P 27-32

In vitro all-trans retinoic acid (ATRA) sensitivity and cellular retinoic acid binding protein (CRABP) levels in relapse leukemic cells after remission induction by ATRA in acute promyelocytic leukemia. Leukemia. 1994. 8 Suppl 2P S16-9

Treatment of mucositis with vitamin E during administration of neutropenic antineoplastic agents. Ann Med Interne (Paris). 1994. 145(6). P 405-8

Effects of sodium ascorbate (vitamin C) and 2-methyl-1,4- naphthoquinone (vitamin K3) treatment on human tumor cell growth in vitro. II. Synergism with combined chemotherapy action. Anticancer Res. 1993 Jan-Feb. 13(1). P 103-6

[Remission of acute promyelocytic leukemia after all-trans-retinoic acid] Harefuah. 1992 Dec 1. 123(11). P 445-8, 507

Abnormal vitamin B6 status in childhood leukemia. Cancer. 1990 Dec 1. 66(11). P 2421-8

Liver (Cirrhosis)

Effect of branched chain amino acid infusions on body protein metabolism in cirrhosis of liver. Gut (1986 Nov) 27 Suppl 1:96-102

Severe recurrent hepatic encephalopathy that responded to oral branched chain amino acids. American Journal of Gastroenterology (USA), 1996, 91/6 (1266-1268)

[Branched-chain amino acids in the treatment of latent porto-systemic encephalopathy. A placebo-controlled double-blind cross-over study]. Z Ernahrungswiss. 1986 Mar. 25(1). P 9-28

A prospective, randomized, double-blind, controlled trial. J Parenter Enteral Nutr. 1985 May-Jun. 9(3). P 288- 95

Prevention of CCL4-induced liver cirrhosis by silymarin. Fundam Clin Pharmacol (1989) 3(3):183-91

Free radicals in tissue damage in liver diseases and therapeutic approach. Tokai J Exp Clin Med (1986) 11 Suppl:121-34

Serum neutral amino acid concentrations in cirrhotic patients with impaired carbohydrate metabolism. Acta Med Okayama. 1983 Aug. 37(4). P 381-4

Is intravenous administration of branched chain amino acids effective in the treatment of hepatic encephalopathy? A multicenter study. Hepatology. 1983 Jul-Aug. 3(4). P 475-80

Branched-chain amino acid-enriched elemental diet in patients with cirrhosis of the liver. A double blind crossover trial. Gastroenterol. 1983 Nov. 21(11). P 644-50

Effect of euglycemic insulin infusion on plasma levels of branched- chain amino acids in cirrhosis. Hepatology. 1983 Mar-Apr. 3(2). P 184-7

Effect of glucose and/or branched chain amino acid infusion on plasma amino acid imbalance in chronic liver failure. J Parenter Enteral Nutr. 1981 Sep-Oct. 5(5). P 414-9

A comparison of the effects of intravenous infusion of individual branched-chain amino acids on blood amino acid levels in man. Clin Sci (Colch). 1981 Jan. 60(1). P 95-100

[Pathogenesis of hepatic encephalopathy (author's transl)] Leber Magen Darm. 1977 Aug. 7(4). P 241-54

Clearance rate of plasma branched-chain amino acids correlates significantly with blood ammonia level in patients with liver cirrhosis. International Hepatology Communications (Ireland), 1995, 3/2 (91-96)

Nutritional treatment of liver cirrhosis with branched chain amino acids. (BCAA) Nutritional support in organ failure: proceedings of the International Symposium, 1990

Branched-chain amino acids - A highly effective substrate of parenteral nutrition for critically ill children with Reye's syndrome. CLIN. NUTR. (USA), 1987, 6/2 (101-104)

References

Ammonia detoxification by accelerated oxidation of branched chain amino acids in brains of acute hepatic failure rats. BIOCHEM. MED. METAB. BIOL. (USA), 1986, 35/3 (367- 375)

Branched chain amino acids in the treatment of latent portosystemic encephalopathy. A double-blind placebo-controlled crossover study. GASTROENTEROLOGY (USA), 1985, 88/4 (887-895)

L-leucine prevent ammonia-induced changes in glutamate receptors in the brain and in visual evoked potentials in the rabbit. J. PARENTER. ENTER. NUTR. (USA), 1984, 8/6 (700-704)

Effects of amino acid infusions on liver regeneration after partial hepatectomy in the rat. J. PARENTER. ENTER. NUTR. (USA), 1986, 10/1 (17-20)

A comparison of the effects of intravenous infusion of individual branched-chain amino acids on blood amino acid levels in man. Clin Sci (ENGLAND) Jan 1981, 60 (1) p95-100

The role of insulin and glucagon in the plasma aminoacid imbalance of chronic hepatic encephalopathy. Z Gastroenterol (GERMANY, WEST) Jul 1979, 17 (7) p469-76

Drug metabolism in cirrhosis. Selective changes in cytochrome P-450 isozymes in the choline-deficient rat model. Biochem Pharmacol (ENGLAND) Jun 1 1986, 35 (11) p1817-24

Action of curcumin on the cytochrome P450-system catalyzing the activation of aflatoxin B1. Chem Biol Interact (IRELAND) Mar 8 1996, 100 (1) p41-51

Inhibition of lipid peroxidation and cholesterol levels in mice by curcumin. Indian J Physiol Pharmacol (INDIA) Oct 1992, 36 (4) p239-43

Induction of glutathione S-transferase activity by curcumin in mice. Arzneimittelforschung (GERMANY) Jul 1992, 42 (7) p962-4

Effect of polyene phosphatidylcholine (Essentiale forte, cps.) in the treatment of steatosis of the liver, focused on the ultrasonographic finding - Preliminary investigation. CAS. LEK. CESK. (Czech Republic), 1994, 133/12 (366- 369)

Relationship between liver cirrhosis death rate and nutritional factors in 38 countries. INT. J. EPIDEMIOL. (United Kingdom), 1988, 17/2 (414-418)

Vitamin B6 status in cirrhotic patients in relation to apoenzyme of serum alanine aminotransferase. CLIN. BIOCHEM. (Canada), 1988, 21/6 (367-370)

Vitamin B6 concentrations in patients with chronic liver disease and hepatocellular carcinoma. BR. MED. J. (UK), 1986, 293/6540 (175)

Choline and human nutrition. ANNU. REV. NUTR. (USA), 1994, 14/- (269-296)

Prostaglandin E2 production by hepatic macrophages and peripheral monocytes in liver cirrhosis patients. LIFE SCI. (USA), 1993, 53/4 (323-331)

Biochemistry of pharmacology of S-adenosyl-L-methionine and rationale for its use in liver disease. DRUGS (New Zealand), 1990, 40/SUPPL. 3 (98-110)

Choline may be an essential nutrient in malnourished patients with cirrhosis. GASTROEN-TEROLOGY (USA), 1989, 97/6 (1514-1520)

Use of polyunsaturated phosphatidyl choline in HBsAg negative chronic active hepatitis: Results of prospective double-blind controlled trial. LIVER (DENMARK), 1982, 2/2 (77-81)

Acetyl-L-carnitine increases cytochrome oxidase subunit I mRNA content in hypothyroid rat liver. FEBS LETT. (Netherlands), 1990, 277/1-2 (191-193)

S-Adenosyl-L-methionine. A review of its pharmacological properties and therapeutic poten-tial in liver dysfunction and affective disorders in relation to its physiological role in cell metab-olism. DRUGS (New Zealand), 1989, 38/3

Lupus

Refer to references under Autoimmune Diseases.

Macular Degeneration (Dry)

Treatment of senile macular degeneration with Ginkgo biloba extract. A preliminary double-blind, drug versus placebo study. PRESSE MED. (FRANCE), 1986, 15/31 (1556-1558)

Hydergine - a new promise in neuro-retinal disorders. AFRO-ASIAN J. OPHTHALMOL. (India), 1989, 8/1

Inhibition of glutathione reductase by flavonoids. A structure-activity study. BIOCHEM. PHAR-MACOL. (United Kingdom), 1992, 44/8

Flavonoids, a class of natural products of high pharmacological potency. BIOCHEM. PHAR-MACOL. (ENGLAND), 1983, 32/7

Results with anthocyanosides from Vaccinium myrtillus equivalent to 25% of anthocyanidines in the treatment of haemorrhagic diathesis due to defective primary haemostasis. GAZZ. MED. ITAL. (ITALY), 1981, 140/10 (445-449)

Studies on vaccinium myrtillus anthocyanosides. I. Vasoprotective and antiinflammatory activity. ARZNEIMITTEL-FORSCH. (GERMANY, WEST), 1976, 26/5

Atrophic macular degeneration. Rate of spread of geographic atrophy and visual loss. OPH-THALMOLOGY (USA), 1989, 96/10

Study of aging macular degeneration in China. JPN. J. OPHTHALMOL. (JAPAN), 1987, 31/3

Subretinal neovascularization in senile macular degeneration. AM. J. OPHTHALMOL. (USA), 1984, 97/2

Delayed macular choriocapillary circulation in age related macular. International Ophthalmology (Netherlands), 1995, 19/1

References

Cystoid macular degeneration in experimental branch retinal vein occlusion. OPHTHAL-MOLOGY (USA), 1988, 95/10

The clinical picture of retinal thrombosis. KLIN. MONATSBL. AUGENHEILKD. (GERMANY, WEST), 1977, 170/2

Results of fluorescence angiography of the posterior pole of the eye. BER.DTSCH.OPH-THAL.GESELLSCH. (GERMANY, WEST), 1975, vol 73

The evoked cortical potential in macular degeneration. J.AMER.GERIAT.SOC. (USA), 1974, 22/12

The development of neovascularization of senile disciform macular degeneration. AMER.J.OPHTHAL. (USA), 1973, 76/1

Macular Degeneration (Wet)

Dietary carotenoids, vitamins A, C, and E, and advanced age-related macular degeneration. Eye Disease Case-Control Study Group. JAMA (UNITED STATES) Nov 9 1994

Evidence by in vivo and in vitro studies that binding of pycnogenols to elastin affects its rate of degradation by elastases. BIOCHEM. PHARMACOL. (ENGLAND), 1984

Studies on the mechanism of early onset macular degeneration in cynomolgus monkeys. II. Suppression of metallothionein synthesis in the retina in oxidative stress. Experimental Eye Research (United Kingdom), 1996, 62/4 (399-408)

Antioxidant enzymes of the human retina: Effect of age on enzyme activity of macula and periphery. Current Eye Research (United Kingdom), 1996, 15/3 (273-278)

Low glutathione reductase and peroxidase activity in age-related macular degeneration. BR. J. OPHTHALMOL. (United Kingdom), 1994, 78/10 (791-794)

Antioxidant enzymes in RBCs as a biological index of age related macular degeneration. ACTA OPHTHALMOL. (Denmark), 1993, 71/2 (214-218)

Oxidative effects of laser photocoagulation. FREE RADIC. BIOL. MED. (USA), 1991, 11/3 (327-330)

Antioxidant status and neovascular age-related macular degeneration. ARCH. OPHTHAL-MOL. (USA), 1993, 111/1 (104-109)

Nutrition in the elderly. ANN. INTERN. MED. (USA), 1988, 109/11 (890-904)

Meningitis

See references Immune Enhancement.

Menopause

Value of micronutrient supplements in the prevention or correction of disturbances accompanying the menopause. REV. FR. GYNECOL. OBSTET. (France), 1990, 85/12 (702-705)

Effect of vitamin B-6 on plasma and red blood cell magnesium levels in premenopausal women. ANN. CLIN. LAB. SCI. (USA), 1981, 11/4 333-336)

Effect of a natural and artificial menopause on serum, urinary and erythrocyte magnesium. UNITED KINGDOM CLIN. SCI. (ENGLAND), 1980, 58/3 (255-257)

Vitamins as therapy in the 1990s. Journal of the American Board of Family Practice (USA), 1995, 8/3 (206-216)

Functional capacity of the tryptophan niacin pathway in the premenarchial phase and in the menopausal age. EGYPT AMER.J.CLIN.NUTR. (USA), 1975, 28/1 (4-9)

Dehydroepiandrosterone sulphate as a source of steroids in menopause. Sulfate de dehidro-epi-androsterona come fuente de esteroides en la menopausia (i). Acta Ginecologica (Spain), 1995, 52/9 (279-284)

Distribution of glutathione S-transferase isoenzymes in human ovary. J. REPROD. FERTIL. (United Kingdom), 1991, 93/2 (303-311)

Changes in circulating steroids with aging in postmenopausal women. OBSTET. GYNECOL. (USA), 1981, 57/5 (624-628)

Adrenal and gonadal steroid hormone deficiency in the etiopathogenesis of rheumatoid arthritis. Journal of Rheumatology (Canada), 1996, 23/SUPPL. 44 (10-12)

The effects of oral dehydroepiandrosterone on endocrine-metabolic parameters in postmenopausal women. J. CLIN. ENDOCRINOL. METAB. (USA), 1990, 71/3 (696- 704)

Catabolic effects and the influence on hormonal variables under treatment with Gynodian-Depot (Reg.trademark) or dehydroepiandrosterone (DHEA) oenanthate. SWEDEN MATURI-TAS (NETHERLANDS), 1981, 3/3-4 (225- 234)

Nutrition and osteoporosis: An analysis of dietary intake in postmenopausal women. Wiener Klinische Wochenschrift (Austria), 1995, 107/14 (418-422)

Magnesium supplementation and osteoporosis. Nutrition Reviews (USA), 1995, 53/3 (71-74)

Calcium, phosphorus and magnesium intakes correlate with bone mineral content in postmenopausal women. GYNECOL. ENDOCRINOL. (United Kingdom), 1994, 8/1 (55-58)

Incident pain caused by collapsed vertebrae in menopause. The logical background to a personal treatment protocol. ITALY MINERVA ANESTESIOL. (ITALY), 1984, 50/11 (573-576)

References

Interaction of family history of breast cancer and dietary antioxidants with breast cancer risk (New York, United States). Cancer Causes and Control (United Kingdom), 1995, 6/5 (407-415)

Altered menstrual cycles in rhesus monkeys induced by lead. FUNDAM. APPL. TOXICOL. (USA), 1987, 9/4 (722-729)

Effect of glucocorticoids and calcium intake on bone density and bone, liver and plasma minerals in guinea pigs. J. NUTR. (USA), 1979, 109/7 (1175-1188)

Relationships between usual nutrient intake and bone-mineral content of women 35-65 years of age: Longitudinal and cross-sectional analysis. AM. J. CLIN. NUTR. (USA), 1986, 44/6 (863-876)

Iron deficiency anemia in postmenopausal women. J.AMER.GERIAT.SOC. (USA), 1976, 24/12 (558-559)

Effect of menopause and estrogen substitutional therapy on magnesium metabolsim. DENMARK MINER. ELECTROLYTE METABOL. (SWITZERLAND), 1984, 10/2 (84-87)

Menstrual Disorders (Premenstrual Syndrome)

Clinical and biochemical effects of nutritional supplementation on the premenstrual syndrome.J. REPROD. MED. (USA), 1987, 32/6 (435-441)

Reduced bone mass in women with premenstrual syndrome. Journal of Women's Health (USA), 1995, 4/2 (161-168)

Calcium-regulating hormones across the menstrual cycle: Evidence of a secondary hyperparathyroidism in women with PMS. Journal of Clinical Endocrinology and Metabolism (USA), 1995, 80/7

Linolenic acid formulations for the treatment of premenstrual syndrome. CURR. OPIN. THER. PAT. (United Kingdom), 1992, 2/12 (2000-2002)

Calcium supplementation in premenstrual syndrome: A randomized crossover trial. J. GEN. INTERN. MED. (USA), 1989, 4/3 (183-189)

Plasma copper, zinc and magnesium levels in patients with premenstrual tension syndrome. ACTA OBSTET. GYNECOL. SCAND. (Denmark), 1994, 73/6 (452-455)

Use of a vitamin-mineral supplement in the management of premenstrual syndrome. BR. J. CLIN. RES. (United Kingdom), 1993, 4/- (219- 224)

Linolenic acid formulations for the treatment of premenstrual syndrome. CURR. OPIN. THER. PAT. (United Kingdom), 1992, 2/12

Oral magnesium successfully relieves premenstrual mood changes. OBSTET. GYNECOL. (USA), 1991, 78/2 (177-181)

Clinical and biochemical effects of nutritional supplementation on the premenstrual syndrome. J. REPROD. MED. (USA), 1987, 32/6 (435-441)

Magnesium and the premenstrual syndrome. ANN. CLIN. BIOCHEM. (UK), 1986, 23/6 (667-670)

The role of essential fatty acids and prostaglandins in the premenstrual syndrome. J. REPROD. MED. (USA), 1983, 28/7 (465-468)

Vitamin B6 in the treatment of the premenstrual syndrome - Review (1). BR. J. OBSTET. GYNAECOL. (United Kingdom), 1991, 98/3 (329-330) BR. J. CLIN. PRACT. (United Kingdom), 1988, 42/11 (448-452)

Migraine

In vivo administration of propranolol decreases exaggerated amounts of serum TNF-alpha in patients with migraine without aura. Possible mechanism of action. Acta Neurol (Napoli); 14(4-6):313-9 1992

Concurrent use of antidepressants and propranolol: case report and theoretical considerations. Biol Psychiatry; 18(2):237-41 1983

Nocturnal melatonin excretion is decreased in patients with migraine without aura attacks associated with menses. Cephalalgia (Norway), 1995, 15/2 (136-139)

Urinary melatonin excretion throughout the ovarian cycle in menstrually related migraine. CEPHALALGIA (Norway), 1994

Nocturnal plasma melatonin levels in migraine: A preliminary report. Headache (UNITED STATES) Apr 1989, 29 (4) p242-5

Octopamine and some related noncatecholic amines in invertebrate nervous systems. INT.REV.NEUROBIOL. (USA), 1976, Vol.19 (173-224)

Nocturnal melatonin excretion is decreased in patients with migraine without aura attacks associated with menses. Cephalalgia (NORWAY) Apr 1995, 15 (2) p136-9; discussion 79

The co-occurrence of multiple sclerosis and migraine headache: the serotoninergic link. Int J Neurosci (ENGLAND) Jun 1994, 76 (3-4) p249-57

Urinary melatonin excretion throughout the ovarian cycle in menstrually related migraine [see comments] Cephalalgia (NORWAY) Jun 1994, 14 (3) p205-9

The influence of the pineal gland on migraine and cluster headaches and effects of treatment with picoTesla magnetic fields. Int J Neurosci (ENGLAND) Nov-Dec 1992, 67 (1-4) p145-71

Nocturnal plasma melatonin levels in migraine: a preliminary report. Headache (UNITED STATES) Apr 1989, 29 (4) p242-5

Is migraine due to a deficiency of pineal melatonin? Ital J Neurol Sci (ITALY) Jun 1986, 7 (3) p319-23

Melatonin in humans physiological and clinical studies. J Neural Transm Suppl (AUSTRIA) 1978, (13) p289-310

Multiple Sclerosis (MS)

Measurement of low-molecular-weight antioxidants, uric acid, tyrosine and tryptophan in plaques and white matter from patients with multiple sclerosis. Eur Neurol (SWITZERLAND) 1992, 32 (5) p248-52

Clinical trials of unsaturated fatty acids in multiple sclerosis. IRCS MED. SCI. (ENGLAND), 1981, 9/12 (1081)

Dietary polyunsaturated fatty acids and depression: When cholesterol does not satisfy. American Journal of Clinical Nutrition (USA), 1995, 62/1 (1-9)

Expression and regulation of brain metallothionein. Neurochem Int (ENGLAND) Jul 1995, 27 (1) p1-22

Indirect evidence for nitric oxide involvement in multiple sclerosis by characterization of circulating antibodies directed against conjugated S-nitrosocysteine. J Neuroimmunol (NETHERLANDS) Jul 1995, 60 (1-2) p117-24

Isoprenoid (coQ10) biosynthesis in multiple sclerosis. Acta Neurol Scand (DENMARK) Sep 1985, 72 (3) p328-35

Abnormality of fatty acid composition of plasma lipid in multiple sclerosis. BRAIN NERVE (TOKYO) (JAPAN), 1979, 31/8 (797-801)

The pineal and regulation of fibrosis: pinealectomy as a model of primary biliary cirrhosis: Roles of melatonin and prostaglandins in fibrosis and regulation of T lymphocytes. MED. HYPOTHESES (ENGLAND), 1979, 5/4 (403-414)

Fatty acid patterns of serum lipids in multiple sclerosis and other diseases. BIOCHEM.SOC.TRANS. (ENGLAND), 1973, 1/1 (141-143)

Alternate usages for medications update. Journal of Neurological and Orthopaedic Medicine and Surgery (USA), 1995 16/3 (167-172)

Magnesium concentration in plasma and erythrocytes in MS. Acta Neurologica Scandinavica (Denmark), 1995, 92/1 (109-111)

Comparative findings on serum IMg2+ of normal and diseased human subjects with the NOVA and KONE ISE's for Mg2+. SCAND. J. CLIN. LAB. INVEST. SUPPL. (United Kingdom), 1994, 54/217

Magnesium concentration in brains from multiple sclerosis patients. ACTA NEUROL. SCAND. (Denmark), 1990, 81/3 (197-200)

References

Zinc, copper and magnesium concentration in serum and CSF of patients with neurological disorders. ACTA NEUROL. SCAND. (Denmark), 1989, 79/5 (373-378)

Multiple sclerosis: Decreased relapse rate through dietary supplementation with calcium, magnesium and vitamin D. MED. HYPOTHESES (UK), 1986, 21/2 (193-200)

Painful tonic seizures in multiple sclerosis. Clinical and electromyographic aspects. MED. CLIN. (BARCELONA) (SPAIN), 1981, 76/10 (454- 456)

On the ion concentration in the cerebrospinal fluid in multiple sclerosis. PSYCHIATR. NEU-ROL. MED. PSYCHOL. (GERMANY, EAST), 1977, 29/8 (482-489)

Evaluation of a nutrition education programme for people with multiple sclerosis. J. HUM. NUTR. DIET. (United Kingdom), 1993, 6/2 (131-147)

Mineral composition of brains of normal and multiple sclerosis victims. PROC. SOC. EXP. BIOL. MED. (USA), 1980, 165/2 (327- 329)

Multiple sclerosis: A diathesis? GAZZ.SANIT. (MILANO) (ITALY), 1973, 22/1 (37-39)

On the causes of multiple sclerosis. MED. HYPOTHESES (United Kingdom), 1993, 41/2 (93-96)

Dietary polyunsaturated fatty acids and depression: when cholesterol does not satisfy. Am J Clin Nutr (UNITED STATES) Jul 1995, 62 (1) p1-9

Lipids and neurological diseases. Med Hypotheses (ENGLAND) Mar 1991, 34 (3) p272-4

Essential fatty acid and lipid profiles in plasma and erythrocytes in patients with multiple sclerosis. Am J Clin Nutr (UNITED STATES) Oct 1989, 50 (4) p801-6

Plasma lipids and their fatty acid composition in multiple sclerosis. Acta Neurol Scand (DEN-MARK) Aug 1988, 78 (2) p152-7

The effect of nutritional counselling on diet and plasma EFA status in multiple sclerosis patients over 3 years. Hum Nutr Appl Nutr (ENGLAND) Oct 1987, 41 (5) p297- 310

[Metabolic aspects of multiple sclerosis] Wien Med Wochenschr (AUSTRIA) Jan 31 1985, 135 (1-2) p20-2

Essential fatty acids in the serum and cerebrospinal fluid of multiple sclerosis patients. Acta Neurol Scand (DENMARK) Mar 1983, 67 (3) p151-63

Multiple sclerosis: the rational basis for treatment with colchicine and evening primrose oil. Med Hypotheses (ENGLAND) Mar 1979, 5 (3) p365-78

Multiple sclerosis: some epidemiological clues to etiology. Acta Neurol Latinoam (URUGUAY) 1975, 21 (1-4) p66-85

Red blood cell and adipose tissue fatty acids in mild inactive multiple sclerosis. Acta Neurol Scand (DENMARK) Jul 1990, 82 (1) p43-50

Multiple sclerosis: effect of gamma linolenate administration upon membranes and the need for extended clinical trials of unsaturated fatty acids. Eur Neurol (SWITZERLAND) 1983, 22 (1) p78-83

The nutritional regulation of T lymphocyte function. Med Hypotheses (ENGLAND) Sep 1979, 5 (9) p969-85

Polyunsaturated fatty acids in treatment of acute remitting multiple sclerosis. Br Med J (ENGLAND) Nov 18 1978, 2 (6149) p1390-1

Effect of prolonged ingestion of gamma-linolenate by MS patients. Eur Neurol (SWITZERLAND) 1978, 17 (2) p67-76

Multiple sclerosis patients express increased levels of beta-nerve growth factor in cerebrospinal fluid. Neurosci Lett (NETHERLANDS) Nov 23 1992, 147 (1) p9- 12

Experimental and clinical studies on dysregulation of magnesium metabolism and the aetiopathogenesis of multiple sclerosis. Magnes Res (ENGLAND) Dec 1992, 5 (4) p295-302

Muscle Building

Ornithine alpha-ketoglutarate in nutritional support. Nutrition (UNITED STATES) Sep-Oct 1991, 7 (5) p313- 22

Anabolic effects of insulin-like growth factor-I (IGF-I) and an IGF-I variant in normal female rats. J Endocrinol (ENGLAND) Jun 1993, 137 (3) p413-21

Arginine needs, physiological state and usual diets. A reevaluation. J Nutr (UNITED STATES) Jan 1986, 116 (1) p36-46

Effects of dietary chromium picolinate supplementation on growth, carcass characteristics, and accretion rates of carcass tissues in growing-finishing swine. J Anim Sci (UNITED STATES) Nov 1995, 73 (11)

Anabolic effects of insulin on bone suggest a role for chromium picolinate in preservation of bone density. Med Hypotheses (ENGLAND) Sep 1995, 45 (3) p241-6

Effect of chromium picolinate on growth, body composition, and tissue accretion in pigs. J Anim Sci (UNITED STATES) Jul 1995, 73 (7) p2033-42

Longevity effect of chromium picolinate—'rejuvenation' of hypothalamic function? Med Hypotheses (ENGLAND) Oct 1994, 43 (4) p253-65

Effects of chromium picolinate on beginning weight training students. Int J Sport Nutr (UNITED STATES) Dec 1992, 2 (4) p343-50

Modulation of immune function and weight loss by L-arginine in obstructive jaundice in the rat. Br J Surg (ENGLAND) Aug 1994, 81 (8) p1199-201

Nutritional ergogenic aids: chromium, exercise, and muscle mass. Int J Sport Nutr (UNITED STATES) Sep 1991, 1 (3) p289-93

References

Efficacy of chromium supplementation in athletes: emphasis on anabolism. Int J Sport Nutr (UNITED STATES) Jun 1992, 2 (2) p111-22

Dietary supplements: Alternatives to anabolic steroids? PHYSICIAN SPORTSMED. (USA), 1992, 20/3 (189-193+196+198)

Direct anabolic effects of thyroid hormone on isolated mouse heart. AM. J. PHYSIOL. (USA), 1983, 14/3 (C328-C333)

Feeding conjugated linoleic acid to animals partially overcomes catabolic responses due to endotoxin injection. Biochem Biophys Res Commun (UNITED STATES) Feb 15 1994, 198 (3 p1107-12)

Muscular Dystrophy

Two successful double-blind trials with coenzyme Q10 (vitamin Q10) on muscular dystrophies and neurogenic atrophies. Biochim Biophys Acta (NETHERLANDS) May 24 1995

Biochemical rationale and the cardiac response of patients with muscle disease to therapy with coenzyme Q10. Proc Natl Acad Sci U S A (UNITED STATES) Jul 1985

[Efficiency of ubiquinone and p-oxybenzoic acid in prevention of E- hypovitaminosis-induced development of muscular dystrophy] Ukr Biokhim Zh (USSR) Sep-Oct 1981, 53 (5) p73-9

Effect of coenzyme Q on serum levels of creatine phosphokinase in preclinical muscular dystrophy. Proc Natl Acad Sci U S A (UNITED STATES) May 1974

[Some indices of energy metabolism in the tissues of mice with progressive muscular dystrophy under the action of ubiquinone] Vopr Med Khim (USSR) May 1974, 20 (3) p276-84

Free radicals, lipid peroxides and antioxidants in blood of patients ith myotonic dystrophy. J Neurol. 1995 Feb. 242(3). P 119-22

Myasthenia Gravis

Humoral and cellular immunity to intrinsic factor in myasthenia gravis. Scand J Haematol; 23(5):442-448 1979

Dietary precursors and brain neurotransmitter formation. Annu Rev Med (UNITED STATES) 1981, 32 p413-25

[The role of nutrition in the synthesis of neurotransmitters and in cerebral functions: clinical implications] Schweiz Med Wochenschr (SWITZERLAND) Sep 26 1981, 111 (39)

Nails

[Gelatin-cystine, keratogenesis and structure of the hair] Boll Soc Ital Biol Sper (ITALY) Jan 31 1983, 59 (1)

NUTRITION — Miscellanea; HEALTH — Miscellanea. Better Nutrition for Today's Living, Sep94, Vol. 56 Issue 9, p8, 1p, 1c

FOOD — Health aspects. Better Nutrition for Today's Living, Sep94, Vol. 56 Issue 9, p8, 1p, 1c

COSMETICS — Marketing. Environmental Nutrition, Mar96, Vol. 19 Issue 3, p1, 2p

SILICA — Physiological effect. Better Nutrition for Today's Living, Dec95, Vol. 57 Issue 12, p30, 1p, 1c

BIOTIN — Therapeutic use. Prevention, Dec94, Vol. 46 Issue 12, p122, 3p, 2c

Neuropathy

Diabetic polyneuropathy: New therapy plan from alpha lipoic acid. Therapiewoche (Germany), 1995, 45/36 (2118)

Oral alpha lipoic acid preparation proves good bioavailability in diabetic polyneuropathy. Frankfurt am Main Germany Therapiewoche (Germany), 1995, 45/23 (1367- 1370)

Therapy with high dose alpha lipoic acid improves the long-term prognosis in diabetic polyneuropathy. TW NEUROL. PSYCHIATR. (Germany), 1994, 8/12 (699-700)

High dose alpha lipoic acid improves the long-term prognosis in diabetic polyneuropathy. THERAPIEWOCHE (Germany), 1994, 44/38 (2247-2248)

Alpha-lipoic acid: A versatile drug which is proved Alpha lipoic acid. Avoidance and therapy of polyneuropathy in diabetes. Z. ALLGEMEINMED. (Germany), 1993, 69/17 (492-494)

Alternative therapeutic principles in the prevention of microvascular and neuropathic complications. Diabetes Res Clin Pract (IRELAND) Aug 1995, 28 Suppl pS201-7

[Preventive treatment of diabetic microangiopathy: blocking the pathogenic mechanisms] Diabete Metab (FRANCE) 1994, 20 (2 Pt 2) p219-28

[Diabetes mellitus—a free radical-associated disease. Results of adjuvant antioxidant supplementation] Z Gesamte Inn Med (GERMANY) May 1993, 48 (5)

[Treatment of diabetic neuropathy with oral alpha-lipoic acid. MMW Munch Med Wochenschr (GERMANY, WEST) May 30 1975

Comparison of the effects of evening primrose oil and triglycerides containing gamma-linolenic acid on nerve conduction and blood flow in diabetic rats. J Pharmacol Exp Ther (UNITED STATES) Apr 1995

References

The effects of gamma-linolenic acid on breast pain and diabetic neuropathy: possible non-eicosanoid mechanisms. Prostaglandins Leukot Essent Fatty Acids (SCOTLAND) Jan 1993

The use of gamma-linolenic acid in diabetic neuropathy. Agents Actions Suppl (SWITZER-LAND) 1992, 37 p120-44

Structural and biochemical effects of essential fatty acid deficiency on peripheral nerve. J Neuropathol Exp Neurol (UNITED STATES) Nov 1980, 39 (6)

Treatment of diabetic neuropathy with gamma-linolenic acid. DIABETES CARE (USA), 1993, 16/1 (8-15)

The effects of gamma-linolenic acid on breast pain and diabetic neuropathy: Possible non-eicosanoid mechanisms. PROSTAGLANDINS LEUKOTRIENES ESSENT. FATTY ACIDS (United Kingdom), 1993, 8/1

The use of gamma-linolenic acid in diabetic neuropathy. AGENTS ACTIONS (Switzerland), 1992, 37/SUPPL. (120-144)

Structural and biochemical effects of essential fatty acid deficiency on peripheral nerve. J. NEUROPATHOL. EXP. NEUROL. (USA), 1980, 39/6 (683-691)

Primary preventive and secondary interventionary effects of acetyl-L- carnitine on diabetic neuropathy in the bio-breeding Worcester rat. J Clin Invest (UNITED STATES) Apr 15 1996, 97 (8) p1900-7

Altered neuroexcitability in experimental diabetic neuropathy: effect of acetyl-L-carnitine. Int J Clin Pharmacol Res (SWITZERLAND) 1992, 12 (5-6)

Acetyl-L-carnitine corrects the altered peripheral nerve function of experimental diabetes. Metabolism: Clinical and Experimental (USA), 1995, 44/5 (677-680)

Diabetic neuropathy in the rat: 1. Alcar augments the reduced levels and axoplasmic transport of substance P Di Giulio A.M.; Lesma E.; Gorio A. RES. (USA), 1995, 40/3

Neural dysfunction and metabolic imbalances in diabetic rats: Prevention by acetyl-L-carnitine. DIABETES (USA), 1994, 43/12 (1469-1477)

Acetyl-L-carnitine prevents substance P loss in the sciatic nerve and lumbar spinal cord of diabetic animals. INT. J. CLIN. PHARMACOL. RES. (Switzerland), 1992, 12/5-6 (243-246)

Altered neuroexcitability in experimental diabetic neuropathy: Effect of acetyl-L-carnitine. INT. J. CLIN. PHARMACOL. RES. (Switzerland), 1992, 12/5-6 (237-241)

Peptide alterations in automatic diabetic neuropathy prevented by acetyl-L-carnitine. CLIN. PHARMACOL. RES. (Switzerland), 1992, 12/5-6 (225-230)

Acetyl-L-carnitine effect on nerve conduction velocity in streptozotocin-diabetic rats. ARZNEIM.-FORSCH. DRUG RES. (Germany), 1993, 43/3 (343-346)

Differential effects of acetyl-L-carnitine, L-carnitine and gangliosides on nerve Na+,K+-ATPase impairment in experimental diabetes. DIABETES NUTR. METAB. CLIN. EXP. (Italy),

1992, 5/1 (31-36)

Treatment of symptomatic diabetic peripheral neuropathy with the anti-oxidant alpha-lipoic acid. A 3-week multicentre randomized controlled trial. Diabetologia (Germany), 1995, 38/12 (1425-1433)

Peptide alterations in autonomic diabetic neuropathy prevented by acetyl-L-carnitine. Int J Clin Pharmacol Res (SWITZERLAND) 1992, 12 (5-6)

Primary preventive and secondary interventionary effects of acetyl-L- carnitine on diabetic neuropathy in the bio-breeding Worcester rat. Journal of Clinical Investigation (USA), 1996, 97/8 (1900-1907)

Obesity

Refer to references under Weight Loss.

Organic Brain Syndrome

Refer to references under Alzheimer's Disease.

Osteoporosis

Is postmenopausal osteoporosis related to pineal gland functions? Int J Neurosci (ENGLAND) Feb 1992, 62 (3-4) p215-25

Glucocorticoid-induced osteoporosis: mechanisms for bone loss; evaluation of strategies for prevention. J Gerontol (UNITED STATES) Sep 1990, 45 (5) pM153-8

Progesterone as a bone-trophic hormone. Endocr Rev (UNITED STATES) May 1990, 11 (2) p386-98

Osteocalcin and its message: relationship to bone histology in magnesium-deprived rats. Am J Physiol (UNITED STATES) Jul 1992, 263 (1 Pt 1) pE107-14

[Influence of active vitamine D3 on bones] Nippon Seikeigeka Gakkai Zasshi (JAPAN) Dec 1979, 53 (12) p1823-37

Relation of magnesium to osteoporosis and calcium urolithiasis. Magnes Trace Elem (SWITZERLAND) 92 1991, 10 (2-4) p281-6

Role of vitamin D, its metabolites, and analogs in the management of osteoporosis. Rheum Dis Clin North Am (UNITED STATES) Aug 1994, 20 (3) p759-75

Anabolic steroids in corticosteroid-induced osteoporosis. Wien Med Wochenschr (AUSTRIA) 1993, 143 (14-15) p395-7

Osteocalcin and its message: relationship to bone histology in magnesium-deprived rats. Am

References

J Physiol (UNITED STATES) Jul 1992, 263 (1 Pt 1) pE107-14

Glucocorticoid-induced osteoporosis: mechanisms for bone loss; evaluation of strategies for prevention. J Gerontol (UNITED STATES) Sep 1990, 45 (5) pM153-8

Nutritional insurance supplementation and corticosteroid toxicity. Med Hypotheses (ENG-LAND) Aug 1982, 9 (2) p145-56

Effects of recombinant human growth hormone (GH) on bone and intermediary metabolism in patients receiving chronic glucocorticoid treatment with suppressed endogenous GH response to GH-releasing hormone. J Clin Endocrinol Metab (UNITED STATES) Jan 1995, 80 (1) p122-9

Human marrow stromal osteoblast-like cells do not show reduced responsiveness to in vitro stimulation with growth hormone in patients with postmenopausal osteoporosis. Calcif Tissue Int (UNITED STATES) Jan 1994, 54 (1) p1-6

Growth hormone and bone. Horm Metab Res (GERMANY) Jul 1993, 25 (7) p335-43

Growth hormone and bone. Horm Res (SWITZERLAND) 1991, 36 Suppl 1 p49-55

Aromatase in bone cell: association with osteoporosis in postmenopausal women. J Steroid Biochem Mol Biol (ENGLAND) Jun 1995, 53 (1-6) p165-74

Biological properties and clinical application of propolis. VIII. Experimental observation on the influence of ethanol extract of propolis (EEP) on the regeneration of bone tissue ARZNEIM.-FORSCH. (GERMANY, WEST) , 1978, 28/1 (35-37)

Pain

Enhancement of a kappa-opioid receptor agonist-induced analgesia by L-tyrosine and L-tryptophan. Eur J Pharmacol (NETHERLANDS) Jun 13 1994, 258 (3) p173-8

L-Tyrosine-induced antinociception in the mouse: involvement of central delta-opioid receptors and bulbo-spinal noradrenergic system. Eur J Pharmacol (NETHERLANDS) Mar 23 1993, 233 (2-3) p255-60

L-dopa induces opposing effects on pain in intact rats: (-)-sulpiride, SCH 23390 or alpha-methyl-DL-p-tyrosine methylester hydrochloride reveals profound hyperalgesia in large antinociceptive doses. J Pharmacol Exp Ther (UNITED STATES) Nov 1992, 263 (2) p470-9

Dietary influences on neurotransmission. Adv Pediatr (UNITED STATES) 1986, 33 p23-47

References

Parathyroid (Hyperparathyroidism)

Calcium, phosphate, vitamin D, and the parathyroid. Pediatric Nephrology (Germany), 1996, 10/3 (364-367)

Vitamin D metabolism in chronic childhood hypoparathyroidism: Evidence for a direct regulatory effect of calcium. J. PEDIATR. (USA), 1990, 116/2 (252-257)

Determinants for serum 1,25-dihydroxycholecalciferol in primary hyperparathyroidism. BONE MINER. (Netherlands), 1989, 5/3 (279-290)

Magnesium hormonal regulation and metabolic interrelations. Regulation hormonale et interrelations metaboliques du magnesium. PRESSE MED. (France), 1988, 17/12 (584-587)

Treatment with active vitamin D (alphacalcidol) in patients with mild primary hyperparathyroidism. ACTA ENDOCRINOL. (Denmark), 1989, 120/2 (250-256)

Intravenous 1,25(OH)2 vitamin D3 therapy in haemodialysis patients: Evaluation of direct and calcium-mediated short-term effects on serum parathyroid hormone concentration. NEPHROL. DIAL. TRANSPLANT. (Germany, Federal Republic of), 1990, 5/6 (457-460)

Parkinson's Disease

Phospholipid in Parkinson's disease: Biochemical and clinical data. ITALY PROG. CLIN. BIOL. RES. (USA), 1980, VOL.39 (205-214)

Efficacy and tolerability of amantadine sulfate in the treatment of Parkinson's disease. Nervenheilkunde (Germany), 1995, 14/2 (76-82)

Bromocriptine lessens the incidence of mortality in L-Dopa-treated parkinsonian patients: Prado-study discontinued. EUR. J. CLIN. PHARMACOL. (Germany), 1992, 43/4 (357- 363)

Nicotinamidadenindinucleotide (NADH): The new approach in the therapy of Parkinson's disease. ANN. CLIN. LAB. SCI. (USA), 1989, 19/1 (38-43)

Levodopa and dopamine agonists in the treatment of Parkinson's disease: Advantages and disadvantages. EUR. NEUROL. (Switzerland), 1994, 34/SUPPL. 3 (20- 28)

Plasma profiles of adrenocorticotropic hormone, cortisol, growth hormone and prolactin in patients with untreated Parkinson's disease. J. NEUROL. (Germany, Federal Republic of), 1991, 238/1

Hypothalamo-pituitary function and dopamine dependence in untreated parkinsonian patients. ACTA NEUROL. SCAND. (Denmark), 1991, 83/3 (145-150)

Effect of dopamine, dimethoxyphenylethylamine, papaverine, and related compounds on mitochondrial respiration and complex I activity. Journal of Neurochemistry (USA), 1996, 66/3 (1174- 1181)

Treatment of Parkinson's disease: From theory to practice. USA POSTGRAD. MED. (USA),

References

1994, 95/5

In vitro oxidation of vitamin E, vitamin C, thiols and cholesterol in rat brain mitochondria incubated with free radicals. USA Neurochemistry International (United Kingdom), 1995, 26/5 (527-535)

Dietary intake and plasma levels of antioxidant vitamins in health and disease: A hospital-based case-control study. India Journal of Nutritional and Environmental Medicine (United Kingdom) 1995, 5/3 (235-242)

Oxidative stress and antioxidant therapy in Parkinson's disease. Progress in Neurobiology (United Kingdom), 1996, 48/1 (1-19)

Co-dergocrine (Hydergine) regulates striatal and hippocampal acetylcholine release through D2 receptors. NEUROREPORT (United Kingdom), 1994, 5/6 (674-676)

Ergot alkaloids and central monoaminergic receptors. J. PHARMACOL. (FRANCE), 1985, 16/SUPPL. 3 (21-27)

Dementia in the aged. PSYCHIATR. CLIN. NORTH AM. (USA), 1982, 5/1 (67-86)

Alterations of electroencephalographic patterns after intravenous administration of hydergine (dihydroergotoxine). ARG.NEURO-PSIQUIAT. (S.PAULO) (BRAZIL), 1973, 31/2

Clinical pharmacodynamics of acetyl-L-carnitine in patients with Parkinson's disease. Int J Clin Pharmacol Res. 1990. 10(1-2). P 139-43

The significance of eye blink rate in parkinsonism: a hypothesis. Int J Neurosci. 1990 Mar. 51(1-2). P 99-103

Mechanisms of action of ECT in Parkinson's disease: possible role of pineal melatonin. Int J Neurosci. 1990 Jan. 50(1-2). P 83-94

Pineal melatonin functions: possible relevance to Parkinson's disease. Int J Neurosci. 1990 Jan. 50(1-2). P 37-53

Locus coeruleus-pineal melatonin interactions and the pathogenesis of the on- off phenomenon associated with mood changes and sensory symptoms in Parkinson's disease. Int J Neurosci. 1989 Nov. 49(1-2). P 95-101

Pineal melatonin and sensory symptoms in Parkinson disease. Ital J Neurol Sci. 1989 Aug. 10(4). P 399-403

[Neuroendocrine and psychopharmacologic aspects of the pineal function. Melatonin and psychiatric disorders] Acta Psiquiatr Psicol Am Lat. 1989 Jan-Jun. 35(1-2). P 71-9

Impact of deprenyl and tocopherol treatment on Parkinson's disease in DATATOP patients requiring levodopa. Parkinson Study Group. Ann Neurol. 1996 Jan. 39(1). P 37-45

In vivo generation of hydroxyl radicals and MPTP-induced dopaminergic toxicity in the basal ganglia. Ann N Y Acad Sci. 1994 Nov 17. 738P 25-36

References

Antioxidant mechanism and protection of nigral neurons against MPP+ toxicity by deprenyl (selegiline) Ann N Y Acad Sci. 1994 Nov 17. 738P 214-21

Parkinson's disease: a chronic, low-grade antioxidant deficiency? Med Hypotheses. 1994 Aug. 43(2). P 111-4

Free radicals in brain metabolism and pathology. Br Med Bull. 1993 Jul. 49(3). P 577-87

Free radicals and their scavengers in Parkinson's disease. Eur Neurol. 1993. 33 Suppl 1P 60-8

Changes in endocrine function after adrenal medullary transplantation to the central nervous system. J. CLIN. ENDOCRINOL. METAB. (USA), 1990, 71/3

Phospholipid in Parkinson's disease: Biochemical and clinical data. ITALY PROG. CLIN. BIOL. RES. (USA), 1980, VOL.39 (205-214)

Efficacy and tolerability of amantadine sulfate in the treatment of Parkinson's disease. Nervenheilkunde (Germany), 1995, 14/2 (76-82)

Bromocriptine lessens the incidence of mortality in L-Dopa-treated parkinsonian patients: Prado-study discontinued. EUR. J. CLIN. PHARMACOL. (Germany), 1992, 43/4 (357- 363)

Nicotinamidadenindinucleotide (NADH): The new approach in the therapy of Parkinson's disease. ANN. CLIN. LAB. SCI. (USA), 1989, 19/1 (38-43)

Levodopa and dopamine agonists in the treatment of Parkinson's disease: Advantages and disadvantages. EUR. NEUROL. (Switzerland), 1994, 34/SUPPL. 3 (20- 28)

Plasma profiles of adrenocorticotropic hormone, cortisol, growth hormone and prolactin in patients with untreated Parkinson's disease. J. NEUROL. (Germany, Federal Republic of), 1991, 238/1

Hypothalamo-pituitary function and dopamine dependence in untreated parkinsonian patients. ACTA NEUROL. SCAND. (Denmark), 1991, 83/3 (145-150)

Effect of dopamine, dimethoxyphenylethylamine, papaverine, and related compounds on mitochondrial respiration and complex I activity. Journal of Neurochemistry (USA), 1996, 66/3 (1174- 1181)

Treatment of Parkinson's disease: From theory to practice. USA POSTGRAD. MED. (USA), 1994, 95/5

In vitro oxidation of vitamin E, vitamin C, thiols and cholesterol in rat brain mitochondria incubated with free radicals. USA Neurochemistry International (United Kingdom), 1995, 26/5 (527-535)

Dietary intake and plasma levels of antioxidant vitamins in health and disease: A hospital-based case-control study. India Journal of Nutritional and Environmental Medicine (United Kingdom) 1995, 5/3 (235-242)

Oxidative stress and antioxidant therapy in Parkinson's disease. Progress in Neurobiology

References

(United Kingdom), 1996, 48/1 (1-19)

Co-dergocrine (Hydergine) regulates striatal and hippocampal acetylcholine release through D2 receptors. NEUROREPORT (United Kingdom), 1994, 5/6 (674-676)

Ergot alkaloids and central monoaminergic receptors. J. PHARMACOL. (FRANCE), 1985, 16/SUPPL. 3 (21-27)

Dementia in the aged. PSYCHIATR. CLIN. NORTH AM. (USA), 1982, 5/1 (67-86)

Alterations of electroencephalographic patterns after intravenous administration of hydergine (dihydroergotoxine). ARG.NEURO-PSIQUIAT. (S.PAULO) (BRAZIL), 1973, 31/2

Clinical pharmacodynamics of acetyl-L-carnitine in patients with Parkinson's disease. Int J Clin Pharmacol Res. 1990. 10(1-2). P 139-43

The significance of eye blink rate in parkinsonism: a hypothesis. Int J Neurosci. 1990 Mar. 51(1-2). P 99-103

Mechanisms of action of ECT in Parkinson's disease: possible role of pineal melatonin. Int J Neurosci. 1990 Jan. 50(1-2). P 83-94

Pineal melatonin functions: possible relevance to Parkinson's disease. Int J Neurosci. 1990 Jan. 50(1-2). P 37-53

Locus coeruleus-pineal melatonin interactions and the pathogenesis of the on- off phenomenon associated with mood changes and sensory symptoms in Parkinson's disease. Int J Neurosci. 1989 Nov. 49(1-2). P 95-101

Pineal melatonin and sensory symptoms in Parkinson disease. Ital J Neurol Sci. 1989 Aug. 10(4). P 399-403

[Neuroendocrine and psychopharmacologic aspects of the pineal function. Melatonin and psychiatric disorders] Acta Psiquiatr Psicol Am Lat. 1989 Jan-Jun. 35(1-2). P 71-9

Impact of deprenyl and tocopherol treatment on Parkinson's disease in DATATOP patients requiring levodopa. Parkinson Study Group. Ann Neurol. 1996 Jan. 39(1). P 37-45

In vivo generation of hydroxyl radicals and MPTP-induced dopaminergic toxicity in the basal ganglia. Ann N Y Acad Sci. 1994 Nov 17. 738P 25-36

Antioxidant mechanism and protection of nigral neurons against MPP+ toxicity by deprenyl (selegiline). Ann N Y Acad Sci. 1994 Nov 17. 738P 214-21

Parkinson's disease: a chronic, low-grade antioxidant deficiency? Med Hypotheses. 1994 Aug. 43(2). P 111-4

Free radicals in brain metabolism and pathology. Br Med Bull. 1993 Jul. 49(3). P 577-87

Free radicals and their scavengers in Parkinson's disease. Eur Neurol. 1993. 33 Suppl 1P 60-8

References

Phobias

[Beta-blocking drugs and anxiety. A proven therapeutic value] Medications beta-bloquantes et anxiete. Un interet therapeutique certain. Encephale (FRANCE) Sep-Oct 1991, 17 (5) p481-92

Effect of beta-receptor blockade on anxiety with reference to the three-systems model of phobic behavior. Neuropsychobiology (SWITZERLAND) 1985, 13 (4) p187- 93

The treatment of social phobia. Real-life rehearsal with nonprofessional therapists. J Nerv Ment Dis (UNITED STATES) Mar 1981, 169 (3) p180-4

Premenstrual Syndrome

Refer to references under Menstrual Disorders-Premenstrual Syndrome.

Prevention Protocols

Increased brain damage after stroke or excitotoxic seizures in melatonin-deficient rats. FASEB Journal (USA), 1996, 10/13 (1546-1551)

Oxidative damage caused by free radicals produced during catecholamine autoxidation: Protective effects of O-methylation and melatonin. Free Radical Biology and Medicine (USA), 1996, 21/2 (241-249)

Oxidative processes and antioxidative defense mechanisms in the aging brain. FASEB Journal (USA), 1995, 9/7 (526-533)

Melatonin, hydroxyl radical-mediated oxidative damage, and aging: A hypothesis. J. PINEAL RES. (Denmark), 1993, 14/4 (151-168)

Neuroimmunotherapy of human cancer with interleukin-2 and the neurohormone melatonin: Its efficacy in preventing hypotension. ANTICANCER RES. (Greece), 1990, 10/6 (1759-1761)

Loss of delta-6-desaturase activity as a key factor in aging. MED. HYPOTHESES (ENGLAND), 1981, 7/9 (1211-1220)

Betaine:homocysteine methyltransferase - A new assay for the liver enzyme and its absence from human skin fibroblasts and peripheral blood lymphocytes. CLIN. CHIM. ACTA (Netherlands), 1991, 204/1-3 (239-250)

Dimethylglycine and chemically related amines tested for mutagenicity under potential nitrosation conditions. MUTAT. RES. (Netherlands), 1989, 222/4 (343-350)

Homocystinuria due to cystathionine beta-synthase deficiency - The effects of betaine treatment in pyridoxine-responsive patients. METAB. CLIN. EXP. (USA), 1985, 34/12 (1115-1121)

Prevention of strychnine-induced seizures and death by the N-methylated glycine derivatives

References

betaine, dimethylglycine and sarcosine. PHARMACOL. BIOCHEM. BEHAV. (USA), 1985, 22/4 (641-643)

Serenoa repens (Permixon (R)). A review of its pharmacology and therapeutic efficacy in benign prostatic hyperplasia. Drugs and Aging (New Zealand), 1996, 9/5 (379-395)

The extract of serenoa repens in the treatment of benign prostatic hyperplasia: A multicenter open study. CURR. THER. RES. CLIN. EXP. (USA), 1994, 55/7 (776-785)

Influence of dietary components on occurrence of and mortality due to neoplasms in male F344 rats. Aging - Clinical and Experimental Research (Italy), 1996, 8/4 (254-262)

Soy isoflavonoids and cancer prevention: Underlying biochemical and pharmacological issues. Advances in Experimental Medicine and Biology (USA), 1996, 401/-(87-100)

A review of the clinical effects of phytoestrogens. Obstetrics and Gynecology (USA), 1996, 87/5 II SUPPL. (897-904)

Perspectives on soy protein as a nonpharmacological approach for lowering cholesterol. Journal of Nutrition (USA), 1995, 125/3 SUPPL. (675S-678S)

Overview: Dietary approaches for reducing cardiovascular disease risks. Journal of Nutrition (USA), 1995, 125/3 SUPPL. (656S-665S)

Protective effects of soy protein on the peroxidizability of lipoproteins in cerebrovascular diseases. Journal of Nutrition (USA), 1995, 125/3 SUPPL. (639S-646S)

Modern applications for an ancient bean: Soybeans and the prevention and treatment of chronic disease. Journal of Nutrition (USA), 1995, 125/3 SUPPL. (567S-569S)

Green tea consumption and serum lipid profiles: A cross-sectional study in Northern Kyushu, Japan. PREV. MED. (USA), 1992, 21/4 (526-531)

Use of soya-beans for the dietary prevention and management of malnutrition in Nigeria. ACTA PAEDIATR. SCAND. SUPPL. (Sweden), 1991, 80/374 (175-182)

Increasing use of soyfoods and their potential role in cancer prevention. J. AM. DIET. ASSOC. (USA), 1991, 91/7 (836-840)

Diet and serum lipids in vegan vegetarians: A model for risk reduction. J. AM. DIET. ASSOC. (USA), 1991, 91/4 (447-453)

Nutritional contributors to cardiovascular disease in the elderly. J. AM. GERIATR. SOC. (USA), 1986, 34/1 (27-36)

Human and laboratory studies on the causes and prevention of gastrointestinal cancer. SCAND. J. GASTROENTEROL. SUPPL. (NORWAY), 1984, 19/104 (15-26)

Preventive nutrition: Disease-specific dietary interventions for older adults. GERIATRICS (USA), 1992, 47/11 (39-49)

Significance of active and passive prevention of cancer, arteriosclerosis and senility. MINER-

References

VA MED. (ITALY), 1982, 73/41 (2867-2872)

Increased brain damage after stroke or excitotoxic seizures in melatonin-deficient rats. FASEB Journal (USA), 1996, 10/13 (1546-1551)

Oxidative processes and antioxidative defense mechanisms in the aging brain. FASEB Journal (USA), 1995, 9/7 (526-533)

Partial restoration of choline acetyltransferase activities in aging and AF64A-lesioned rat brains by vitamin E. NEUROCHEM. INT. (United Kingdom), 1993, 22/5 (487-491)

Do antioxidant micronutrients protect against the development and progression of knee osteoarthritis?. Arthritis and Rheumatism (USA), 1996, 39/4 (648-656)

Dietary flavonoids, antioxidant vitamins, and incidence of stroke: The Zutphen study. Archives of Internal Medicine (USA), 1996, 156/6 (637-642)

Free radicals, oxidative stress, oxidized low density lipoprotein (LDL), and the heart: Antioxidants and other strategies to limit cardiovascular damage. Connecticut Medicine (USA), 1995, 59/10 (579-588)

Causes and prevention of premature aging. GERIATRIKA (Spain), 1994, 10/7 (19-24)

Antioxidant vitamins and disease - Risks of a suboptimal supply. THER. UMSCH. (Switzerland), 1994, 51/7 (467-474)

Tracking the daily supplement. TODAY'S LIFE SCI. (Australia), 1994, 6/3 (24-31)

Preventive nutrition: Disease-specific dietary interventions for Older adults. GERIATRICS (USA), 1992, 47/11 (39-49)

Experimental approaches to nutrition and cancer: Fats, calories, vitamins and minerals. MED. ONCOL. TUMOR PHARMACOTHER. (United Kingdom), 1990, 7/2-3 (183-192)

Vitamin D requirements for the elderly. CLIN. NUTR. (USA), 1986, 5/3 (121-129)

Vitamin D deficiency and hip fractures. TIJDSCHR. GERONTOL. GERIATR. (NT), 1985, 16/6 (239-245)

The physiologic and pharmacologic factors protecting the lens transparency and the update approach to the prevention of experimental cataracts: A review. METAB. PEDIATR. SYST. OPHTHALMOL. (USA), 1983, 7/2 (115-124)

Prostate Cancer (Early Stage)

Rationale for the use of genistein-containing soy matrices in chemoprevention trials for breast and prostate cancer. Journal of Cellular Biochemistry (USA), 1995, 58/SUPPL. 22

Phytoestrogens are partial estrogen agonists in the adult male mouse. Environmental Health Perspectives (USA), 1995, 103/SUPPL. 7

References

Soy intake and cancer risk: A review of the in vitro and in vivo data. NUTR. CANCER (USA), 1994, 21/2 (113-131)

Plasma concentrations of phyto-oestrogens in Japanese men. LANCET (United Kingdom), 1993, 342/8881 (1209-1210)

Urinary excretion of lignans and isoflavonoid phytoestrogens in Japanese men and women consuming a traditional Japanese diet. AM. J. CLIN. NUTR. (USA), 1991, 54/6

How is individual risk for prostate cancer assessed? Hematology/Oncology Clinics of North America (USA), 1996, 10/3

Control of LNCaP proliferation and differentiation: Actions and interactions of androgens, 1alpha,25-dihydroxycholecalciferol, all-trans retinoid acid, 9-cis retinoic acid, and phenylacetate. Prostate (USA), 1996, 28/3 (182-194)

1,25-Dihydroxy-16-ene-23-yne-vitamin D3 and prostate cancer cell proliferation in vivo. Urology (USA), 1995, 46/3 (365-369)

Recent advances in hormonal therapy for cancer. Current Opinion in Oncology (USA), 1995, 7/6

Endocrine control of prostate cancer. Cancer Surveys (USA), 1995, 23/- (43-62)

Vitamin D and prostate cancer. Advances in Experimental Medicine, 1995, 375/-

Actions of vitamin D3 analogs on human prostate cancer cell lines: Comparison with 1,25-dihydroxyvitamin D3. ENDOCRINOLOGY (USA), 1995, 136/1 (20-26)

Vitamin D and cancer. REV. FR. ENDOCRINOL. CLIN. NUTR. METAB. (France), 1994, 35/4-5

Human prostate cancer cells: Inhibition of proliferation by vitamin D analogs. ANTICANCER RES. (Greece), 1994, 14/3 A (1077-1081)

Vitamin D and prostate cancer: 1,25 Dihydroxyvitamin D3 receptors and actions in human prostate cancer cell lines. ENDOCRINOLOGY (USA), 1993, 132/5 (1952-1960)

Is vitamin D deficiency a risk factor for prostate cancer? (hypothesis). ANTICANCER RES. (Greece), 1990, 10/5 A (1307-1312)

The in vitro response of four antisteroid receptor agents on the hormone-responsive prostate cancer cell line LNCaP. Oncology Reports (Greece), 1995, 2/2 (295-298)

Combination treatment in M1 prostate cancer. CANCER (USA), 1993, 72/12 SUPPL. (3880-3885)

Antiandrogenic drugs. CANCER (USA), 1993, 71/3 SUPPL. (1046-1049)

The effects of flutamide on total DHT and nuclear DHT levels in the human prostate. PROSTATE (USA), 1981, 2/3 (309-314)

Endocrine profiles during administration of the new non-steroidal anti-androgen Casodex in prostate cancer. CLIN. ENDOCRINOL. (United Kingdom), 1994, 41/4 (525-530)

Antiandrogenic drugs. CANCER (USA), 1993, 71/3 SUPPL. (1046-1049)

Prostate Cancer (Metastasized/Late Stage)

Refer to references under Cancer Treatment.

Prostate Enlargement
(Benign Prostatic Hypertrophy)

NOTE: PERMIXON and SERENOA REPENS are synonyms for SAW PALMETTO EXTRACT.

The extract of serenoa repens in the treatment of benign prostatic hyperplasia: A multicenter open study. CURR. THER. RES. CLIN. EXP. (USA), 1994, 55/7 (776- 785)

Prostaserene (R). Treatment for BPH. DRUGS FUTURE (Spain), 1994, 19/5 (452-453)

The effect of Permixon on androgen receptors. ACTA OBSTET. GYNECOL. SCAND. (Sweden), 1988, 65/6

Pharmacological combinations in the treatment of benign prostatic hypertrophy. J. UROL. (France), 1993, 99/6 (316-320)

Inhibition of androgen metabolism and binding by a liposterolic extract of 'Serenoa repens B' in human foreskin fibroblasts. J. STEROID BIOCHEM. (ENGLAND), 1984, 20/1 (515-519)

Testosterone metabolism in primary cultures of human prostate epithelial cells and fibroblasts. J Steroid Biochem Mol Biol (ENGLAND) Dec 1995, 55 (3-4) p375-83

The effect of Permixon on androgen receptors. Acta Obstet Gynecol Scand (SWEDEN) 1988, 67 (5) p397-9

Binding of Permixon, a new treatment for prostatic benign hyperplasia, to the cytosolic androgen receptor in the rat prostate. J Steroid Biochem (ENGLAND) Jan 1984, 20 (1) p521-3

Inhibition of androgen metabolism and binding by a liposterolic extract of Serenoa repens B in human foreskin fibroblasts. J Steroid Biochem (ENGLAND) Jan 1984, 20 (1) p515-9

Testosterone metabolism in primary cultures of human prostate epithelial cells and fibroblasts. Journal of Steroid Biochemistry and Molecular Biology (United Kingdom), 1995, 55/3-4 (375-383)

Human prostatic steroid 5alpha-reductase isoforms - A comparative study of selective inhibitors. Journal of Steroid Biochemistry and Molecular Biology (United Kingdom) 1995, 54/5-6 (273-279)

The lipidosterolic extract from Serenoa repens interferes with prolactin receptor signal. Journal of Biomedical Science (Switzerland), 1995, 2/4 (357-365)

References

Lack of effects of a lyposterolic extract of Serenoa repens on plasma levels of testosterone, follicle-stimulating hormone, and luteinizing hormone. CLIN. THER. (USA), 1988, 10/5 (585-588)

Serenoa repens capsules: A bioequivalence study. ACTA TOXICOL. THER. (Italy), 1994, 15/1 (21-39)

Rectal bioavailability and pharmacokinetics in healthy volunteers of serenoa repens new formulation. ARCH. MED. INTERNA (Italy), 1994, 46/2 (77-86)

Clinical controlled trial on therapeutical bioequivalence and tolerability of Serenoa repens oral capsules 160 mg or rectal capsules 640 mg. ARCH. MED. INTERNA (Italy), 1994, 46/2 (61-75)

Evidence that serenoa repens extract displays an antiestrogenic activity in prostatic tissue of benign prostatic hypertrophy patients. EUR. UROL. (Switzerland), 1992, 21/4 (309-314)

Liposterolic extract of Serenoa Repens in management of benign prostatic hypertrophy. UROLOGIA (Italy), 1988, 55/5 (547-552)

Lack of effects of a lyposterolic extract of Serenoa repens on plasma levels of testosterone, follicle-stimulating hormone, and luteinizing hormone. CLIN. THER. (USA), 1988, 10/5 (585-588)

Binding of permixon, a new treatment for prostatic benign hyperplasia, to the cytosolic androgen receptor in the rat prostate. J. STEROID BIOCHEM. (ENGLAND), 1984, 20/1 (521-523)

Effect of Pygeum africanum extract on A23187-stimulated production of lipoxygenase metabolites from human polymorphonuclear cells. J Lipid Mediat Cell Signal. 1994 May. 9(3). P 285-90.

Combined extracts of Urtica dioica and Pygeum africanum in the treatment of benign prostatic hyperplasia: double-blind comparison of two doses. Clin Ther. 1993 Nov-Dec. 15(6). P 1011-20

[Urological and sexual evaluation of treatment of benign prostatic disease using Pygeum africanum at high doses]. Arch Ital Urol Nefrol Androl. 1991 Sep. 63(3). P 341-5

[Efficacy of Pygeum africanum extract in the medical therapy of urination disorders due to benign prostatic hyperplasia: evaluation of objective and subjective parameters. A placebo-controlled double-blind multicenter study] Wien Klin Wochenschr. 1990 Nov 23. 102(22). P 667-73

Pulmonary Insufficiencies

Refer to references under Emphysema and Chronic Obstructive Pulmonary Disease.

Retinopathy

A deficiency of vitamin B6 is a plausible molecular basis of the retinopathy of patients with diabetes mellitus. Biochem Biophys Res Commun. 1991 Aug 30. 179(1). P 615-9

Pharmacological prevention of diabetic microangiopathy, MECANISMES PATHOGENIQUES, DIABETE METABOL. (France), 1994, 20/2 BIS (219-228)

Clinical study of vitamin influence in diabetes mellitus. Journal of the Medical Society of Toho University (Japan), 1996, 42/6

Erythrocyte and plasma antioxidant activity in type I diabetes mellitus. Presse Medicale (France), 1996, 25/5 (188-192)

Lipid peroxidation in insulin-dependent diabetic patients with early retina degenerative lesions: Effects of an oral zinc supplementation. European Journal of Clinical Nutrition (United Kingdom), 1995, 49/4 (282-288)

Angioid streaks associated with abetalipoproteinemia. OPHTHALMIC GENET. (Netherlands), 1994, 15/3-4 (151- 159)

Comparison of gamma-glutamyl transpeptidase in retina and cerebral cortex, and effects of antioxidant therapy. CURR. EYE RES. (United Kingdom), 1994, 13/12 (891- 896)

Status of antioxidants in patients with diabetes mellitus with and without late complications. AKTUEL. ERNAHR.MED. KLIN. PRAX. (Germany), 1994, 19/3 (155-159)

Vitamins for seeing. COMPR. THER. (USA), 1990, 16/4 (62)

The regional distribution of vitamins E and C in mature and premature human retinas. INVEST. OPHTHALMOL. VISUAL SCI. (USA), 1988, 29/1 (22-26)

Oral vitamin E supplements can prevent the retinopathy of abetalipoproteinaemia. BR. J. OPHTHALMOL. (UK), 1986, 70/3 (166-173)

The role of taurine in developing rat retina. Ophtalmologie (France), 1995, 9/3 (283-286)

Taurine: Review and therapeutic applications (Part I). J. FARM. CLIN. (Spain), 1990, 7/7 (580-600)

Supplemental taurine in diabetic rats: Effects on plasma glucose and triglycerides. BIOCHEM. MED. METAB. BIOL. (USA), 1990, 43/1 (1-9+8)

Taurine deficiency retinopathy in the cat. J. SMALL ANIM. PRACT. (ENGLAND), 1980, 21/10 (521- 534)

[Clinical experimentation with pyridoxylate in treatment of various chorioretinal degenerative disorders (50 cases)]. Bull Soc Ophtalmol Fr. 1969 Dec. 69(12). P 1145-50

Rationales for micronutrient supplementation in diabetes. Med Hypotheses. 1984 Feb. 13(2). P 139-51

Magnesium and potassium in diabetes and carbohydrate metabolism. Review of the present status and recent results. Magnesium. 1984. 3(4-6). P 315-23

Seasonal Affective Disorder (SAD)

Seasonal affective disorder and season-dependent abnormalities of melatonin suppression by light. Lancet (1990 Sep 22) 336(8717):703-6. (For additional references on treating seasonal affective disorder, refer to Depression, above.)

Skin Aging

Skin photosensitizing agents and the role of reactive oxygen species in photoaging. J. PHOTOCHEM. PHOTOBIOL. B BIOL. (Switzerland), 1992, 14/1-2 (105-124)

An in vitro model to test relative antioxidant potential: Ultraviolet- induced lipid peroxidation in liposomes. ARCH. BIOCHEM. BIOPHYS. (USA), 1990, 283/2 (234-240)

Diminished stimulation of hyaluronic acid synthesis by PDGF, IGF-I or serum in the senescence phase of skin fibroblasts in vitro. Z. GERONTOL. (Germany), 1994, 27/3 (177-181)

Ultrastructural study of hyaluronic acid before and after the use of a pulsed electromagnetic field, electrorydesis, in the treatment of wrinkles. INT. J. DERMATOL. (Canada), 1994, 33/9 (661-663)

Hyaluronic acid in cutaneous intrinsic aging. INT. J. DERMATOL. (Canada), 1994, 33/2 (119-122)

Stimulation of cell proliferation by hyaluronidase during in vitro aging of human skin fibroblasts. EXP. GERONTOL. (USA), 1993, 28/1 (59-68)

Topical retinoic acid treatment of photoaged skin: Its effects on hyaluronan distribution in epidermis and on hyaluronan and retinoic acid in suction blister fluid. ACTA DERM.-VENEREOL. (Norway), 1992, 72/6 (423-427)

Werner's syndrome: Biochemical and cytogenetic studies. ARCH. DERMATOL. (USA), 1985, 121/5 (636-641)

Urinary acidic glycosaminoglycans in Werner's syndrome. EXPERIENTIA (SWITZERLAND), 1982, 38/3 (313-314)

Non-enzymatic degradation of acid-soluble calf skin collagen by superoxide ion: Protective effect of flavonoids. BIOCHEM. PHARMACOL. (ENGLAND), 1983, 32/1 (53-58)

In vitro cytotoxic effects of enzymatically induced oxygen radicals in human fibroblasts:

References

Experimental procedures and protection by radical scavengers. TOXICOL. VITRO (United Kingdom), 1989, 3/2 (103-109)

Antiviral activity of plant components. 1st Communication: flavonoids. ANTIVIRALE WIRKUNG VON PFLANZENINHALTSSTOFFEN. 1. MITTEILUNG: FLAVONOIDE. ARZNEIM.-FORSCH. (GERMANY, WEST), 1978, 28/3 (347-350)

Therapy of radiation damage in mice with O (L hydroxyethyl) rutoside. STRAHLENTHERAPIE (GERMANY, WEST), 1973, 145/6 (731-734)

Anti-ageing active principals by the oral route. Myth or reality? NOUV. DERMATOL. (France), 1994, 13/6 (423-425)

Topical 8% glycolic acid and 8% L-lactic acid creams for the treatment of photodamaged skin: A double-blind vehicle-controlled clinical trial. Archives of Dermatology (USA), 1996, 132/6 (631-636)

Alpha hydroxy acids in the cosmetic treatment of photo-induced skin ageing. Journal of Applied Cosmetology (Italy), 1996, 14/1 (1-8)

Effects of alpha-hydroxy acids on photoaged skin: A pilot clinical, histologic, and ultrastructural study. Journal of the American Academy of Dermatology (USA), 1996, 34/2 I (187- 195)

Topical gelatin-glycine and alpha-hydroxy acids for photoaged skin. J. APPL. COSMETOL. (Italy), 1994, 12/1 (1-10)

Antioxidants, fat and skin cancer. Skin Cancer (Portugal), 1995, 10/2 (97-101)

An in vitro model to test relative antioxidant potential: Ultraviolet- induced lipid peroxidation in liposomes. ARCH. BIOCHEM. BIOPHYS. (USA), 1990, 283/2 (234-240)

Photoprotective effect of superoxide scavenging antioxidants against ultraviolet radiation-induced chronic skin damage in the hairless mouse. Photodermatology Photoimmunology Photomedicine (Denmark), 1990, 7/2 (56-62)

Impairment of enzymic and nonenzymic antioxidants in skin by UVB irradiation. J. INVEST. DERMATOL. (USA), 1989, 93/6 (769-773)

Low levels of essential fatty acids are related to impaired delayed skin hypersensitivity in malnourished chronically ill elderly people. EUR. J. CLIN. INVEST. (United Kingdom), 1994, 24/9 (615-620)

Two concentrations of topical tretinoin (retinoic acid) cause similar improvement of photoaging but different degrees of irritation: A double- blind, vehicle-controlled comparison of 0.1% and 0.025% tretinoin creams. Archives of Dermatology (USA), 1995, 131/9 (1037-1044)

Topical tretinoin (retinoic acid) treatment for liver spots associated with photodamage. NEW ENGL. J. MED. (USA), 1992, 326/6 (368-374)

The effects of an abrasive agent on normal skin and on photoaged skin in comparison with topical tretinoin. BR. J. DERMATOL. (United Kingdom), 1990, 123/4 (457-466)

References

Aging and the skin. POSTGRAD. MED. (USA), 1989, 86/1 (131-144)

Topical tretinoind and photoaged skin. CUTIS (USA), 1989, 43/5 (476-482)

Stress

Refer to references under Anxiety.

Stroke (Hemorrhagic)

[Effect of piracetam on inorganic phosphates and phospholipids in the blood of patients with cerebral infarction in the earliest period of the disease]. Neurol Neurochir Pol (POLAND) Nov-Dec 1991, 25 (6)

Effect of piracetam on recovery and rehabilitation after stroke: A double- blind, placebo-controlled study. CLIN. NEUROPHARMACOL. (USA, 1994, 17/4 (320-331)

Ergoloids (Hydergine) and ischaemic strokes; Efficacy and mechanism of action. Journal of International Medical Research (United Kingdom), 1995, 23/3 (154-160)

Satellite symposium 'Piracetam and acute stroke : Pass' within the framework of the 3rd International Conference on stroke, 18-21 October 1995 in Prague satelliten-symposium 'Piracetam and acute stroke: Pass' im rahmen der 3. International Conference on stroke, 18.-21. Oktober 1995, Prag. Nervenheilkunde (Germany, 1996, 15/1

The nootropic agent piracetam in the treatment of acute stroke.NOOTROPIKA. PIRACETAM BEIM AKUTEN SCHLAGANFALL. TW Neurologie Psychiatrie (Germany, 1996, 10/1-2 (81)

Cerebroprotective effect of piracetam: The acute and chronic administrations of piracetam during short-term and long-term transient ischaemia. Turkish Journal of Medical Sciences (Turkey), 1995, 24/SUPPL.(39)

Stroke (Thrombotic)

Vitamin E plus aspirin compared with aspirin alone in patients with transient ischemic attacks. American Journal of Clinical Nutrition (USA), 1995, 62/6 SUPPL.

Poor plasma status of carotene and vitamin C is associated with higher mortality from ischemic heart disease and stroke: Basel Prospective Study. CLIN. INVEST. (Germany), 1993, 71/1 (3-6)

The treatment of acute cerebral ischemia. Ginkgo: Free radical scavenger and PAF antagonist. THERAPIEWOCHE (Germany), 1994, 44/24 (1394-1396) CODEN: THEWA

Efficiency of ginkgo biloba extract (EGb 761) in antioxidant protection against myocardial ischemia and reperfusion injury. Biochemistry and Molecular Biology International (Australia), 1995, 35/1 (125-134)

References

Magnesium content of erythrocytes in patients with vasospastic angina. CARDIOVASC. DRUGS THER. (USA), 1991, 5/4 (677-680)

Neuroprotective properties of Ginkgo biloba - Constituents. Z. PHYTOTHER. (Germany), 1994, 15/2 (92-96)

Variant angina due to deficiency of intracellular magnesium. CLIN. CARDIOL. (USA), 1990, 13/9 (663-665)

Magnesium and sudden death. S. AFR. MED. J. (SOUTH AFRICA), 1983, 64/18 (697-698)

Magnesium deficiency produces spasms of coronary arteries: Relationship to etiology of sudden death ischemic heart disease. SCIENCE (USA), 1980, 208/4440 (198-200)

Effect of vitamin E on hydrogen peroxide production by human vascular endothelial cells after hypoxia/reoxygenation. Free Radical Biology and Medicine (USA), 1996, 20/1 (99-105)

On the mechanism of the anticlotting action of vitamin E quinone. Proceedings of the National Academy of Sciences of the United States of America (USA), 1995, 92/18 (8171-8175)

Vitamin E may enhance the benefits of aspirin in preventing stroke. American Family Physician (USA), 1995, 51/8 (1977

Antioxidant vitamins and disease - Risks of a suboptimal supply. THER. UMSCH. (Switzerland), 1994, 51/7 (467-474)

Vitamin E consumption and the risk of coronary disease in women. NEW ENGL. J. MED. (USA), 1993, 328/20 (1444-1449)

Increased risk of cardiovascular disease at suboptimal plasma concentrations of essential antioxidants: An epidemiological update with special attention to carotene and vitamin C. AM. J. CLIN. NUTR. (USA), 1993, 57/5 SUPPL. (787S-797S)

Lipid peroxide, phospholipids, glutathione levels and superoxide dismutase activity in rat brain after ischaemia: Effect of ginkgo biloba extract. Pharmacological Research (United Kingdom), 1995, 32/5 (273-278)

Protection of hypoxia-induced ATP decrease in endothelial cells by ginkgo biloba extract and bilobalide. Biochemical Pharmacology (United Kingdom), 1995, 50/7 (991-999)

Lipid peroxidation in experimental spinal cord injury. Comparison of treatment with Ginkgo biloba, TRH and methylprednisolone. Research in Experimental Medicine (Germany), 1995, 195/2 (117-123)

Effects of natural antioxidant Ginkgo biloba extract (EGb 761) on myocardial ischemia-reperfusion injury. FREE RADIC. BIOL. MED. (USA), 1994, 16/6 (789-794)

Experimental model of cerebral ischemia. Preventive activity of Ginkgo biloba extract.Rapin J.R.; Le Poncin-Lafitte M. SEM. HOP. (FRANCE), 1979, 55/43-44 (2047-2050)

On brain protection of co-dergocrine mesylate (Hydergine (R)) against hypoxic hypoxidosis of

References

different severity: Double-blind placebo-controlled quantitative EEG and psychometric studies. INT. J. CLIN. PHARMACOL. THER. TOXICOL. (Germany, Federal Republic of), 1990, 28/12 (510-524)

Pharmacodynamics of the cerebral circulation. Effects of ten drugs on cerebral blood flow and metabolism in cerebrovascular insufficiency. PATH.BIOL. (PARIS) (FRANCE), 1974, 22/9 (815-825)

Effects of ionic and nonionic contrast media on clot structure, platelet function and thrombolysis mediated by tissue plasminogen activator in plasma clots. Haemostasis (Switzerland), 1995, 25/4 (172-181)

Thrombolytic therapy: Recent advances. Treatment of myocardial infarction. APPL. CARDIOPULM. PATHOPHYSIOL. (Netherlands), 1991/92, 4/3 (193-204)

Selective decrease in lysis of old thrombi after rapid administration of tissue-type plasminogen activator. J. AM. COLL. CARDIOL. (USA), 1989, 14/5 (1359-1364)

Antioxidant Curcuma extracts decrease the blood lipid peroxide levels of human subjects. Age (USA), 1995, 18/4 (167-169)

Inhibition of tumor necrosis factor by curcumin, a phytochemical. Biochemical Pharmacology (United Kingdom), 1995, 49/11 (1551-1556)

Inhibitory effect of curcumin, an anti-inflammatory agent, on vascular smooth muscle cell proliferation. EUR. J. PHARMACOL. (Netherlands), 1992, 221/2-3 (381-384)

Change of fatty acid composition, platelet aggregability and RBC function in elderly subjects with administration of low dose fish oil concentrate and comparison with those in younger subjects. JPN. J. GERIATR. (Japan), 1994, 31/8 (596-603)

Premature Carotid Atherosclerosis: Does It Occur in Both Familial Hypercholesterolemia and Homocystinuria? Ultrasound Assessment of Arterial Intima-Media Thickness and Blood Flow Velocity. Stroke, May 1994;25(5):943-950.

Fibrinogen, Arterial Risk Factor in Clinical Practice.Clinical Hemorrheology, 1994;14(6):739-767

Fibrinogen and Cardiovascular Disorders. Quarterly Journal of Medicine, 1995;88:155-165.

Can Lowering Homocysteine Levels Reduce Cardiovascular Risk? The New England Journal of Medicine, February 2, 1995;332(5):328-329.

Fibrinogen, Arterial Risk Factor in Clinical Practice.Potron,G., et al. Clinical Hemorrheology, 1994;14(6):739-767

The Lipoprotein(a). Significance and Relation to Atherosclerosis.Heller, F.R., et al. ACTA Clinica Belgica, 1991;46(6):371-383.

Surgical Precautions

Refer to references under Anesthesia and Surgical Precautions.

Thyroid Deficiency

Soy protein, thyroid regulation and cholesterol metabolism. Journal of Nutrition (USA), 1995, 125/3 SUPPL. (619S-623S)

Comparative pharmacology of the thyroid hormones. ANN. THORAC. SURG. (USA), 1993, 56/1 SUPPL. (S2-S8)

Primary hypothyroidism in an adult patient with protein-calorie malnutrition: A study of its mechanism and the effect of amino acid deficiency. METAB. CLIN. EXP. (USA), 1988, 37/1 (9-14)

Preferential formation of triiodothyronine residues in newly synthesized (14C)tyrosine-labeled thyroglobulin molecules in follicles reconstructed in a suspension culture of hog thyroid cells. MOL. CELL. ENDOCRINOL. (Ireland), 1988, 59/1-2 (117- 124)

Importance of the content and localization of tyrosine residues for thyroxine formation within the N-terminal part of human thyroglobulin den. European Journal of Endocrinology (Norway), 1995, 132/5 (611-617)

Melatonin and the endocrine role of the pineal organ. ARGENTINA CURR.TOPICS EXP.ENDOCRIN. (USA), 1974, Vol. 2 (107-128)

Brief report: Circadian melatonin, thyroid-stimulating hormone, prolactin, and cortisol levels in serum of young adults with autism. Israel Journal of Autism and Developmental Disorders (USA), 1995, 25/6 (641-654)

Effects of melatonin and thyroxine replacement on thyrotropin, luteinizing hormone, and pro-lactin in male hypothyroid hamsters. ENDOCRINOLOGY (USA), 1985, 117/6 (2402-2407)

Influence of phytogenic substances with thyreostatic effects in combination with iodine on the thyroid hormones and somatomedin level in pigs. EXP. CLIN. ENDOCRINOL. (GERMANY, EAST), 1985, 85/2 (183-190)

Importance of the content and localization of tyrosine residues for thyroxine formation within the N-terminal part of human thyroglobulin. European Journal of Endocrinology (Norway), 1995, 132/5 (611-617)

Preferential formation of triiodothyronine residues in newly synthesized (14C)tyrosine-labeled thyroglobulin molecules in follicles reconstructed in a suspension culture of hog thyroid cells. MOL. CELL. ENDOCRINOL. (Ireland), 1988, 59/1-2 (117- 124)

Primary hypothyroidism in an adult patient with protein-calorie malnutrition: A study of its mechanism and the effect of amino acid deficiency. METAB. CLIN. EXP. (USA), 1988, 37/1 (9-14)

References

Comparative pharmacology of the thyroid hormones. ANN. THORAC. SURG. (USA), 1993, 56/1 SUPPL. (S2-S8)

Tinnitus

[Hydergine in pathology of the inner ear] Hydergina en patologia del oido interno. An Otorrinolaringol Ibero Am (1990) 17(1):85-98 (Published in Spanish)

Tinnitus rehabilitation in sensorineural hearing loss. Based on 400 patients. Otorinolaringologia (Italy), 1994, 44/5 (227-229)

The value of rheological, vasoactive and metabolically active substances in the initial treatment of acute acoustic trauma. HNO (GERMANY, WEST), 1986, 34/10 (424-428)

Trental and Cavinton in the therapy of cochleovestibular disorders. CESK. OTOLARYNGOL. (CZECHOSLOVAKIA), 1984, 33/4 (264-267)

Prospects of using Cavinton in Meniere's disease. VESTN. OTORINOLARINGOL. (USSR), 1980, 42/3 (18-22)

Results of combined low-power laser therapy and extracts of Ginkgo biloba in cases of sensorineural hearing loss and tinnitus. In: Adv Otorhinolaryngol (1995) 49:101-4

Trauma

Effect of dietary vitamin C on compression injury of the spinal cord in a rat mutant unable to synthesize ascorbic acid and its correlation with that of vitamin E. Japan Spinal Cord (United Kingdom), 1996, 34/4 (234- 238)

Effect of allopurinol, sulphasalazine, and vitamin C on aspirin induced gastroduodenal injury in human volunteers. United Kingdom Gut (United Kingdom), 1996, 38/4 (518-524

Hemodynamic effects of delayed initiation of antioxidant therapy (beginning two hours after burn) in extensive third-degree burns. Journal of Burn Care and Rehabilitation (USA), 1995, 16/6 (610-615)

Dietary intake and plasma levels of antioxidant vitamins in health and disease: A hospital-based case-control study. Journal of Nutritional and Environmental Medicine (United Kingdom), 1995, 5/3

Vitamin C and pressure sores.Journal of Dermatological Treatment (United Kingdom), 1995, 6/3

Supplementation with vitamins C and E suppresses leukocyte oxygen free radical production in patients with myocardial infarction. European Heart Journal (United Kingdom), 1995, 16/8 (1044-1049)

Antioxidant therapy using high dose vitamin C: Reduction of postburn resuscitation fluid vol-

References

ume requirements. World Journal of Surgery (USA), 1995, 19/2 (287-291)

Vitamin C reduces ischemia-reperfusion injury in a rat epigastric island skin flap model. ANN. PLAST. SURG. (USA), 1994, 33/6 (620-623)

An experimental study on the protection against reperfusion myocardial ischemia by using large doses of vitamin C. CHIN. J. CARDIOL. (China), 1994, 22/1 (52-54+80)

Vitamins as radioprotectors in vivo. I. Protection by vitamin C against internal radionuclides in mouse testes: Implications to the mechanism of damage caused by the auger effect. USA RADIAT. RES. (USA), 1994, 137/3 (394-399)

Experimental studies on the treatment of frostbite in rats. INDIAN J. MED. RES. SECT. B BIO-MED. RES. OTHER THAN INFECT. DIS. (India), 1993, 98/AUG. (178-184)

The effects of high-dose vitamin C therapy on postburn lipid peroxidation. USA J. BURN CARE REHABIL. (USA), 1993, 14/6 (624- 629)

Effect of antioxidant vitamin supplementation on muscle function after eccentric exercise. EUR. J. APPL. PHYSIOL. OCCUP. PHYSIOL. (Germany), 1993, 67/5 (426-430)

Vitamin C as a radioprotector against iodine-131 in vivo. J. NUCL. MED. (USA), 1993, 34/4 (637-640)

Effects of high-dose vitamin C administration on postburn microvascular fluid and protein flux. REHABIL. (USA), 1992, 13/5 (560-566)

Modification of the daily photoreceptor membrane shedding response in vitro by antioxidants. INVEST. OPHTHALMOL. VISUAL SCI. (USA), 1992, 33/10 (3005-3008)

Ascorbate treatment prevents accumulation of phagosomes in RPE in light damage. INVEST. OPHTHALMOL. VISUAL SCI. (USA), 1992, 33/10 (2814-2821)

Topical vitamin C protects porcine skin from ultraviolet radiation-induced damage. BR. J. DERMATOL. (United Kingdom), 1992, 127/3 (247- 253)

The synergism of gamma-interferon and tumor necrosis factor in whole body hyperthermia with vitamin C to control toxicity. MED. HYPOTHESES (United Kingdom), 1992, 38/3 (257-258)

Tirilazad mesylate protects vitamins C and E in brain ischemia- reperfusion injury. J. NEU-ROCHEM. (USA), 1992, 58/6 (2263-2268)

Vitamin C supplementation in the patient with burns and renal failure. J. BURN CARE REHA-BIL. (USA), 1992, 13/3 (378-380)

High-dose vitamin C therapy for extensive deep dermal burns. USA BURNS (United Kingdom), 1992, 18/2 (127-131)

Metabolic and immune effects of enteral ascorbic acid after burn trauma. BURNS (United Kingdom), 1992, 18/2 (92-97)

Reduced fluid volume requirement for resuscitation of third-degree burns with high-dose vitamin C. J. BURN CARE REHABIL. (USA), 1991, 12/6 (525-532)

Biochemical basis of ozone toxicity. FREE RADIC. BIOL. MED. (USA), 1990, 9/3 (245-265)

Decreases in tissue levels of ubiquinol-9 and -10, ascorbate and alpha-tocopherol following spinal cord impact trauma in rats. USA NEUROSCI. LETT. (Netherlands), 1990, 108/1-2 (201-206)

Nutritional considerations for the burned patient. SURG. CLIN. NORTH AM. (USA), 1987, 67/1 (109-131)

Nutritional considerations for the burned patient. SURG. CLIN. NORTH AM. (USA), 1987, 67/2 (109-131)

Ascorbic acid metabolism in trauma. INDIAN J. MED. RES. (INDIA), 1982, 75/5 (748-751)

Multiple pathologic fractures in osteogenesis imperfecta. ORTHOPADE (GERMANY, WEST), 1982, 11/3 (101-108)

Effect of zinc supplementation in fracture healing. INDIAN J. ORTHOP. (INDIA), 1980, 14/1 (62-71)

Treatment results of spinal cord injuries in the Swiss paraplegic centre of Basle. PARAPLEGIA (EDINB.) (SCOTLAND), 1976, 14/1 (58-65)

Effect of piracetam on electroshock induced amnesia and decrease in brain acetylcholine in rats. INDIAN J. EXP. BIOL. (India), 1993, 31/10 (822-824)

Use of piracetam in treatment of head injuries. Observations in 903 cases. CLIN. TER. (ITALY), 1985, 114/6 (481-487)

Urinary Tract Infections

Inhibition of bacterial adherence by cranberry juice: potential use for the treatment of urinary tract infections. J Urol (1984 May) 131(5):1013-6

Anti-Escherichia coli adhesin activity of cranberry and blueberry juices [letter]. N Engl J Med (1991 May 30) 324(22):1599

Effect of cranberry juice on urinary pH. Nurs Res (1979 Sep-Oct) 28(5):287-90

Inhibitory activity of cranberry juice on adherence of type 1 and type P fimbriated Escherichia coli to eucaryotic cells. Antimicrob Agents Chemother (1989 Jan) 33(1):92-8

An examination of the anti-adherence activity of cranberry juice on urinary and nonurinary bacterial isolates. Microbios (1988) 55(224-225):173-81

Valvular Insufficiency/Heart Valve Defects

Refer to references under Congestive Heart Failure/Cardiomyopathy

Vertigo

[Clinical trial of the use of the combination of piracetam and dihydroergocristine in vertigo from different causes] An Otorrinolaringol Ibero Am (SPAIN) 1989, 16 (3)

Treatment of vertigo syndrome with Nootropil] Otolaryngol Pol (POLAND) 1988, 42 (5) p312-7

The use of piracetam in vertigo. S Afr Med J (SOUTH AFRICA) Nov 23 1985, 68 (11) p806-8

The efficacy of piracetam in vertigo. A double-blind study in patients with vertigo of central origin. Arzneimittelforschung (GERMANY, WEST) 1980, 30 (11)

Piracetam in the treatment of post-concussional syndrome. A double-blind study. Eur Neurol (SWITZERLAND) 1978, 17 (1) p50-5

[Evaluation of the therapeutic effectiveness of a piracetam plus dihydroergocristine combination in the treatment of vertigo] Acta Otorrinolaringol Esp (SPAIN) Jul-Aug 1988, 39 (4)

[Hydergine in pathology of the inner ear] An Otorrinolaringol Ibero Am (1990) 17(1):85-98

[The elimination of chemotherapy side effects in pulmonary tuberculosis patients] Vrach Delo (USSR) Apr 1990, (4) p71-3

The treatment of minocycline-induced brainstem vertigo by the combined administration of piracetam and ergotoxin. Acta Otolaryngol Suppl (Stockh) (SWEDEN) 1989, 468

Weight Loss

Magnesium and carbohydrate metabolism. THERAPIE (France), 1994, 49/1 (1-7)

Disorders of magnesium metabolism. Endocrinology and Metabolism Clinics of North America (USA), 1995, 24/3

Magnesium deficiency produces insulin resistance and increased thromboxane synthesis. HYPERTENSION (USA), 1993, 21/6 II (1024-1029)

Magnesium and glucose homeostasis. DIABETOLOGIA (Germany, Federal Republic of), 1990, 33/9 (511-514)

Effect of thyroxine supplementation on the response to perfluoro-n-decanoic acid (PFDA) in rats. J. TOXICOL. ENVIRON. HEALTH (USA), 1988, 24/4 (491- 498)

The role of thyroid hormones and insulin in the regulation of energy metabolism. AM. J. CLIN. NUTR. (USA), 1983, 38/6 (1006-1017)

References

The effect of triiodothyronine on weight loss and nitrogen balance of obese patients on a very low calorie liquid formula diet. INT. J. OBESITY (ENGLAND), 1981, 5/3 (279-282)

The effect of a low-calorie diet alone and in combination with triiodothyronine therapy on weight loss and hypophyseal thyroid function in obesity. INT. J. OBESITY (ENGLAND), 1983, 7/2 (123-131)

The effect of triiodothyronine on weight loss, nitrogen balance and muscle protein catabolism in obese patients on a very low calorie diet. NUTR. REP. INT. (USA), 1981, 24/1 (145-151)

Effect of triiodothyronine on some metabolic responses of obese patients. AMER.J.CLIN.NUTR. (USA), 1973, 26/7 (715-721)

The variability of weight reduction during fasting: Predictive value of thyroid hormone measurements. INT. J. OBESITY (ENGLAND), 1982, 6/1 (101-111)

The effects of triiodothyronine on energy expenditure, nitrogen balance and rates of weight and fat loss in obese patients during prolonged caloric restriction. INT. J. OBESITY (EN), 1985, 9/6 (433-442)

Desiccated thyroid in a nutritional supplement. J. FAM. PRACT. (USA), 1994, 38/3 (287-288)

Factors determining energy expenditure during very-low-calorie diets. AM. J. CLIN. NUTR. (USA), 1992, 56/1 SUPPL. (224S-229S)

Resting metabolic rate, body composition and thyroid hormones. Short term effects of very low calorie diet. HORM. METAB. RES. (Germany, Federal Republic of), 1990, 22/12 (632-635)

Decrease in resting metabolic rate during rapid weight loss is reversed by low dose thyroid hormone treatment. METAB. CLIN. EXP. (USA), 1986, 35/4 (289-291)

Relationship between the changes in serum thyroid hormone levels and protein status during prolonged protein supplemented caloric deprivation. CLIN. ENDOCRINOL. (OXFORD) (ENGLAND), 1985, 22/1 (1-15)

Thyroid hormone changes in obese subjects during fasting and a very-low-calorie diet. INT. J. OBESITY (ENGLAND), 1981, 5/3 (305-311)

The role of Tsub 3 and its receptor in efficient metabolisers receiving very-low-calorie diets. INT. J. OBESITY (ENGLAND), 1981, 5/3 (283-286)

Effects of total fasting in obese women. III. Response of serum thyroid hormones to thyroxine and triiodothyronine administration. ENDOKRINOLOGIE (GERMANY, EAST), 1979, 73/2 (221-226)

Thyroidal hormone metabolism in obesity during semi-starvation. CLIN. ENDOCRINOL. (OXFORD) (ENGLAND), 1978, 9/3 (227-231)

Clinical characteristics of hyperthyroidism. A study of 100 patients. REV.CUBA.MED. (CUBA),

References

1973, 12/1 (39-52)

The effect of triiodothyronine (Tsub 3) on protein turnover and metabolic rate. INT. J. OBESITY (ENGLAND), 1985, 9/6 (459-463)

Soy protein, thyroid regulation and cholesterol metabolism. Journal of Nutrition (USA), 1995, 125/3 SUPPL.

Overview of proposed mechanisms for the hypocholesterolemic effect of soy. Journal of Nutrition (USA), 1995, 125/3 SUPPL.

Endocrinological response to soy protein and fiber in mildly hypercholesterolemic men. NUTR. RES. (USA), 1993, 13/8 (873-884)

Response of hormones modulating plasma cholesterol to dietary casein or soy protein in minipigs. J. NUTR. (USA), 1990, 120/11 (1387-1392)

Dietary protein effects on cholesterol and lipoprotein concentrations: A review. J. AM. COLL. NUTR. (USA), 1986, 5/6 (533-549)

Comparison of dietary casein or soy protein effects on plasma lipids and hormone concentrations in the gerbil (Meriones unguiculatus). J. NUTR. (USA), 1986, 116/7 (1165-1171)

Hypolipidemic effect of casein vs. soy protein in the hyperlipidemic hypothyroid chick model. NUTR. REP. INT. (USA), 1980, 21/4 (497-503)

Characterization of the insulin resistance of glucose utilization in adipocytes from patients with hyper- and hypothyroidism. Acta Endocrinol (Copenh) (DENMARK) Oct 1988

Thyroid hormone action on intermediary metabolism. Part I: respiration, thermogenesis and carbohydrate metabolism. Klin Wochenschr (GERMANY, WEST) Jan 2 1984

Relative roles of the thyroid hormones and noradrenaline on the thermogenic activity of brown adipose tissue in the rat. J Endocrinol (ENGLAND) Jun 1995, 145

Age-related differences in body weight loss in response to altered thyroidal status. Exp Gerontol (ENGLAND) 1990, 25 (1)

Long-term weight regulation in treated hyperthyroid and hypothyroid subjects. Am J Med (UNITED STATES) Jun 1984, 76 (6)

Chromium improves insulin response to glucose in rats. Metabolism (UNITED STATES) Oct 1995, 44 (10)

Enhancing central and peripheral insulin activity as a strategy for the treatment of endogenous depression—an adjuvant role for chromium picolinate? Med Hypotheses (ENGLAND) Oct 1994, 43 (4)

Homologous physiological effects of phenformin and chromium picolinate. Med Hypotheses (ENGLAND) Oct 1993, 41 (4)

Chromium in human nutrition: a review. J Nutr (UNITED STATES) Apr 1993, 123 (4)

Use of the artificial beta cell (ABC) in the assessment of peripheral insulin sensitivity: effect of chromium supplementation in diabetic patients. Gen Pharmacol (ENGLAND) 1984, 15 (6)

Wound Healing
(Surgical Wounds, Trauma, Burns)

Nutritional intake and status of clients in the home with open surgical wounds. J Community Health Nurs (UNITED STATES) 1990, 7 (2)

High-dose vitamin C therapy for extensive deep dermal burns. Burns (ENGLAND) Apr 1992, 18 (2)

Yeast Infections

Refer to references under Candida Infection.

275

Index

74, 76, 91, 145, 147
Bezafibrate 67, 96
Bifido bacteria 43
Bilberry 24, 44-45, 92
Bioflavonoids 8
Biostim 80, 87
Biotin 43
Black currant seed 20, 22
Bladder conditions 31
Blood clots 14, 24-25, 45, 65
Blood pressure 21, 51
Blood PTH test 38
Blood Testing 31
Blurred vision 143
Borage oil 8, 20, 22, 27
Brain cell injury 4
Brain hormones 49
Branched-chain amino acid complex 91
Breast cancer 31-32, 37, 41, 61-62
Bromelain 28, 47, 67, 96
Bromocriptine 113, 121
Bronchial constriction 23
Bursitis 21, 34
Buspar 15
Cachexia (catabolic wasting) 44
Caffeine 17, 146
Calcium ascorbate 126
Calcium ion exchange 6
Calcium oxalate formation 89
Calcium-protein bindings 6
Calcium 34, 38, 42, 45, 65, 82, 88, 109, 111
Cancer chemotherapy 34
Cancer Profile tests (CA Profile) 34
Cancer Radiation Therapy 34
Cancer Surgery 35
Cancer treatment protocol 35-38
Cancer 7, 21, 25, 75, 86, 93-94, 98
Candida (fungal, yeast) infections 42-43
Capoten 83
Caprylic acid 43, 69
Cardiac arrhythmia 17
Cardiomyopathy 51
Cardiovascular disease 46, 66, 93
Carnitine 17
Casodex 120, 122, 125
Castration 123
Catabolic wasting 44
Cataract 25, 44-45
CD4 (T-helper cells) 81
CEA or carcinoembryonic antigen test 34
Cellular cyclical adenosine monophosphate 51
Centrophenoxine 5, 10-11
Cerebral aneurysm 45
Cerebral artery disease 65
Cerebral atherosclerosis 128

Cerebral hemorrhage 45
Cerebrovascular disease 23, 45, 48
Chelation therapy 73-74, 94
Chemotherapy 32, 35, 85
Chitosan 138
Chlorophyll extract 69
Chloroplex 93
Cholesterol Reduction 46
Cholesterol 23, 25, 102
Cholinergic neurons, and Alzheimer's disease 9
Choline 5-6, 52, 59, 91, 108
Chondroitin sulfates 19, 22
Chondroprotective agents 19
Choriocarcinoma 36
Chromium picolinate 56-57, 84, 88, 94, 107, 136, 138
Chromium polynicotinate 88
Chromium 56-58, 84, 135-136, 138
Chronic fatigue syndrome 15, 49
Chronic obstructive pulmonary disease 59
Chronic pain 3
Cigarette smoking 66
Cimetidine (Tagamet) 29
Circadian rhythm 88-89
Cirrhosis 50, 72-73, 78
Clinical depression 146
Clotting factors 45
Clotting time 45
Coenzyme Q10 5-6, 11, 13-14, 17, 24-25, 34, 38, 49, 51-52, 60, 69, 76, 82, 85, 91, 106-107, 114
Cognex 11
Cognitex 6, 11, 26, 108
Cognitive Enhancement 50
Cognitive functions, decline in 5
Collagen 20, 45
Colon cancer 37
Colon 52
Common cold 50, 75
Concentrated fish oil (Mega-EPA) 8
Cardiomyopathy 51
Congestive heart failure 16-17, 51, 91, 105
Conjugated linoleic acid (CLA) 33, 44
Constipation 52
Contact dermatitis 30
Contraceptives 62
Copper 139-140
Coronary artery disease 23
Corticosteroids 18
Cortisol 4, 16, 40, 97
Cranberry juice 132
Cranex Cranberry Juice Concentrate 132
Cruciferous vegetables 63
Curcumin 46-47, 91, 94
Cyclic AMP 23
Cyproterone acetate (Androcur/Diane) 29

Index

Index

Index

Index

Index

Index

Total Estrogen 97
Toxic free radicals in the liver 3
Toxins 8
TPA 129
Transient ischemic attack 23
Transurethral resection 125
Trauma 131
Tretinoin (Retin-A) 31
TriEst 64, 103
Triglycerides 23, 47-48, 66
Tryptophan 88
Tumor Marker Test 38
Tylenol 3
Tyrosine kinase 90
Tyrosine 49, 54, 112, 130, 147
Udo's Choice Essential Fatty Acids 12
Udo's Choice Flax Oil 105
Udo's Choice Oil Blend 26
Udo's Choice Ultimate Oil 38
Ulcers 21
Ultraviolet (UV) sunlight 45, 126
Urinary Tract Infections 132
Uterine cancer 61
Valerian 88, 148
Valine 44, 91
Valium 88
Valvular Insufficiency/Heart Valve Defects 132
Vanadyl sulfate 57-58, 94
Vasopressin 11
Vasotec 83
Vertigo 132
Vesanoid 90-91
Viral hepatitis 46
Vitamin A liquid drops 17, 143
Vitamin A toxicity 143
Vitamin A 17, 32, 34, 37-38, 41, 66, 73-74, 90-91, 93, 109, 145, 147-148
Vitamin B-complex 92
Vitamin B1 7, 13, 84, 91
Vitamin B2 13, 91
Vitamin B5 6, 52, 91
Vitamin B6 13, 24-25, 56, 63, 67, 84, 88, 91, 105-106, 125
Vitamin B12 10-11, 13, 76, 88, 106, 109
Vitamin C 3-4, 7-8, 12, 22-23, 39, 45, 50, 52, 56, 59, 67, 69, 71-72, 74-75, 83-84, 91, 94, 97, 109, 126, 131, 140
Vitamin D 65
Vitamin D3 17, 32, 34, 37-38, 42, 90-91, 108, 110-111, 113, 122
Vitamin E 6-7, 14, 17, 22, 24, 34, 63, 66-67, 69, 71, 91, 107, 113, 126, 131
Viva Drops 45, 92
Weight Loss 133-134
Wound-Healing (Wounds, Trauma, Burns) 138

Xanax 15
Yeast Fighters 43
Yeast infections 42, 140
Zantac 60
Zeaxanthin 93
Zinc lozenges 50
Zinc 69, 71, 92-93, 138, 140
Zocor 48

Join the Life Extension Foundation
for Information That Can Save Your Life

For Just $75, you can join the Life Extension Foundation and receive:

- *Life Extension* magazine mailed to you every month. *Life Extension* magazine keeps you informed about medical breakthroughs from around the world, and tells you how to obtain them.

- Discounts on blood testing, hormone therapies, offshore medications and advanced nutrient formulas that more than pay for your membership fee.

- The Directory of Life Extension nutrients and drugs . . . a compendium of nutrients and medicines used to prevent diseases and slow aging.

- The Physician's Guide to Life Extension Drugs . . . a complete guide to safe and effective offshore drugs.

- The Directory of Innovative Medical Clinics, a listing of medical clinics that are using innovative therapies to treat cancer, Alzheimer's disease and aging.

- The Directory of Innovative Medical Doctors, a listing of physicians throughout the U.S. who practice innovative medicine.

As a member of the Life Extension Foundation, you will receive the most advanced information in the world about improving your health, treating your chronic disease(s), and slowing down aging.

To join the Foundation for optimal health and longevity, call **1-800-841-5433**, or join on the web at www.lef.org. You may also mail the coupon below.

Yes! I want to join the most aggressive health maintenance organization in the world . . . The Life Extension Foundation.

Enclosed is my $75 membership fee.

Mail to: Life Extension Foundation
P.O. Box 229120
Hollywood, FL 33022-9120

Name: _____

Address: _____

City/State/Zip: _____